From Death to Birth

Mortality Decline and Reproductive Change

Mark R. Montgomery and Barney Cohen, Editors

Committee on Population

Commission on Behavioral and Social Sciences and Education

National Research Council

NATIONAL ACADEMY PRESS
Washington, D.C.   1998

NATIONAL ACADEMY PRESS • 2101 Constitution Ave., NW • Washington, DC   20418

NOTICE: The project that is the subject of this report was approved by the Governing Board of the National Research Council, whose members are drawn from the councils of the National Academy of Sciences, the National Academy of Engineering, and the Institute of Medicine. The members of the committee responsible for the report were chosen for their special competences and with regard for appropriate balance.

This report has been reviewed by a group other than the authors according to procedures approved by a Report Review Committee consisting of members of the National Academy of Sciences, the National Academy of Engineering, and the Institute of Medicine.

This activity was funded by the Office of Population of the U.S. Agency for International Development, the Andrew W. Mellon Foundation, and the William and Flora Hewlett Foundation.

Library of Congress Cataloging-in-Publication Data

From death to birth : mortality decline and reproductive change / Mark
 R. Montgomery and Barney Cohen, editors.
   p. cm.
  "Committee on Population, Commission on Behavioral and Social
Sciences and Education, National Research Council."
  Includes bibliographical references.
  ISBN 0-309-05896-1 (pbk.)
  1. Mortality. 2. Fertility, Human. I. Montgomery, Mark, 1953-
. II. Cohen, Barney, 1959- . III. National Research Council
(U.S.). Committee on Population.
HB1321.F76 1997
304.6'3—dc21   97-33802

From Death to Birth: Mortality Decline and Reproductive Change is available for sale from the National Academy Press, 2101 Constitution Avenue, NW, Lock Box 285, Washington, DC 20055. Call 800-624-6242 or 202-334-3313 (in the Washington Metropolitan Area). Order electronically via Internet at **http://www.nap.edu.**

---

* through May 1997
** through June 1997

iii

CONTRIBUTORS

MARTHA AINSWORTH, The World Bank, Washington, D.C.

P.N. MARI BHAT, Institute of Economic Growth, Delhi, India

BARNEY COHEN, Committee on Population, National Research Council

BARTHÉLÉMY KUATE DEFO, Department of Demography, University of Montreal

DEON FILMER, The World Bank, Washington, D.C.

ELIZABETH FRANKENBERG, RAND, Santa Monica, California

PATRICK R. GALLOWAY, Department of Demography, University of California, Berkeley

LAURENCE M. GRUMMER-STRAWN, Centers for Disease Control and Prevention, U.S. Department of Health and Human Services, Atlanta, Georgia

MICHAEL R. HAINES, Department of Economics, Colgate University

EUGENE A. HAMMEL, Departments of Anthropology and Demography, University of California, Berkeley

RONALD D. LEE, Departments of Demography and Economics, University of California, Berkeley

ZUGUO MEI, Centers for Disease Control and Prevention, U.S. Department of Health and Human Services, Atlanta, Georgia

MARK R. MONTGOMERY, Department of Economics, State University of New York, Stony Brook, and The Population Council, New York

LUIS ROSERO-BIXBY, Office of Population Research, Princeton University, and Institute of Health Research, University of Costa Rica

INNOCENT SEMALI, Muhimbili University College of Health Sciences, University of Dar es Salaam, Tanzania

PAUL W. STUPP, Centers for Disease Control and Prevention, U.S. Department of Health and Human Services, Atlanta, Georgia

KENNETH I. WOLPIN, Department of Economics, University of Pennsylvania

Preface

The Committee on Population was established by the National Research Council in 1983 to bring the knowledge and methods of the population sciences to bear on major issues of science and public policy. The committee's mandate is to conduct scientific assessments of major population issues and to provide a forum for discussion and analysis of important public policy issues related to population.

The Committee on Population has a long history of activities in world population issues. In anticipation of the United Nations International Conference on Population and Development in 1994, representatives of national academies of science from around the world met in New Delhi, India, in a "science summit" on World Population. In a joint statement, 58 of the World's scientific academies challenged "scientists, engineers, and health professionals" to "study and provide advice on . . . factors that affect reproductive behavior, family size, and successful family planning" (p. 11). In response, the committee has organized a range of different activities designed to increase knowledge of these important demographic variables. In 1994, the committee organized a Panel on Reproductive Health; its report, published in 1997, assesses the state of knowledge of reproductive health problems in developing countries and proposes research and program priorities designed to improve global reproductive health. And, since 1995, the committee has organized a series of workshops to review what is known about the determinants of fertility transition in developing countries.

The papers in this volume were first presented at such a workshop, held in November 1995, which was designed to bring together researchers from a variety of different disciplines to discuss what is known about how changes in infant and child mortality risk affect reproductive outcomes. Given that the balance of mortality and fertility rates determines the rate of population growth, which in turn has important implications for social and economic welfare, it is perhaps surprising that it has been almost 20 years since there has been a systematic examination of these crucial demographic variables. Many demographic changes have occurred over this period. Considerable variability has been recorded in countries' routes to the fertility transition, but the cause of such variation, and particularly the role of government policy towards population and family planning, remains an open question. Casual observation might suggest that a decline in mortality is the most important prerequisite for a decline in fertility, but the research base for this conclusion is surprisingly thin.

The Committee on Population thanks all those who helped in this activity from its inception, through the workshop, to the final publication of this volume. Primary organization and planning for the workshop and this report was overseen by committee member Mark Montgomery, aided by several other current and former members, including Caroline Bledsoe, John Casterline, Anne Pebley, and Ron Rindfuss. They were assisted by several members of the committee's staff: the work took place under the general direction of John Haaga, director of the Committee on Population; Trish DeFrisco skillfully handled all administrative duties; Winfield Swanson and Elaine McGarraugh adroitly edited the manuscript; and Trang Ta prepared the final version of the manuscript for publication. Key to all the work was Barney Cohen, who managed the project from its inception to this publication, with intelligence, humor, and, above all, patience.

The committee also gratefully acknowledges the United States' Agency for International Development, the Andrew W. Mellon Foundation, and the William and Flora Hewlett Foundation for their generous financial support.

Finally, we are indebted to all the workshop participants for their willingness to participate and to contribute their special knowledge.

Ronald D. Lee, *Chair*
Committee on Population

Contents

From
Death
to
Birth

1

Introduction

Barney Cohen and Mark R. Montgomery

BACKGROUND

The twentieth century has witnessed a remarkable expansion in the average length of human life. Significant differentials in mortality remain, to be sure, and these testify to the continued presence of political and socioeconomic barriers to effective health care. The differentials should not, however, obscure the larger achievement. In developed countries, the oldest generation living today was born in an era in which nearly one child in five failed to survive to his or her fifth birthday. In developing countries, for the most part, mortality risks are now far lower than they were at the turn of the century in the wealthier societies of the West.

This profound change in the human condition has had far-reaching implications, unsettling long-established habits of thought and behavior. As early as mid-century, Notestein (1945, 1953) recognized and began to emphasize one particular implication: the effects of mortality decline on the motivation for high fertility. The initial formulations of demographic transition theory gave prominence to this theme and it continues to serve as a unifying feature in models of fertility and related demographic behavior (Mason, 1997). Even when first articulated, the mechanisms by which mortality reduction might bring about fertility decline were understood to be complex, involving both individual- and societal-level responses. Subsequent demographic research has done much to clarify the individual-level relationships, and in so doing has added new considerations.

In 1975, a scientific meeting organized by the Committee for International Coordination of National Research in Demography synthesized and codified what had been learned. The resulting volume, *The Effects of Infant and Child Mortal-*

ity on Fertility (Preston, 1978a), stands as a landmark in demographic research. It enumerated four mechanisms by which child mortality might affect fertility. First, parental expectations of child loss might be expressed in *insurance* or "hoarding" behavior, causing fertility to be higher than if survival were assured. In the event of an infant or child death, two additional mechanisms could come into play: *lactation interruption* effects and *behavioral replacement* strategies. Fourth, the Preston volume made a place for *societal-level effects*, those having to do with institutional forces that had long served to maintain high fertility in the face of high mortality, and which would therefore continue to shape the fertility response to mortality decline.

Having summarized the key mechanisms, the 1978 volume went on to refine the methodological tools with which the strength of the individual-level effects might be measured. The volume also presented an array of applications to both aggregate- and individual-level data, which provided evidence on the likely magnitude of the fertility response. These theoretical and methodological developments were set out in compelling, lucid, and vivid terms. Interestingly, the net effect was to dissipate much of the momentum for further research.

In retrospect, the ensuing lull in research appears all the more curious. Preston's introduction to the 1978 volume pointed toward new intellectual territory into which demographers had not yet ventured (Preston, 1978b). He argued for a deeper consideration of the societal-level mechanisms, including the place of nuptiality, and emphasized the role of mortality perceptions. Yet neither line of research was pursued. The new tools of hazard-rate modeling were just then coming onto the demographic scene, accompanied by a dramatic expansion of individual-level data in the form of World Fertility Surveys and the later Demographic and Health Surveys. Armed with these tools and new resources, researchers were soon much better equipped to understand the multiple determinants of birth interval dynamics and to explore the effects of high fertility and close birth spacing on mortality. Yet relatively little attention was given to the possibility that earlier estimates of the effects of mortality on fertility might be contaminated by reverse causation. Continued advances in the availability of historical demographic data also invited a reexamination of the Western experience, but on this front, too, progress was slow (although see Chesnais, 1992). New theoretical and empirical research in economics began to underscore the importance of health to economic productivity and growth and put increasing emphasis on the trade-off between such investments in human capital and the level of fertility (Becker et al., 1990; Mincer, 1996). Apart from the review by Lloyd and Ivanov (1988), however, no systematic effort was mounted to draw together such important but rather disparate lines of research.

In the early 1990s, a spirited debate broke out in which the long-term benefits produced by child health programs were brought into question. In a series of provocative articles, King (1990, 1991, 1992) argued that in certain cases, programs aimed at reducing infant and child mortality might do no more than exacerbate the problems of sustainable development. For the poorest countries in the world, King said, the rapid increase in population generated as a direct result of saving lives had the potential to undermine biological support systems to the point that death rates might begin to climb. King termed this phenomenon a "demographic trap" (see King, 1990, 1991; Hammarskjöld et al., 1992).

Other writers sharply disagreed, arguing in the first place that health programs can and should be justified on their own terms (Taylor, 1991; UNICEF, 1991). Moreover, it was said, policies and programs aimed directly at high fertility will tend to be more effective when parents can be confident that their children will survive (Freedman, 1963; Taylor et al., 1976). In addition, the potential feedback benefits of fertility decline were cited, these having to do with the role of lower and better-spaced fertility in reducing the risks of maternal, infant, and child mortality. In the view of King's critics, health and family planning programs have the potential to set off a series of responses that could culminate in a more-than-compensating fertility decline over the long term. The possibility of such responses in fertility can be glimpsed in recent cross-country analyses of mortality-fertility relations in low-income countries (Schultz, 1994a,b)[1] and in new analyses of the historical record (Galloway et al., in this volume).

To be sure, if attention were to be confined to the lactation interruption and behavioral replacement effects, such overcompensating fertility responses could be dismissed as implausible on empirical grounds. Citing numerous early studies that found the responsiveness of individual fertility to the loss of a child to be much less than one-for-one, Preston (1978b) concluded that, on average, an additional child death in a family would lead to something less than an additional birth. If the lactation interruption and replacement effects were indeed the only mechanisms at work, then reductions in infant and child mortality would, by themselves, tend to increase the rate of population growth. The possibility of more-than-compensating effects thus rests on the insurance motivation and on a longer-term series of feedbacks whose causal basis is yet to be fully understood.

---

[1]Schultz used data from 62 low-income countries in 1972, 1982, and 1988 to investigate the relationship between fertility and mortality at the macro level. In his analysis (Schultz, 1994b:27):

> Declines in the level of child mortality in developing countries are not associated with increases in population growth, because coordinated fertility decline fully offset this demographic effect of improvements in child nutrition and survival. In this time period, improvements in child health are associated with slower population growth.

Schultz found that female educational attainment was the most important determinant associated with both lower child mortality and lower fertility.

THE NEED FOR REASSESSMENT

The recent policy debate, and more generally the lack of systematic research over the past 20 years, would suggest that a thorough reassessment of the theory and evidence is in order. This volume is based on a set of papers presented at a scientific meeting organized in November 1995 by the U.S. National Academy of Sciences' Committee on Population and convened in Washington, D.C. It attempts to contribute to the debate by advancing the demographic literature on three fronts: theoretical, methodological, and empirical.

Given the current state of the research and policy debate, several tasks faced the authors of this volume. The first imperative was simply to document, more precisely than had previously been possible, the various pathways that have been taken by mortality and fertility in the developing countries and in selected historical settings. When the full empirical record is assembled, it is seen to encompass a remarkable diversity of experience. Many countries have adhered to the simple scheme of demographic transition in which mortality declines first and fertility decline then follows with a lag. Even here, however, the lags in response are highly variable and are themselves worthy of consideration. Some countries (e.g., Costa Rica, see Rosero-Bixby, in this volume) experienced decades of profound mortality decline without any apparent fertility response. In a few others, fertility decline seems to have preceded mortality decline.

The very diversity of developing country mortality and fertility declines suggests that there can be nothing automatic or self-sustaining about the effects of mortality decline on fertility. This diversity should also put to rest the notion that mortality decline can be linked to fertility decline by way of simple necessary or sufficient conditions. It seems that a particular configuration of social, political, and economic forces may be required for any given country to embark on transition, but the outlines of that configuration may be difficult to discern in advance.

A second task facing the authors was to assess, with new data and techniques, the robustness of the lactation interruption and replacement effects that Preston had described earlier. Given the debate within the policy community, it was important to determine whether, taken together, these effects could not reasonably be expected to induce more-than-compensating fertility responses. In this volume, a considerable amount of statistical and methodological ingenuity is expended in securing precise estimates of the lactation and replacement effects. The conclusion reached by this new research is that the earlier findings are indeed robust.

This brings to the forefront the remaining task that faced the authors: to better understand the role played by insurance (or hoarding) effects. If the lactation and replacement effects are less than compensating, the net reproduction rate will fall in response to mortality decline only if the insurance effects are powerful. Such insurance effects are very difficult to detect with aggregate data, or indeed, with any demographic data that are routinely collected. Something of their influence is presumably expressed in the coefficients of community mortality measures employed in individual fertility regressions, but even this is too crude a measuring device. The essence of the insurance effect resides in the combination of individual experience and social structure that shapes individual perceptions of mortality and forms the basis of their expectations. It is closely linked to the perceived potency of human agency as against fatalistic views of the world, and likewise to the transition from family building by fate to family building by design that Lloyd and Ivanov (1988) have emphasized. Remarkably little demographic research has addressed these fundamental concerns.

In the remainder of this introductory chapter, we review the research developments since the landmark Preston (1978a) volume. We offer our views as to why the relationship linking mortality decline to fertility is likely to resist simplification and easy generalization. We then document the astonishing diversity of mortality and fertility transitions that have taken place in developing countries over the past 40 years. The penultimate section of this chapter previews the contribution of the remaining chapters in the volume. The final section offers brief conclusions and draws out some implications for policy.

THE RECENT RESEARCH RECORD

Since the 1978 Preston volume, research on the effects of mortality on fertility has proceeded in three directions. First, some researchers have continued to search for statistically significant thresholds of life expectancy or socioeconomic development that, when attained, provide motivation for couples to limit their fertility (see, for example, Cutright, 1983; Cutright and Hargens, 1984; Bulatao, 1985).[2] Such studies have generally failed to identify meaningful thresholds for fertility decline, although measures of social development often appear to be more closely associated to declines in fertility than are measures of economic development (Cleland, 1993).

Second, the emergence of detailed micro-level data from developing countries has supported a new generation of studies of both the lactation interruption and replacement effects (A.I. Chowdhury et al., 1992; A.K.M.A. Chowdhury et al., 1976; Balakrishnan, 1978; Park et al., 1979; de Guzman, 1984; Mauskopf and

---

[2]Cutright and Hargens (1984) analyzed a pooled regression of crude birth rates from 20 Latin American countries for four points in time. They found statistically significant threshold levels of literacy and life expectancy that are independent of lagged measures of literacy and life expectancy, measures of economic and family planning program development, and period controls. Bulatao (1985) analyzed data from 124 developing countries and concluded that no fertility transition has been observed in any developing country until life expectancy has reached 53 years. In a similar analysis, Ross and Frankenberg (1993) concluded that fertility is unlikely to decline until life expectancy rises to 50-60 years.

Wallace, 1984; Mensch, 1985; Santow and Bracher, 1984; Nur, 1985; Rao and Beaujot, 1986; Johnson and Sufian, 1992).[3] These micro-level studies have confirmed that women who experience the death of one or more of their children tend to have higher subsequent fertility than women whose children survived. Birth intervals tend to be considerably shorter following the death of a child, with much of this due to the interruption of lactation and the removal of its contraceptive protection. When adjustments are made for duration of exposure and other demographic and socioeconomic factors, the residual replacement effect estimates have tended to be rather small. In marked contrast to studies of lactation and replacement effects, relatively few micro-level analyses have attempted to link fertility change to community-level changes in mortality, although Pebley et al. (1979) and Rashad et al. (1993) are exceptions.

Economists, interested in both conceptual and statistical issues, have pursued two related lines of research. Wolpin (1984) and Sah (1991) further refined the dynamic theory that underlies modern economic models of insurance and replacement effects. Others developed multivariate techniques to circumvent some of the problems that plague bivariate analyses (Schultz, 1976; Williams, 1977; Olsen, 1980; Trussell and Olsen, 1983; Wolpin, 1984; Yamada, 1985; Chowdhury, 1988; Pitt, 1994). Subsequent empirical work, often using linked macro- and micro-level data, generated a set of estimates of both the breastfeeding and behavioral effects that are similar in magnitude and range to those reported in the studies mentioned above (Hashimoto and Hongladarom, 1981; Lee and Schultz, 1982; Anderson, 1983; Olsen and Wolpin, 1983; Okojie, 1991; Benefo and Schultz, 1996; Panis and Lillard, 1993; Maglad, 1993, 1994).

As noted above, surprisingly few attempts have been made over the past two decades to weave these diverse strands of research into a coherent whole. A notable exception is the comprehensive 1988 review by the United Nations Population Division (United Nations Secretariat, 1988; Lloyd and Ivanov, 1988). This thoughtful synthesis clarified much about the evolution of the relationship between mortality and fertility over the course of the demographic transition. As Lloyd and Ivanov argued, the demographic transition is in essence a transition in family strategies: the reactive, largely biological family-building decision rules appropriate to highly uncertain environments come eventually to be supplanted by more deliberate and forward-looking strategies that require longer time horizons. We take up several of the themes raised by Lloyd and Ivanov in the following sections.

---

[3]Most such studies have used data that were collected under the World Fertility Survey program, although some rely on census, panel, or ad hoc demographic surveys. Surprisingly, until the publication of this volume, analyses of data from the Demographic and Health Surveys on this question have been almost nil.

THE DIFFICULTIES IN ANALYZING THE
MORTALITY-FERTILITY RELATIONSHIP

Perceptions and Agency

Women in pretransitional societies often express no clear personal preference about the number of children they will bear (see, for example, Knodel et al., 1987; van de Walle, 1992). This lack of preference is sometimes termed "fatalistic," but on closer inspection can be understood as a rational stance vis-à-vis an uncertain and contingent environment. Child survival is only one of many uncertainties that must be faced in deciding family productive and reproductive strategies (Castle, 1994).

As improvements in child survival begin to occur in such settings, they may reshape parental views in subtle but profound ways. Parents may begin to conceive of the possibility of influencing the size of their own families, instead of leaving such matters to chance or to the higher powers. Lloyd and Ivanov (1988) termed this a "transitional effect," whereas UNICEF refers to it as the "confidence factor" (UNICEF, 1991).

Demographers know the concept as Coale's first precondition for fertility transition, that fertility behavior must lie within the "calculus of conscious choice" (Coale, 1973). In their review, Lloyd and Ivanov hypothesized that the emergence of conscious family planning, and the speed of its diffusion, depends on both the age pattern of mortality in childhood and the degree to which risks can be reduced by parental actions. Heavy infant but light child mortality makes child survival more secure and predictable following infancy. When new health behaviors are adopted, and these innovative health decisions are shown to exert a perceptible influence on mortality risks, parents may be led to consider new, more self-conscious strategies of family building in general.

The standard methods of economic and demographic inquiry are not at all well suited to measuring such fundamental changes in psychological context. Perceptions of mortality risks and of the efficacy of health interventions are doubtless very difficult to elicit. Parents may not be able to articulate precisely why they feel as they do, or be able to connect logically mortality risks to fertility decisions in the schematic fashion that social scientists would prefer (see Knodel et al., 1987, and Castle, 1994 for examples). In pretransitional settings, it would surely prove difficult to extract meaningful information about the long-standing preferences, beliefs, and modes of behavior that the participants themselves have taken as given and not much examined.

Some evidence on these matters is available in the historical record for the United States. For the period from the late eighteenth to the early twentieth centuries (Preston and Haines, 1991; Dye and Smith, 1986; Vinovskis, 1991) there are fascinating qualitative accounts of both continuity and change in mortality perceptions. The materials of Dye and Smith, largely drawn from women's diaries, attest to an ever-present concern throughout the period with the possibility of child death. Adults also seemed to be intensely aware of the risks facing themselves. Indeed, Vinovskis argues that adult mortality perceptions were much inflated in relation to the empirical realities, in part because of the interests of religious institutions in keeping their members focused on the afterlife.

Dye and Smith (1986) show that over the course of the nineteenth century, childrearing came to be increasingly child centered in nature and became a task increasingly assigned to mothers rather than one distributed among siblings, kin, and other caretakers. Until the very end of the nineteenth century, however, this transition in the definition of the quality of child care presented mothers with a dilemma: They were being entrusted with safeguarding their children, and yet, where mortality was concerned, lacked any effective means of doing so. The result was an increasing tension between socially defined responsibilities and technically constrained options. When the necessary medical breakthroughs were finally made, according to Dye and Smith, women responded in both personal and political terms. In personal terms, they enthusiastically adopted the new medical techniques and adhered to advice; in political terms, they channeled their pent-up energies to the creation of the Children's Bureau and other government and public health institutions.

Although this account of the U.S. experience is only impressionistic, it raises certain themes that have otherwise received very little research attention in demographic circles. There is the issue of perceptions of mortality risks as against the empirical risks themselves. There is the distinction between high risks and risks that, although high, might be controlled. There is an evolving definition and redefinition of child quality, in which parental health investments, newly perceived to be effective, eventually come to play a role. Finally, the decisive actions are played out not only at the individual level, but also at the level of political and public health institutions. All these factors figure into the development of family-building strategies that stress design over fate, emphasize deeper investment in child quality, and lead ultimately to lower fertility. The particular circumstances were perhaps unique to one historical era in the United States, but in broad outline have parallels elsewhere (e.g., Caldwell, 1986; Caldwell et al., 1983; Caldwell and Caldwell, 1987).

Preferences and Unwanted Fertility

The fertility response to mortality decline cannot be easily disentangled from other factors that affect fertility preferences in general (whether for the number of children, their sex composition, or their spacing) and the costs (whether monetary, health related, or linked to spousal bargaining) that are associated with the means of fertility control. Although debate continues about the measurement, meaning, and depth of fertility preferences, one aspect is clear: Child replacement effects are likely to be stronger among families that have not yet exceeded their ideal family size and weaker among families that have already experienced at least one unwanted birth. A notable feature of demographic research over the past decade is the increasing appreciation of unwanted and unintended fertility (see Bongaarts, 1997, for a review). The emergence of replacement effects is thus linked, directly or indirectly, to the factors that shape fertility preferences, govern the costs of fertility regulation, and thereby affect the proportion of families that have yet to reach, or have already exceeded, their desired family sizes. To a lesser extent, perhaps, insurance strategies are also affected by these factors.

Alternative Strategies Can Coexist

A further consideration is that the strategies of insurance and replacement behavior, although conceptually distinct, have common roots in household constraints, preferences, and perceptions (see Wolpin, in this volume). A range of such strategies can coexist within any given community or be adopted by a given family at different points in its reproductive career (Preston, 1978b; Lloyd and Ivanov, 1988). Moreover, by constraining the options that are open to parents, the program environment may affect their mix of strategies. For example, parents might seek to combine replacement and insurance behavior where reversible methods of contraception are unavailable (Bhat, in this volume).

The Nature of the Relationship Changes Over Time

In an earlier era, differences in fertility levels among developing countries seem mainly to have reflected differences in social customs concerning such matters as age at first marriage, divorce and remarriage, the length of breast-feeding, sanctions on postpartum abstinence, and coital frequency. These social and cultural influences in pretransition settings served to restrain fertility to levels well below its biological maximum (Bongaarts, 1975). The ensuing decline in fertility can be viewed as a shift away from such "natural" fertility regimes toward more self-conscious, parity-specific birth control, although changes in age at first marriage—associated with the rising educational achievements of women—have also played a significant role (Cleland, 1993). Not surprisingly, therefore, the relative importance of mortality effects also varies over the course of the transition (Preston, 1975; Park et al., 1979; Frankenberg, in this volume; Lloyd and Ivanov, 1988).

Preston (1975) suggests that the extent to which dead children are replaced in a family is approximately U-shaped, with populations at the highest and lowest developmental levels exhibiting the strongest effects. Over the course of development, he argues, the importance of the lactation interruption effect tends to be reduced in relative terms, and the significance of behavioral responses proportionately enhanced, as societies increasingly adopt parity-specific controls over childbearing. Furthermore, as mortality conditions improve and the demand for surviving children falls, parents are more likely to abandon pure insurance strategies and substitute for them various forms of replacement behavior. Hence, over the course of the demographic transition, the dominant mechanism changes from a biological relationship associated with the truncation of breastfeeding to behavioral replacement, passing through an intermediate stage in which insurance strategies could be expected to hold sway.[4]

The Link to Human Capital Investments

We noted above the role that could be played in demographic transitions by redefinitions of the norms governing child care and investments in the human capital of children, with the emerging norms helping to reduce mortality and, in addition, to raise the costs of continued high fertility. Among several forms of human capital investment, the potential link between mortality and the motivation for investments in children's schooling merits special consideration.

Why might high mortality risks threaten children's schooling? The demographic reality is that the great majority of deaths occurring under age 20 are those that occur before school age. Even in high-mortality environments, the death of a school-age child is a relatively rare event. It would thus be unusual for parental investments to be rendered fruitless by the death of a school child. Unless there is a decided mismatch between parental perceptions of mortality and the demographic realities, the roots of an association would need to be sought elsewhere.

One possibility is that the conditions producing high infant and child mortality are also responsible for significant morbidity among school-age children. Such morbidities would undermine children's energies and abilities to learn, thereby reducing the payoffs that parents could expect to receive from their schooling investments. Another possibility is that when higher parental fertility is occasioned by higher child mortality, school-aged children are more often called upon to serve as caretakers for their younger siblings or to assist their mothers in household tasks. These additional duties may reduce the time that children have available for schoolwork or even for school attendance, which again could erode learning abilities and reduce the expected returns to additional parental investments.

The perceived risks of adult mortality may play a role as well. Looking to the future, and perhaps exaggerating the risks that they face, parents may fear that they may not be able to sustain the resource flows needed to embark on what might be, in context, an ambitious program of human capital investment in their children. Not willing to risk the returns for themselves over the near term, and being reluctant to raise their children's hopes only to have them later dashed, parents might well conclude that a less ambitious strategy is in order. Moreover,

---

[4]In China, an extreme variant of the replacement mechanism—sex-selective abortion—is emerging as a result of widespread availability of ultrasound and other diagnostic techniques (Zeng Yi et al., 1993; Goodkind, 1996).

one would expect that parental discount factors—those subjective utility parameters that summarize how all future events are downweighted in salience by comparison to the present—would themselves be lower in highly uncertain environments. The link between high mortality, environmental uncertainty in general, and time orientation deserves serious study. Ainsworth et al. (in this volume) take up the issues in connection with mortality from AIDS.

Statistical Estimation Problems

In addition to the conceptual problems that have been described above, attempts to isolate the effects of improved child survival on fertility face numerous methodological difficulties (Schultz, 1976; Williams, 1977; Brass and Barrett, 1978). For example, unmeasured third factors may well affect both fertility and mortality, thus obscuring the true relationship between them. When micro-level data are used, the discreteness of fertility measures and the nonlinearity of the replacement effect induce an artificial correlation between fertility and child mortality that can also affect estimates of behavioral relationships (Williams, 1977). When macro-level time series data are used, the time dimension of the analysis raises questions of autocorrelation (Brass and Barrett, 1978), which would threaten the basis for inference. Furthermore, in many developing countries, estimates of fertility and mortality rates have been adjusted using indirect estimation techniques that contain implicit assumptions about the nature of other demographic conditions embedded within them (Brass and Barrett, 1978).

Perhaps the most difficult estimation issue, however, is that causality between improved child survival and fertility runs in two directions (Galloway et al., in this volume). It is now well established that the probabilities of survival are lower for children born to teenagers, to older women, and to women of high parity or closely spaced births (Hobcraft et al., 1983, 1985; Hobcraft, 1992). Hence, reductions in the number of births, particularly high-risk births, can be expected to affect infant and child mortality rates.[5] To circumvent this problem, economists have long argued for the use of structural equations models (Schultz, 1988). Such models require researchers to impose crucial identifying restrictions. Except in unusual cases, however, neither theory nor specific knowledge of the relevant processes is sufficient to guide the choice of instruments (Schultz, 1988; Bhat, in this volume). Estimates of the effects of child mortality on fertility tend to be disturbingly sensitive to such key details of model specification.[6]

---

[5]The direction of effect, however, is not always obvious (see the exchanges in Trussell and Pebley, 1984; Bongaarts, 1987, 1988; Trussell, 1988).

[6]When put to the test, structural models often fail to reject the hypothesis that child mortality is exogenous (see, for example, Benefo and Schultz, 1996; Maglad, 1993; Panis and Lillard, 1993). This may well reflect the low power of the tests involved, but could also indicate that fears of statistical endogeneity have been exaggerated.

MORTALITY AND FERTILITY TRENDS
OVER THE PAST 40 YEARS

With all this as background, we now turn to a review of the empirical evidence. Figure 1-1 presents a graphical representation of the varied evolution of fertility-mortality pathways over some 40 years (1950-1990) in specific countries in Latin America, sub-Saharan Africa, Asia, and the Middle East. Conversion of these data into rates of population growth is not always straightforward, as one must also take into account the age structure of the population, changes in mortality at other ages, and population momentum. Figure 1-2 depicts changes in population growth rates for these countries over the same period.

Latin America

Two recent reviews of fertility and mortality transitions have concluded that no single dominant pattern of population change in Latin America exists, and, indeed, "to invoke the image of a unique experience, even if only for descriptive purposes, is highly misleading" (Palloni, 1990:128; see also Guzman, 1994). Population trends in the region are the product of a complex set of historical, social, and economic forces (Palloni, 1990). This rich social context includes marked differences between countries in (1) the official ideology toward population issues; (2) the extent of influence of the Catholic Church; (3) the prevalence of consensual unions; (4) the extent of international migration flows, particularly after World War II; (5) the timing of the introduction of modern family planning services; (6) levels of female education and rates of labor force participation between countries; and (7) ethnic composition.

Mortality decline preceded fertility decline across Latin America. Mortality decline in some countries was already well under way during the 1930s, that is, before the introduction of medical innovations to the region, thanks to general improvements in living standards (Palloni, 1990). After World War II, and particularly between 1945 and 1965, life expectancy in the region increased dramatically as socioeconomic development complemented the introduction of medicines such as sulfa drugs and penicillin to treat infectious diseases and the introduction of vaccines against measles, diphtheria, tetanus, and typhoid (Palloni, 1981; Merrick, 1991).

Fertility began to decline throughout Latin America at approximately the same historical moment—in the 1960s—despite quite different prevailing levels of mortality. At the onset of fertility decline, the rate of infant mortality ranged from under 65 per 1,000 in Paraguay and Panama to over 150 per 1,000 in Haiti and Bolivia (Guzman, 1994). Mexico and Bolivia were the only two notable late starters, with fertility declines that began in the early 1970s (Guzman, 1994). The Latin American decline in fertility resulted almost entirely from a decline in marital fertility associated with increased use of modern contraception, although later marriage and abortion also played a role (Palloni, 1990; Merrick, 1991).

Although fertility has fallen across the region, the speed of decline has varied dramatically. In some countries, the fertility transition is now almost complete; in others, meanwhile, it seems to have barely begun. By analyzing the specific experiences of individual Latin American countries, Guzman (1994) identified no fewer than four distinct patterns of fertility decline. These range from countries that have completed or almost completed their transition to low fertility (Argentina, Uruguay, Chile, and Cuba) to countries where the fertility transition has been delayed and childbearing remains high, with more than five children per woman in 1985-1990 (Bolivia, Guatemala, Honduras, and Nicaragua).

In his review of fertility and mortality decline in Latin America, Palloni (1990) concluded that exogenous changes in socioeconomic development and family planning program efforts are less than adequate as explanations for mortality and fertility decline. In his view, future analysis of demographic change in the region should specifically allow for endogenous mortality-fertility interaction effects (Palloni, 1990:144). Although the relatively short duration of breast-feeding in the region implies that the lactation interruption effect must be small, analyses of pooled cross-sectional time series data reveal a surprisingly strong correspondence between infant mortality and fertility in Latin America, a relationship that is diluted as the length of time considered is increased (Palloni, 1989, cited in Palloni, 1990).

Sub-Saharan Africa

Fertility in sub-Saharan Africa remains the highest in the world. The slow speed with which sub-Saharan African countries have adopted family planning has led to a great deal of debate as to whether Africa is more resistant to fertility change than are other parts of the world. A few countries, notably Kenya, Botswana, and Zimbabwe, began their transitions toward lower fertility in the early 1990s. More recently, Demographic and Health Surveys (DHS) have recorded apparent declines in fertility in a variety of countries across the continent, including Côte d'Ivoire, Ghana, southern Malawi, southern Namibia, southwest Nigeria, Rwanda, Senegal, northern Tanzania, and Zambia.

From his comprehensive review of published studies on mortality-fertility dynamics in Africa, Kuate Defo (in this volume) concludes that aggregate-level studies have usually failed to document any clear effect of mortality decline on fertility whereas individual-level studies have consistently found a significant fertility response to child loss. Nevertheless, Caldwell et al. (1992) have noted that Botswana, Kenya, and Zimbabwe all enjoy infant mortality rates below 70 per 1,000 whereas most countries in the region face rates of over 100. Arguing that African parents are more sensitive to the risk of losing a child because of an extreme fear of family extinction, Caldwell et al. suggest that achieving these

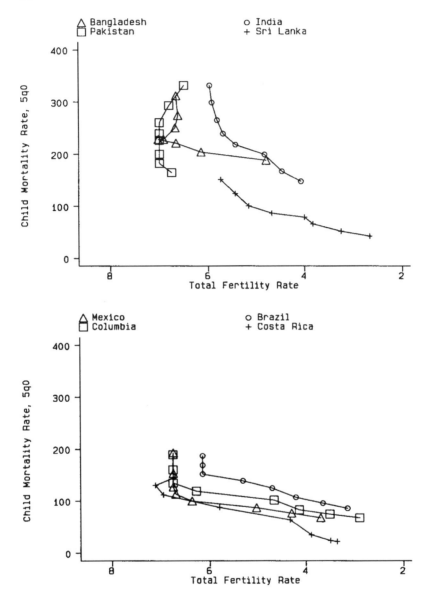

FIGURE 1-1 Alternative mortality-fertility pathways, 1950-1990. NOTE: Each line depicts one country's experience over the period from 1950 to 1990. Because the transition has been from high to low levels of mortality and fertility, time is represented by

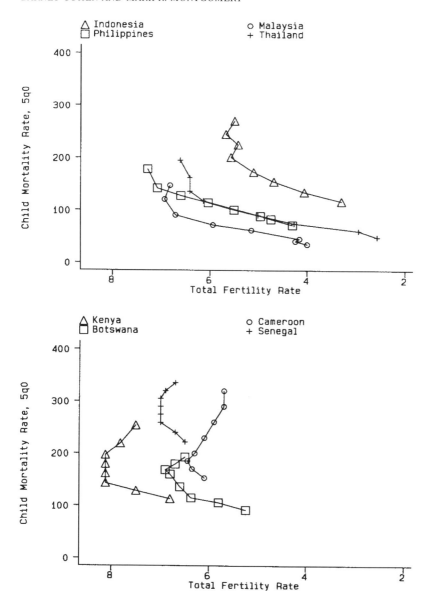

going from left to right along any line. Hence the far left point of any line represents the period 1950-1955. Each subsequent point represents the country's position in the next period. The far right-hand point represents a country's position in 1985-1990.

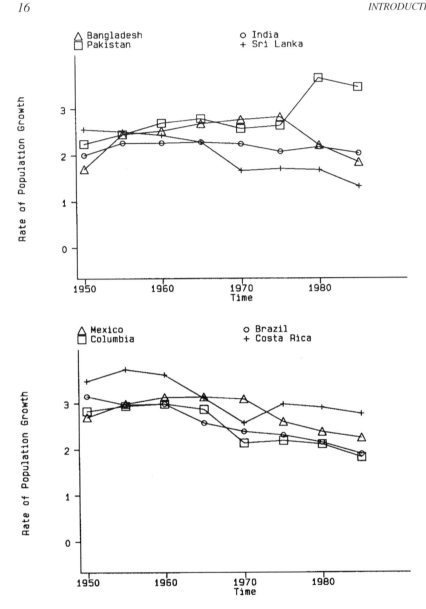

FIGURE 1-2 Rates of population growth, 1950-1990.

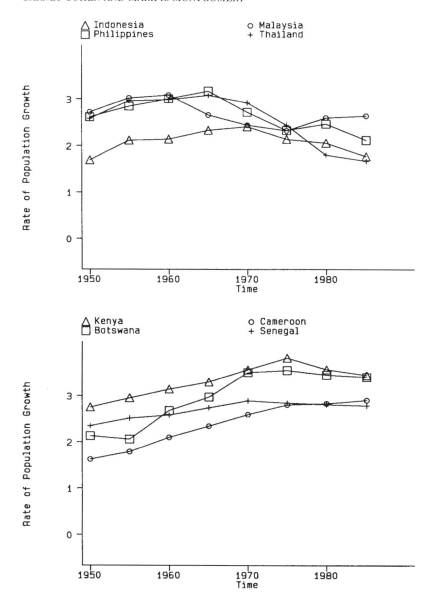

minimum goals for child survival may prove to be "the necessary condition for African fertility decline" (Caldwell et al., 1992:212).

Mortality rates in West Africa have long been higher than those of East or southern Africa (Hill, 1991, 1993), and indications of incipient decline in fertility at the national level have been fewer. Yet recent data have revealed the first signs of fertility decline in Senegal. Here, child mortality has been falling rapidly, but it is not yet low; female education remains low; and the national family planning program is as yet quite weak (Pison et al., 1995). The apparent relationship between mortality and fertility decline in Senegal can be questioned, not least because Senegal's fertility decline appears to be atypical. Fertility decline has been concentrated almost entirely among women under age 30, the result of a trend toward later marriage and later first birth (Pison et al., 1995). Little of this decline appears to be attributable either to an increase in the use of modern contraception or to a decrease in ideal family size (Pison et al., 1995).

Any investigation into the association between fertility and mortality in Africa must take into account the consequences of the AIDS epidemic, whose widespread and severe consequences are becoming increasingly apparent throughout much of society. There is a staggering amount of literature being generated on AIDS in Africa, yet almost none of it has addressed the epidemic's impact on birth rates (but see Ainsworth et al., in this volume). After reviewing the effects of testing and counseling programs on subsequent reproductive behavior, Setel (1995) concludes that little or no evidence indicates that women who are HIV positive will accelerate childbearing upon learning of their diagnosis. A few studies indicate that HIV-positive women, particularly those closer to completing their reproductive goals and those who receive counseling as part of a couple, have somewhat lower fertility than do women who are told that they are HIV negative. The only other published study to date, which suggests that HIV epidemics are most likely to exert downward pressure on fertility, fails to account for the possibility that couples can make compensating adjustments to their desired family size or to decisions regarding the timing or spacing of children (Gregson, 1994). This latter effect already appears to be evident in Tanzania (Ainsworth et al., in this volume) and should be of increasing importance as levels of contraceptive use rise across the continent.

Asia and the Middle East

Asia has been described as "more diverse than . . . any other region in the world" (Rele and Alam, 1993).[7] Fertility decline in Asia has occurred under a variety of economic, political, and sociocultural regimes and under quite differ-

---

[7]As evidence of this, pretransition fertility levels have varied widely across the region, with total fertility rates ranging from 5.5 to 7.0, as a result of differences in nuptiality patterns, postpartum practices, and other unspecified factors (see Casterline, 1994; Caldwell, 1993, and references therein).

ent infant and child mortality environments. The changes have been complex and, for the most part, are explainable only in hindsight. Most of the fertility decline in the region has been associated with increases in the use of modern contraception within marriage, although some of the decline has also been linked to changes in marriage patterns (Casterline, 1994). Since the late 1970s, the decline in fertility in Asia has been sufficiently great to offset the contemporaneous decline in mortality, resulting in a slowdown in the region's rate of population growth.

In East Asia, fertility declines in China, South Korea, and Taiwan began in the 1960s, a point in time when all three countries remained predominantly rural, although the circumstances under which the declines occurred differed a great deal. In China, an aggressive government policy was among the major factors inducing fertility decline (Tien, 1984; Wolf, 1986; Rele and Alam, 1993). In South Korea and Taiwan, fertility transitions were more spontaneous, as rapid economic modernization and social transformation gave couples the motivation to restrict fertility and governments played significant supporting roles by providing family planning information and subsidized services (Gunnarsson, 1992; Coale and Freedman, 1993).

In Southeast Asia, the fertility transition began in earnest in the early 1970s.[8] Once again, the onset of fertility transition appeared in different countries under quite different conditions and did not always evolve in the manner predicted by demographic transition theory. Several countries' fertility transitions seem to have commenced in advance of significant social and economic development. For example, in Thailand fertility rates began to decline even as much of the country remained at only a modest level of economic development; subsequent changes in reproductive behavior do not correlate closely with socioeconomic or sociocultural changes, which have evidently occurred at a substantially slower pace. The change in reproductive behavior and attitudes in Thailand has been so rapid and so pervasive that it has permeated almost all broad segments of Thai society within a period of some 15 years (Knodel et al., 1987).[9]

In the Philippines, after a fall from 6.5 children per woman in 1960 to 5.2 children per woman in 1975, the decline in fertility slowed. In 1984, women in the Philippines were still having 4.8 children, a level well above what might have been predicted on the basis of earlier trends, the relatively high educational

---

[8]The one major exception to this generalization is Singapore. In Singapore, fertility began to decline in the mid-1950s and by the late 1970s had fallen below replacement levels, where it has remained ever since (Rele and Alam, 1993). In other countries, such as Vietnam, the fertility transition is still under way (Goodkind, 1995; Phai et al., 1996).

[9]Summarizing the evidence, Knodel et al. (1987:120) conclude that "It is difficult to imagine that had infant and child mortality remained at the levels of several decades ago that fertility would have fallen to the current levels. . . . Nevertheless, direct evidence of improved child survival contributing to the decline of fertility in Thailand is largely lacking."

attainments of Filipino women, and other improvements in socioeconomic conditions. Part of the explanation lies in the fact that the Filipino government has long been reluctant to take an aggressive approach to family planning, perhaps because political leaders have felt themselves hindered by the strongly pronatalist influence of the Roman Catholic Church (Alam and Leete, 1993a).

In Malaysia, life expectancy at birth was considerably higher than in much of the region by the early 1950s, and fertility decline began relatively early—in the late 1950s—and continued at an increasingly rapid pace for almost 20 years. By 1975, fertility in Malaysia had fallen to some 67 percent of its pretransition level (Hirschman, 1980). But, just at the point when most demographers would have predicted that Malaysian fertility would further decline to replacement levels, fertility among the majority Malay community began instead to rise. Such was not the case among either the Chinese or the Indian community, and ethnic differences in fertility in Malaysia have thus become increasingly pronounced (Hirschman, 1986; Leete and Ann, 1993). Instead of falling predictably in response to increased education, urbanization, and living standards, the Malaysian fertility decline effectively stalled at around four children per woman. The explanations that have been proposed for this phenomenon include a resurgence in Islamic values and marked shifts in government policy (Leete and Ann, 1993; Cleland, 1993).

South-central Asia has recorded major differences in the timing of fertility transitions both between and within countries. In Sri Lanka, for example, where late age at first marriage for women has traditionally kept fertility rates relatively low, fertility declined rapidly in the late 1960s and early 1970s. By 1974, the total fertility rate stood at some 3.4 children per woman (Alam and Leete, 1993a). Within India, quite possibly the world's most heterogeneous country in regard to ethnic diversity, economic status, religious beliefs, and class divisions, the fertility transition is at quite different stages in different states within the country. In Bangladesh, fertility has been falling dramatically over the past two decades even though it is a country that "appears to possess no features that are conducive to fertility decline, except for a strong, persistent government commitment to reducing population growth" (Cleland et al., 1994:xi).[10] By contrast, the fertility transition in Pakistan and Nepal has barely begun (Shah and Cleland, 1993).

The Middle East provides a final example of a region where the pace of the transition from high to low mortality and fertility varies enormously among

---

[10]According to the latest World Development Report, Bangladesh is the 12th poorest country in the world (World Bank, 1995). The vast majority of the rural population is engaged in agriculture (principally at the subsistence level), mortality in the country remains relatively high, and the status of women is relatively low; levels of female literacy and participation rates for females outside of the home are both low. By most economic and social indicators, Pakistan could be said to be ahead of Bangladesh (Cleland, 1993), and it enjoys slightly lower levels of child and infant mortality than Bangladesh (Mitra et al., 1994; National Institute of Population Studies [Pakistan], 1992).

countries, urban and rural populations, and different ethnic groups (Omran and Roudi, 1993). Despite rapidly declining mortality, fertility appears to have fallen only slightly from its 1950s levels in Jordan, Oman, Syria, and Yemen. Elsewhere, such as in Saudi Arabia, Qatar, or the United Arab Emirates, oil revenues have raised standards of living and ushered in high-quality medical care, but these changes have translated into only modest declines in fertility. Where fertility is declining, it is declining at much higher levels of socioeconomic development than in Latin America or Asia. Possible explanations for this phenomenon include the region's unique political and cultural context in which reproductive decisions are made (Weeks, 1988; Cleland, 1993). In the Middle East, issues of politics, religion, national security, and economics are all inextricably linked, and population policies vary widely across the region (Cleland, 1993).

THE SIGNIFICANCE OF THE RESEARCH IN THIS VOLUME

The chapters in this volume contribute to the theoretical, methodological, and empirical literature on three broad fronts: by refining the mechanisms through which mortality decline can affect fertility; by providing a reassessment of the historical record; and by supplying new evidence from detailed case studies in developing countries.

Theory and Evidence on the Strength of Various Mechanisms

Lactation Interruption Effects

Until now, demographers have not systematically exploited the largest demographic database from developing countries—the Demographic and Health Surveys—to examine the strength of the lactation interruption and replacement effects. The chapter by Laurence Grummer-Strawn, Paul Stupp, and Zuguo Mei effectively fills this gap. The authors use proportional hazard models to examine whether the length of the interval between two births is affected by whether or not an index child was alive at the time of the next child's conception. They find that mean birth intervals are some 32 percent longer if the index child survives than if he or she dies in infancy. Premature truncation of breastfeeding explains, on average, about 65 percent of this difference, with other mechanisms, such as reduced coital frequency or differences in contraceptive use, presumably accounting for the residual. Interestingly, intensive breastfeeding appears to influence both the time to resumption of menses and the length of the period from their resumption to the next conception, the latter reflecting the presence of anovulatory cycles after the return of menses or reduced fecundability. These results add weight to earlier studies, confirming that breastfeeding is an important factor affecting differences in birth interval lengths in both populations that use contraception and in those that do not. Using better and more sophisticated techniques, and applying them to a wider array of data, the authors have strongly reinforced earlier conclusions about the strength of this effect.

Insurance and Replacement Effects

Kenneth Wolpin's chapter reviews recent theoretical insights into micro-level decision making from the field of economics. Economic models of reproductive behavior have progressed considerably from the static lifetime formulations to complex sequential decision-making models. These advances have enabled economists to estimate increasingly more sophisticated and realistic models of human behavior. Wolpin's chapter underscores a point that has been insufficiently appreciated—that insurance and replacement effects have common roots in individual preferences, perceptions, and constraints—and guides the reader through an illuminating dynamic formulation. In addition to summarizing the potential contributions of such models to demographic research, Wolpin carefully analyzes the statistical problems that researchers face when trying to estimate replacement and insurance effects.

Economic models of rational decision-making behavior typically assume that parents know within some bounds the likelihood of their children's survival. Such an assumption may be untenable for rural semiliterate populations in many developing countries. For example, Mark Montgomery argues that in a changing demographic environment, parents may not be equipped with any direct knowledge of the probabilities of their children's survival. This suggests the need to understand how mortality perceptions are formed. Are perceptions influenced principally by direct experience or observed experience; or is the decisive factor the knowledge acquired in school, through the media, or from health personnel in the community? What time lags are involved? What psychological weight do people place on extreme cases of mortality as compared with the norm?

Montgomery's review of the cognitive and social psychological literature on judgment and belief updating casts doubt on the hypothesis that people act as if they were Bayesian statisticians. Rather, they tend to depart in systematic ways from Bayesian predictions. For example, they adhere too closely to preconceived notions, resist change, give insufficient weight to certain types of information, and allow negative events to exert an undue influence. Montgomery's chapter points to the need to make use of psychological models of how people learn and make decisions in environments of pervasive uncertainty.

One of the mechanisms about which very little is yet known is the insurance or hoarding mechanism. One approach is to investigate environments where mortality conditions are changing very rapidly. Martha Ainsworth, Deon Filmer, and Innocent Semali take this approach in their chapter in which they examine the impact of AIDS mortality on individual fertility in Tanzania, where the adverse consequences of the epidemic are becoming increasingly apparent. Their effort is notable in attempting to link adult mortality, as well as child mortality, to fertility decisions.

For the most part, models of the demographic impact of the AIDS epidemic have ignored the possibility that individuals might alter their fertility in response to deteriorating mortality conditions. This is clearly a dubious assumption. Using data from one high-prevalence region and two national surveys of Tanzania, the authors find that higher community levels of child mortality are associated with higher fertility, whereas higher community levels of adult mortality are associated with lower fertility aspirations and lower recent fertility.

Reassessment of Historical Events

Casual observation of the demographic transition in nineteenth century Europe suggests that the mortality decline preceded the fertility decline, leading researchers to theorize a causal link between the two. Mortality declined sharply, largely because of improvements in living standards, sanitation, and medical progress. Fertility also fell, mainly as a result of the termination of childbearing within marriage. Methods such as coitus interruptus or withdrawal, together with periodic abstinence and some abortion, accounted for much of the decline. Detailed analyses of European data from the Princeton European Fertility Project showed that high levels of development and low levels of child mortality were sufficient to initiate a decline in marital fertility, but that no single threshold level of development or mortality could be identified. Empirical evidence from Europe indicated that fertility declined under a wide variety of social, economic, and demographic conditions. The transition also appeared to move quickly through areas with common dialects or similar cultural characteristics, regardless of socioeconomic or demographic conditions, suggesting that diffusion or cultural factors must have played a key role (Knodel and van de Walle, 1986). In some cases the declines in fertility were gradual, whereas in others, they were remarkably rapid (Coale and Treadway, 1986).

The decline in mortality usually, but not always, preceded the onset of family limitation (Coale, 1973; van de Walle, 1986). As Chesnais (1992) and others have emphasized, conclusions about timing depend on the measure of mortality that is employed. Infant mortality declined before marital fertility in only about half the administrative districts in Germany and in all but one province in Belgium (Knodel, 1974; Lesthaeghe, 1977). In the case of Belgium, Lesthaeghe concludes "[m]ost probably, other factors were already conditioning marital fertility in the direction of a decline before the weight of an infant mortality reduction could be felt" (1977:176). In England, while child mortality was in decline from the 1860s, infant mortality began to decline after 1900, several decades after the onset of the decline in marital fertility (Teitelbaum, 1984). Thus, the historical evidence suggests that declines in infant mortality rate do not always precede declines in fertility (van de Walle, 1986). Instead, both declines appear to have occurred over the course of modernization. At the same time, however, replacement effects probably strengthened as family limitation spread (Knodel, 1982).

In their chapter, Patrick Galloway, Ronald Lee, and Eugene Hammel argue that previous studies have often failed to account explicitly for the fact that mortality and fertility are jointly determined. The formulation of an appropriate causal model is difficult, requiring both unusual care and richer data than needed in other areas of demographic research. Galloway and colleagues argue that the complications necessitate the use of two-stage estimation techniques. Using data from Prussia over the period 1875-1910, the authors find that declines in infant mortality are positively associated with declines in fertility.[11] In reanalyzing the European macro evidence, Galloway et al. stress two additional points. First, the time frame for the analysis is critical: In the long term, macro-economic or macro-societal mechanisms operate to ensure that fertility and mortality are more or less in equilibrium. In the very short run such mechanisms are ineffective. Conditions that produce short-run high mortality probably also produce short-run low fertility. Hence, the key question is what happens over the medium term, which Galloway et al. define as 5-30 years. Second, levels of fertility and mortality are less informative than are changes in these variables over time. Studies of changes are less vulnerable to contamination by persistent unobserved heterogeneity.

To date, very little work on this topic has been focused on the United States, perhaps because macro-level time series data indicate that fertility decline preceded mortality decline by at least 70 years. Thus, declines in mortality could not have prompted the onset of family limitation, although mortality could well have influenced the subsequent speed and depth of the transition. In his chapter, Michael Haines examines the strength of replacement and hoarding effects in the United States in the early twentieth century, using public-use micro samples from the 1900 and 1910 censuses. Haines finds that between 10 and 30 percent of all child deaths in the United States at the turn of the century were directly replaced by subsequent births; high death rates also induced considerable hoarding behavior. These findings resemble those reported in studies of contemporary populations in developing countries at low levels of socioeconomic development (see Preston, 1975).

---

[11]Note that even in cases in which the direction and strength of the effect can be identified, this might not determine the net effect of health improvements on total fertility. This is because the underlying level of natural fertility cannot be assumed to remain constant over time. Hence, as shown by the authors in a related paper, improvements in child mortality had little net effect on fertility in Prussia over the period 1875-1910. Improvements in general health increased the level of natural fertility at the same time as the desired number of births decreased (Lee et al., 1994).

Further Evidence from Developing Countries

The past 40 years or so have witnessed a remarkable trend in the demography of many developing countries—unprecedented declines in infant and child mortality throughout the world and, in most places, a dramatic shift from high fertility and little parity-specific control to a situation in which family limitation has come within the "calculus of conscious choice." The factors responsible for fertility decline are still not fully understood. As we have seen, heterogeneity between and within the various regions of the world has been conspicuous in several dimensions: the initial levels of fertility; the socioeconomic and demographic conditions prevailing at the onset of fertility declines; the date of the onset and the speed of the declines once under way; the extent of the declines (i.e., the ultimate levels of fertility achieved); the role of government policy toward population and family planning; and, most important in the context of this volume, the role of prior mortality declines. The four case studies in this volume are drawn from three continents and four countries at very different stages of their fertility transitions. Collectively, they confirm the importance of social, political, and economic context. The history of the family planning programs in these countries appears particularly important.

Cameroon

Fertility in sub-Saharan Africa remains the highest in the world. Many women are unable to articulate their desired family size and, when they do, their answers often imply a demand for children that exceeds or presses close on the biological limits. Significant advances have been made over the past 20 years in the availability of solid demographic data from the region as well as in methods of demographic analysis. Barthélémy Kuate Defo's chapter takes advantage of both developments.

Kuate Defo proposes a semiparametric multistate duration methodology that uses hazard models to estimate a reduced-form birth process. The elegant aspect of the methodology is that it allows for the possibility of testing for the significance of woman-specific unobservables. Not surprisingly, given the low prevalence of contraception in Cameroon, Kuate Defo finds that maternal characteristics exert weak effects on fertility outcomes, and the strongest differences in reproductive behavior associated with a child death are found among women at high parities. On further inspection, Kuate Defo finds that the parity-specific effects on timing to conception operate through the timing of the first child's death. By separating the effects of a death at each successive parity, Kuate Defo shows that the death of a first child has a differentially large, lasting, and significant influence over the remainder of a woman's reproductive life. The author attributes this to the special significance of the first born in traditional Cameroonian culture.

Indonesia

Fertility has been declining in Indonesia for more than two decades—from some 5.6 births per woman in the late 1960s to 2.9 births per woman in 1991-1994 (Indonesia/DHS, 1995). The decline began at a time when levels of child mortality were still relatively high and economic development, school attendance, and rates of urbanization relatively low. Significantly, however, the government of Indonesia switched from firm opposition to fertility control to a recognition of the disadvantages of continued rapid population growth and made a strong commitment to reducing fertility (Alam and Leete, 1993b).[12] Observers of this period of Indonesian history express little doubt that the government family planning program was a central ingredient in the country's fertility transition and that it speeded the process of decline, especially among the rural poor (Freedman et al., 1981; McNicoll and Singarimbun, 1983; Sanderson and Tan, 1995).[13]

This is the context for Elizabeth Frankenberg's chapter and her meticulous analysis of the effect of improved child survival under a regime of falling fertility. Frankenberg finds that replacement has been less than complete in Indonesia but that the effect has strengthened over time. Frankenberg's chapter also contributes to the methodological debate by proposing a difference-in-differences approach to analyzing birth intervals so as to control for unobserved heterogeneity due to family-specific fixed effects. Using this model, she finds evidence that the death of a child leads to small changes in the length of subsequent birth intervals relative to when the child does not die. The size of the changes are conditional on the sex composition of surviving children.

India

India is the second most populous country in the world and probably the most heterogeneous with respect to its inhabitants' ethnic diversity, economic status, religious beliefs, linguistic divisions, cultural heritage, class divisions, and beliefs and traditions (International Institute for Population Sciences [Bombay], 1995). The sheer size of the country allows macro-level relationships to be

---

[12]In the late 1960s, the Indonesian government initiated a vigorous family planning program that created a network for the distribution of subsidized contraceptives, ran campaigns to promote their use, and maintained strong links with local government and community groups in an effort to pressure couples to regulate their fertility (McNicoll and Singarimbun, 1983; Warwick, 1986; Cleland, 1993).

[13]During the mid-1980s fertility decline resulted from increased contraceptive use induced primarily by economic development and by improved education and economic opportunities for females (Gertler and Molyneaux, 1994).

examined at the state and district levels. Given such vast cultural diversity, it should not be surprising to learn that fertility transition is at quite different stages in different Indian states. For example, in states such as Goa in the west or Kerala in the south, fertility is already below replacement; elsewhere in the country, such as in Uttar Pradesh, fertility remains close to five children per family. About 10 percent of the variation in fertility between northern and southern Indian states can be attributed to differences in levels of child survival.

Examining data at various levels of aggregation, Mari Bhat argues for a structural shift in the relationship between mortality and fertility in India in the 1970s, indicating that family-building strategies probably changed as fertility began to decline. Bhat shows how the speed at which reproductive behaviors adjust to changing mortality environments is determined partly by the nature of family planning programs. In India, the government's near-exclusive reliance on sterilization as a family planning method prevented couples from adopting a pure replacement strategy and forced a dependence on the insurance mechanism. Nevertheless, the strength of the replacement effect increased over time.

Costa Rica

The case study of Costa Rica provides further evidence that at the macro level, declines in mortality can be only weakly connected to declines in fertility. Rather, the strength of the relationship in Costa Rica varies over time and over the course of the transition. Using county-level data from 89 counties, Luis Rosero-Bixby finds that, once one has controlled for other indicators of socioeconomic development, there is little indication that low infant mortality rates exert much influence on fertility rates. Consequently, Rosero-Bixby concludes that although improved child survival may facilitate fertility declines, and low survival chances may delay the transition, there is no critical mortality threshold to be overcome.

During focus group interviews, women in Costa Rica who had lived through the fertility transition indicated that the prevailing level of child mortality was not at the forefront of their thinking. Nevertheless, other comments suggested that improved child survival could have been a key reason leading such women to question culturally determined reproductive behavior. For example, for many women the first exposure to family planning came at health centers. Perhaps, apart from learning about birth control at these clinics, favorable experiences with modern medicine predisposed women to make use of other health services, such as contraception. Furthermore, the time and labor burden associated with having larger families as a result of improved child survival made Costa Rican women more likely to question earlier culturally determined reproductive norms.

DISCUSSION

Twenty years ago, the most recent data available to assess the relationship between mortality and fertility were from 1975. Since then, substantial improvements in life expectancy have been recorded, state-sponsored family planning programs were initiated and grew toward maturity, and fertility began to fall across Latin America and Asia. In this chapter, we have described the recent demographic situation with our principal focus being on the demographic changes of the past two decades. The recent empirical record provides an outer core of knowledge on the complex interrelationship between mortality and fertility.

Outside West Africa, virtually all developing countries have by now experienced some order of joint decline of mortality and fertility. Their fertility declines are the product of diverse social, economic, political, and cultural changes and are shaped as well by a response to programs and mortality change. The precise nature and specific contribution of each of these factors varies from one society to another. Thus, at the macro level, a search for a simple and universal rule linking the timing of mortality and fertility declines would seem to be futile.

At the micro level, what effect do mortality experiences and expectations have on reproductive behavior? Numerous empirical studies have documented that the death of a child reduces the probability that its parents will adopt contraception and increases the likelihood of additional births. This is because deaths and the expectation of deaths produce both behavioral and biological fertility responses. Investigations of such effects depend crucially on the level (family versus aggregate) and time frame of the analysis (Casterline, 1995). Furthermore, as the chapters in this volume clearly demonstrate, the nature of the mortality-fertility relationship changes over the course of the demographic transition as couples take greater control of their reproductive decisions and outcomes.

More has been learned about some mechanisms than about others. The lactation interruption effect of a child's death on fertility is now far better understood than are the behavioral effects. The lactation mechanism is most important in populations where breastfeeding is practiced widely but it remains important even in populations that use modern contraception (Lloyd and Ivanov, 1988). As for the behavioral effects, most is known about replacement behavior, whether studied by way of parity progression ratios or simultaneous equation models. The chapters in this volume focus mainly on such replacement effects. These studies strongly second the conclusion of the original Preston volume, that replacement is less than complete (Knodel, 1995).

The mechanisms about which we continue to know the least are the insurance effect and the "transition" or "confidence" effect. As noted above, research into these mechanisms has been hampered by serious problems of conceptualization and measurement, as well as by a lack of data. Progress in understanding the insurance effect will require linking fertility change to community-level changes in mortality; it will also require better models of individual decision making and social learning. These were areas that Brass and Barrett (1978) regarded as being out of reach in the mid-1970s, but ones that may benefit from recent work on diffusion theory (see, for example, Casterline et al., 1987; Montgomery and Casterline, 1996).

To learn more about the onset of fertility declines, it is vital to understand the transitional effect. Much of the pretransition literature points to the lack of parity-specific control; either parents were unaware of the means to regulate their fertility, saw little point in such regulation, or were constrained by social institutions. Lloyd and Ivanov (1988) hypothesized that differences in the age pattern of improvements in child survival could affect the size of the fertility response; this important hypothesis remains untested.

Perhaps the most important policy implication of this work is for the interactions among mortality, fertility, and family planning services. Twenty years of lively debate in the demographic literature have yet to lay to rest the question of whether family planning programs make an important independent contribution to fertility decline (see, for example, Freedman and Berelson, 1976; Mauldin and Berelson, 1978; Cutright and Kelly, 1981; Lapham and Mauldin, 1987; Bongaarts et al., 1990; Pritchett, 1994a,b; Bongaarts, 1994; Knowles et al., 1994). The research on mortality-fertility relationships reported in this volume shows that the strength of the behavioral response can be affected by the extent and quality of family planning services. For example, Bhat (in this volume) demonstrates how the lack of reversible contraception has dampened the responsiveness of fertility to improvements in child survival in India. In Costa Rica, Rosero-Bixby (in this volume) found that, even in settings with moderately high levels of infant mortality, the greater the supply of family planning services, the greater the likelihood of fertility-limiting behavior. There is no evidence to suggest either that child survival programs must precede family planning programs or vice versa. Rather, the research discussed here suggests that child survival and family planning programs play important complementary roles.

ACKNOWLEDGMENTS

This chapter has benefited from the discussion of participants at a seminar entitled "Reevaluating the Link between Infant and Child Mortality and Fertility," which was organized by the Committee on Population in November 1995. Nevertheless, the views and opinions in this chapter are solely those of the authors and are not meant to reflect those of the National Research Council or the other seminar participants. We are grateful to Caroline Bledsoe, Patrick Galloway, John Haaga, Ken Hill, Bill House, Carolyn Makinson, and Faith Mitchell for their comments on an earlier draft.

REFERENCES

Alam, I., and R. Leete

1993a   Pauses in fertility trends in Sri Lanka and the Philippines? Pp. 83-95 in R. Leete and I. Alam, eds., *The Revolution in Asian Fertility: Dimensions, Causes, and Implications.* Oxford, England: Clarendon Press.

1993b   Variations in fertility in India and Indonesia. Pp. 148-172 in R. Leete and I. Alam, eds., *The Revolution in Asian Fertility: Dimensions, Causes, and Implications.* Oxford, England: Clarendon Press.

Anderson, K.H.

1983   The determinants of fertility, schooling, and child survival in Guatemala. *International Economic Review* 24(3):567-589.

Balakrishnan, T.R.

1978   Effects of child mortality on subsequent fertility of women in some rural and semi-urban areas of certain Latin American countries. *Population Studies* 32(1):135-145.

Becker, G., K. Murphy, and R. Tamura

1990   Human capital, fertility and economic growth. *Journal of Political Economy* 98(5, part 2):S12-S37.

Benefo, K., and T.P. Schultz

1996   Fertility and child mortality in Côte d'Ivoire and Ghana. *The World Bank Economic Review* 10(1):123-158.

Bongaarts, J.

1975   Why high birth rates are so low. *Population and Development Review* 1(2):289-296.

1987   Does family planning reduce infant mortality rates? *Population and Development Review* 13(2):323-334.

1988   Does family planning reduce infant mortality? Reply. *Population and Development Review* 14(1):188-190.

1994   The impact of population policies: Comment. *Population and Development Review* 20(3):616-620.

1997   Trends in Unwanted Childbearing in the Developing World. Paper presented at the Annual Meetings of the Population Association of America, Washington, D.C., March 27-29.

Bongaarts, J., W.P. Mauldin, and J.F. Phillips

1990   The demographic impact of family planning programs. *Studies in Family Planning* 21(6):299-310.

Brass, W., and J.C. Barrett

1978   Measurement problems in the analysis of linkages between fertility and child mortality. Pp. 209-233 in S.H. Preston, ed., *The Effects of Infant and Child Mortality on Fertility.* New York: Academic Press.

Bulatao, R.A.

1985   Fertility and Mortality Transition. World Bank Staff Working Paper no. 681. The World Bank, Washington, D.C.

Caldwell, J.C.

1986   Routes to low mortality in poor countries. *Population and Development Review* 12(2):171-220.

1993   The Asian fertility revolution: Its implications for transition theories. Pp. 299-316 in R. Leete and I. Alam, eds., *The Revolution in Asian Fertility: Dimensions, Causes, and Implications.* Oxford, England: Clarendon Press.

Caldwell, J.C., and P. Caldwell

1987   The cultural context of high fertility in sub-Saharan Africa. *Population and Development Review* 13(3):409-437.

Caldwell, J.C., P. Reddy, and P. Caldwell
1983   The social component of mortality decline: An investigation in South India employing alternative methodologies. *Population Studies* 37(2):185-205.

Caldwell, J.C., I.O. Orubuloye, and P. Caldwell
1992   Fertility decline in Africa: A new type of transition? *Population and Development Review* 18(2):211-242.

Casterline, J.B.
1994   Fertility transition in Asia. Pp. 69-86 in T. Locoh and V. Hertrich, eds., *The Onset of Fertility Transition in Sub-Saharan Africa*. Liège, Belgium: Derouaux Ordina Editions for International Union for the Scientific Study of Population (IUSSP).

1995   Remarks made at National Academy of Sciences' Workshop on Reevaluating the Effects of Infant and Child Mortality on Fertility, Washington, D.C., November 6-7. The Population Council, New York.

Casterline, J.B., M.R. Montgomery, and R.L. Clark
1987   *Diffusion Models of Fertility Control: Are There New Insights?* Population Studies and Training Center (PSTC) Working Paper Series 87-06. Providence, R.I.: PSTC, Brown University.

Castle, S.
1994   The Effect of Repeated Child Deaths on Child Care Practices among the Malian Fulani and the Implications for Demographic Research. Paper presented at the 1994 Annual Meetings of the Population Association of America, Miami, Fla., May 5-7.

Chesnais, J.-C.
1992   *The Demographic Transition: Stages, Patterns and Economic Implications*. Oxford, England: Clarendon Press.

Chowdhury, A.I., V. Fauveau, and K.M.A. Aziz
1992   Effects of child survival on contraceptive use in Bangladesh. *Journal of Biosocial Sciences* 24(4):427-432.

Chowdhury, A.K.M.A., A.R. Khan, and L.C. Chen
1976   The effect of child mortality experience on subsequent fertility: In Pakistan and Bangladesh. *Population Studies* 30(1):249-261.

Chowdhury, A.R.
1988   The infant mortality-fertility debate: Some international evidence. *Southern Economic Journal* 54(3):666-674.

Cleland, J.
1993   Different pathways to demographic transition. Pp. 229-247 in F. Graham-Smith, ed., *Population—The Complex Reality*. London: The Royal Society.

Cleland, J., J.F. Phillips, S. Amin, and G.M. Kamal
1994   *The Determinants of Reproductive Change in Bangladesh: Success in a Challenging Environment*. Washington, D.C.: The World Bank.

Coale, A.J.
1973   The demographic transition. Pp. 53-72 in *International Union for the Scientific Study of Population (IUSSP) Proceedings*, Vol. 1. International Population Conference, Liège, 1973. Liège, Belgium: IUSSP.

Coale, A.J., and R. Freedman
1993   Similarities in the fertility transition in China and three other East Asian populations. Pp. 208-238 in R. Leete and I. Alam, eds., *The Revolution in Asian Fertility: Dimensions, Causes, and Implications*. Oxford, England: Clarendon Press.

Coale, A.J., and R. Treadway
1986   A summary of the changing distribution of overall fertility, marital fertility, and the proportion married in the provinces of Europe. Pp. 31-181 in A.J. Coale and S.C. Watkins, eds., *The Decline of Fertility in Europe*. Revised Proceedings of a Conference on the Princeton European Fertility Project. Princeton, N.J.: Princeton University Press.

Cutright, P.
1983   The ingredients of recent fertility decline in developing countries. *International Family Planning Perspectives* 9:101-109.

Cutright, P., and L. Hargens
1984   The threshold hypothesis: Evidence from less developed Latin American countries, 1950 to 1980. *Demography* 21(4):459-473.

Cutright, P., and W.R. Kelly
1981   The role of family planning programs in fertility declines in less developed countries, 1958-1977. *International Family Planning Perspectives* 7(4):145-151.

de Guzman, E.A.
1984   The effects of infant mortality on fertility in the Philippines. Pp. 123-130 in L.T. Engracia, C. Mejia-Raymundo, and J.B. Casterline, eds., *Fertility in the Philippines: Further Analysis of the Republic of the Philippines Fertility Survey 1978.* Voorburg, Netherlands: International Statistical Institute.

Dye, N., and D. Smith
1986   Mother love and infant death, 1750-1920. *Journal of American History* 73:329-353.

Freedman, R.
1963   Norms for family size in underdeveloped areas. *Proceedings of the Royal Society* 159(B): 220-245.

Freedman, R., and B. Berelson
1976   The record of family planning programs. *Studies in Family Planning* 7(1):1-40.

Freedman, R., S. Khoo, and B. Supraptilah
1981   Use of modern contraceptives in Indonesia: A challenge to conventional wisdoms. *International Family Planning Perspectives* 7(1):3-15.

Gertler, P.J., and J.W. Molyneaux
1994   How economic development and family planning programs combined to reduce Indonesian fertility. *Demography* 31(1):33-63.

Goodkind, D.M.
1995   Vietnam's one-or-two child policy in action. *Population and Development Review* 21(1): 85-111.
1996   On substituting sex preference strategies in East Asia: Does prenatal sex selection reduce postnatal discrimination? *Population and Development Review* 22(1):111-125.

Gregson, S.
1994   Will HIV become a major determinant of fertility in sub-Saharan Africa? *Journal of Development Studies* 30(3):650-679.

Gunnarsson, C.
1992   Economic and demographic transition in East Asia: Economic modernization vs family planning in Taiwan. Pp. 81-101 in M. Hammarskjöld, B. Egerö, and S. Lindberg, eds., *Population and the Development Crisis in the South: Proceedings for a Conference in Båstad, April 17-18, 1991.* Lund, Sweden: University of Lund, Programme on Population and Development in Poor Countries (PROP).

Guzman, J.M.
1994   The onset of fertility decline in Latin America. Pp. 43-67 in T. Locoh and V. Hertrich, eds., *The Onset of Fertility Transition in sub-Saharan Africa.* Liège, Belgium: Derouaux Ordina Editions for the International Union for the Scientific Study of Population (IUSSP).

Hammarskjöld M., B. Egerö, and S. Lindberg
1992   *Population and the Development Crisis in the South: Proceedings from a Conference in Båstad, April 17-18, 1991.* Lund, Sweden: University of Lund, Programme on Population and Development in Poor Countries (PROP).

Hashimoto, M., and C. Hongladarom
1981   Effects of child mortality on fertility in Thailand. *Economic Development and Cultural Change* 29(4):781-794.

Hill, A.
1991   Infant and child mortality levels, trends, and data deficiencies. Pp. 37-74 in R.G. Feachem and D.T. Jamison, eds., *Disease and Mortality in Sub-Saharan Africa*. New York: Oxford University Press for the World Bank.
1993   Trends in childhood mortality. Pp. 153-217 in K.A. Foote, K.H. Hill, and L.G. Martin, eds., *Demographic Change in Sub-Saharan Africa*. Committee on Population, National Research Council. Washington, D.C.: National Academy Press.

Hirschman, C.
1980   Demographic trends in peninsular Malaysia, 1947-1975. *Population and Development Review* 6(1):103-125.
1986   The recent rise in Malay fertility: A new trend or a temporary lull in a fertility transition? *Demography* 23(2):161-184.

Hobcraft, J.
1992   Fertility patterns and child survival: A comparative analysis. *Population Bulletin of the United Nations* 33:1-31.

Hobcraft, J., J.W. McDonald, and S. Rutstein
1983   Child-spacing effects on infant and early child mortality. *Population Index* 49(4):585-618.
1985   Demographic determinants of infant and early child mortality: A comparative analysis. *Population Studies* 39(3):363-385.

Indonesia/DHS
1995   *Demographic and Health Survey 1994*. Jakarta, Indonesia: Central Bureau of Statistics (CBS) [Indonesia], State Ministry of Population/National Family Planning Coordinating Board (NFPCB) and Ministry of Health (MOH). Calverton, Md.: Macro International, Inc.

International Institute for Population Sciences [Bombay]
1995   *National Family Health Survey (MCH and Family Planning), India, 1992-93*. Bombay: International Institute for Population Sciences (IIPS).

Johnson, N.E., and A.J.M. Sufian
1992   Effect of son mortality on contraceptive practice in Bangladesh. *Journal of Biosocial Sciences* 24(1):9-16.

King, M.
1990   Health is a sustainable state. *Lancet* 336:664-667.
1991   The demographic trap. *Lancet* 337:307-308.
1992   Escaping the demographic trap. Pp. 38-44 in M. Hammarskjöld, B. Egerö, and S. Lindberg, eds., *Population and the Development Crisis in the South: Proceedings for a Conference in Båstad, April 17-18, 1991*. Lund, Sweden: University of Lund, Programme on Population and Development in Poor Countries (PROP).

Knodel, J.
1974   *The Decline of Fertility in Germany, 1871-1939*. Princeton, N.J.: Princeton University Press.
1982   Child mortality and reproductive behavior in German village populations in the past: A micro-level analysis of the replacement effect. *Population Studies* 36(2):177-200.
1995   Remarks made at National Academy of Sciences' Workshop on Reevaluating the Effects of Infant and Child Mortality on Fertility, Washington, D.C., November 6-7.

Knodel, J., and E. van de Walle
1986   Lessons from the past: Policy implications of historical fertility studies. Pp. 390-419 in A.J. Coale and S.C. Watkins, eds., *The Decline of Fertility in Europe*. Revised Proceedings of a Conference on the Princeton European Fertility Project. Princeton, N.J.: Princeton University Press.

Knodel, J., A. Chamratrithirong, and N. Debavalya
1987   *Thailand's Reproductive Revolution: Rapid Fertility Decline in a Third-World Setting.*
        Madison: University of Wisconsin Press.
Knowles, J.C., J.S. Akin, and D.K. Guilkey
1994   The impact of population policies: Comment. *Population and Development Review*
        20(3):611-615.
Lapham, R.J., and W.P. Mauldin
1987   The effects of family planning on fertility: Research findings. Pp. 647-680 in R.J.
        Lapham and G.B. Simmons, eds., *Organizing for Effective Family Planning Programs.*
        Committee on Population, National Research Council. Washington, D.C.: National Acad-
        emy Press.
Lee, B.S., and T.P. Schultz
1982   Implications of child mortality reductions for fertility and population growth in Korea.
        Journal of Economic Development 71(1):21-44.
Lee, R.D., P.R. Galloway, and E.A. Hammel
1994   Fertility decline in Prussia: Estimating influences on supply, demand, and degree of
        control. *Demography* 31(2):347-373.
Leete, R., and T.B. Ann
1993   Contrasting fertility trends among ethnic groups in Malaysia. Pp. 128-147 in R. Leete
        and I. Alam, eds., *The Revolution in Asian Fertility: Dimensions, Causes, and Implica-
        tions.* Oxford, England: Clarendon Press.
Lesthaeghe, R.J.
1977   *The Decline of Belgian Fertility, 1800-1970.* Princeton, N.J.: Princeton University Press.
Lloyd, C.B., and S. Ivanov
1988   The effects of improved child survival on family planning practice and fertility. *Studies
        in Family Planning* 19(3):141-161.
Maglad, N.E.
1993   *Socioeconomic Determinants of Fertility and Child Mortality in Sudan.* Economic Growth
        Center Discussion Paper no. 686. New Haven, Conn.: Yale University.
1994   Fertility in rural Sudan: The effect of landholding and child mortality. *Economic Devel-
        opment and Cultural Change* 42(4):761-772.
Mason, K.
1997   Explaining Fertility Transitions. Presidential address to the 1997 Annual Meetings of the
        Population Association of America, Washington D.C., March 27-29.
Mauldin, W.P., and B. Berelson
1978   Conditions of fertility decline in developing countries, 1965-1975. *Studies in Family
        Planning* 9(5):89-147.
Mauskopf, J., and T.D. Wallace
1984   Fertility and replacement: Some alternative stochastic models and results for Brazil.
        Demography 21(4):519-536.
McNicoll, G., and M. Singarimbun, eds.
1983   *Fertility Decline in Indonesia: Analysis and Interpretation.* Committee on Population
        and Demography report no. 20, National Research Council. Washington, D.C.: National
        Academy Press.
Mensch, B.S.
1985   The effect of child mortality on contraceptive use and fertility in Colombia, Costa Rica,
        and Korea. *Population Studies* 39(2):309-327.
Merrick, T.
1991   Population pressures in Latin America. *Population Bulletin* 41(3).
Mincer, J.
1996   Economic development, growth of human capital, and the dynamics of the wage struc-
        ture. *Journal of Economic Growth* 1:29-48.

Mitra, S.N., M.N. Ali, S. Islam, A.R. Cross, and T. Saha
  1994   *Bangladesh Demographic and Health Survey, 1993-1994*. Dhaka, Bangladesh: National Institute of Population Research and Training (NIPORT) and Mitra and Associates. Calverton, Md.: Macro International, Inc.
Montgomery, M.R., and J.B. Casterline
  1996   Social influence, social learning, and new models of fertility. *Population and Development Review* 22(Suppl.):151-175.
National Institute of Population Studies [Pakistan]
  1992   *Pakistan Demographic and Health Survey, 1990/1991*. Islamabad: National Institute of Population Studies. Columbia, Md.: IRD/Macro International, Inc.
Notestein, F.
  1945   Population—the long view. Pp. 37-57 in T.W. Schultz, ed. *Food for the World*. Chicago, Ill.: University of Chicago Press.
  1953   Economic problems of population change. Pp. 13-31 in *Proceedings of the Eighth International Conference of Agricultural Economists*. London: Oxford University Press.
Nur, O.E.M.
  1985   An analysis of the child survival hypothesis in Jordan. *Studies in Family Planning* 16(4):211-218.
Okojie, C.E.E.
  1991   Fertility response to child survival in Nigeria: An analysis of microdata from Bendel State. *Research in Population Economics* 7:93-112.
Olsen, R.J.
  1980   Estimating the effect of child mortality on the number of births. *Demography* 17(4):429-443.
Olsen, R.J., and K.I. Wolpin
  1983   The impact of exogenous child mortality on fertility: A waiting time regression with dynamic regressors. *Econometrica* 51(3):731-749.
Omran, A.R., and F. Roudi
  1993   The middle east population puzzle. *Population Bulletin* 48(1).
Palloni, A.
  1981   Mortality in Latin America: Emerging patterns. *Population and Development Review* 7(4):623-649.
  1990   Fertility and mortality decline in Latin America. *Annals of the American Academy of Political and Social Science* 510:126-144.
Panis, C.W.A., and L.A. Lillard
  1993   *Timing of Child Replacement Effects on Fertility in Malaysia*. RAND Labor and Population Program Working Paper Series 93-13. Santa Monica, Calif.: RAND.
Park, C.B., S.H. Han, and M.K. Choe
  1979   The effect of infant death on subsequent fertility in Korea and the role of family planning. *American Journal of Public Health* 69(6):557-565.
Pebley, A.R., H. Delgado, and E. Brinemann
  1979   Fertility desires and child mortality experience among Guatemalan women. *Studies in Family Planning* 10(4):129-136.
Phai, N.V., J. Knodel, M.V. Cam, and H. Xuyen
  1996   Fertility and family planning in Vietnam: Evidence from the 1994 Inter-censal Demographic Survey. *Studies in Family Planning* 27(1):1-17.
Pison, G., K.H. Hill, B. Cohen, and K.A. Foote, eds.
  1995   *Population Dynamics of Senegal*. Committee on Population, National Research Council. Washington, D.C.: National Academy Press.
Pitt, M.M.
  1994   Women's Schooling, Selective Fertility and Child Mortality in Sub-Saharan Africa. Unpublished manuscript, Department of Economics, Brown University, Providence, R.I.

Preston, S.H.
　1975　Health programs and population growth. *Population and Development Review* 1(2):189-199.
　1978a　*The Effects of Infant and Child Mortality on Fertility.* New York: Academic Press.
　1978b　Introduction. Pp. 1-18 in S.H. Preston, ed., *The Effects of Infant and Child Mortality on Fertility.* New York: Academic Press.

Preston, S.H., and M. Haines
　1991　*Fatal Years: Child Mortality in Late Nineteenth-Century America.* Princeton, N.J.: Princeton University Press.

Pritchett, L.H.
　1994a　Desired fertility and the impact of population policies. *Population and Development Review* 20(1):1-55.
　1994b　The impact of population policies: Reply. *Population and Development Review* 20(3):621-630.

Rao, K.V., and R. Beaujot
　1986　Effect of infant mortality on subsequent fertility in Pakistan and Sri Lanka. *Journal of Biosocial Science* 18(3):297-303.

Rashad, H., M. El Bahy, and S. Attia
　1993　*Linking Fertility Changes to Community Level Changes in Mortality: The Egyptian Case.* Amman, Jordan: The Jordanian Printing Press for UNICEF.

Rele, J.R., and I. Alam
　1993　Fertility transition in Asia: The statistical evidence. Pp. 15-37 in R. Leete and I. Alam, eds., *The Revolution in Asian Fertility: Dimensions, Causes, and Implications.* Oxford, England: Clarendon Press.

Ross, J.A., and E. Frankenberg
　1993　*Findings From Two Decades of Family Planning Research.* New York: The Population Council.

Sah, R.K.
　1991　The effects of child mortality changes on fertility choice and parental welfare. *Journal of Political Economy* 99(3):582-606.

Sanderson, W.C., and J-P. Tan
　1995　*Population in Asia.* World Bank regional and sectoral studies series. Washington D.C.: The World Bank.

Santow, G., and M.D. Bracher
　1984　Child death and time to the next birth in Central Java. *Population Studies* 38(2):241-253.

Schultz, T.P.
　1976　Interrelationships between mortality and fertility. Pp. 239-289 in R.G. Ridker, ed., *Population and Development.* Baltimore, Md.: Johns Hopkins University Press.
　1988　Economic demography and development: New directions in an old field. Pp. 416-458 in G. Ranis and T.P. Schultz, eds., *The State of Development Economics: Progress and Perspectives.* Oxford, England: Basil Blackwell.
　1994a　Human capital, family planning, and their effects on population growth. *American Economic Review* 84(2):255-260.
　1994b　*Sources of Fertility Decline in Modern Economic Growth: Is Aggregate Evidence on the Demographic Transition Credible?* New Haven, Conn.: Yale University.

Setel, P.
　1995　The effects of HIV and AIDS on fertility in East and Central Africa. *Health Transition Review* 5(Suppl.):179-189.

Shah, I.H., and J.G. Cleland
　1993　High fertility in Bangladesh, Nepal, and Pakistan: Motives and means. Pp. 175-207 in R. Leete and I. Alam, eds., *The Revolution in Asian Fertility: Dimensions, Causes, and Implications.* Oxford, England: Clarendon Press.

Taylor, C.E.
1991   Letter to the editor. *Lancet* 337:51.
Taylor, C.E., J.S. Newman, and N.U. Kelly
1976   The child survival hypothesis. *Population Studies* 30(2):263-278.
Teitelbaum, M.S.
1984   *The British Fertility Decline: Demographic Transition in the Crucible of the Industrial Revolution.* Princeton, N.J.: Princeton University Press.
Tien, H.Y.
1984   Induced fertility transition: Impact of population policies and socioeconomic change in the People's Republic of China. *Population Studies* 38(3):385-400.
Trussell, J.
1988   Does family planning reduce infant mortality? An exchange. *Population and Development Review* 14(1):171-178.
Trussell, J., and R. Olsen
1983   Evaluation of the Olsen technique for estimating the fertility response to child mortality. *Demography* 20(3):391-405.
Trussell, J., and A.R. Pebley
1984   The potential impact of changes in fertility on infant, child, and maternal mortality. *Studies in Family Planning* 15(6):267-280.
UNICEF
1991   *The State of the World's Children, 1991.* New York: Oxford University Press for UNICEF.
United Nations Secretariat
1988   Interrelationships between child survival and fertility. *Population Bulletin of the United Nations* 25:27-50.
van de Walle, E.
1992   Fertility transition, conscious choice, and numeracy. *Demography* 29(4):487-502.
van de Walle, F.
1986   Infant mortality and the European demographic transition. Pp. 201-233 in A.J. Coale and S.C. Watkins, eds., *The Decline of Fertility in Europe.* Revised Proceedings of a Conference on the Princeton European Fertility Project. Princeton, N.J.: Princeton University Press.
Vinovskis, M.
1991   Angels' heads and weeping willows: Death in early America. Pp. 209-231 in G. Moran and M. Vinovskis, eds., *Religion, Family and the Life Course: Explorations in the Social History of Early America.* Ann Arbor: University of Michigan Press.
Warwick, D.P.
1986   The Indonesian Family Planning Program: Government influence and client choice. *Population and Development Review* 12(3):453-490.
Weeks, J.R.
1988   The demography of Islamic Nations. *Population Bulletin* 43(4).
Williams, A.D.
1977   Measuring the impact of child mortality on fertility: A methodological note. *Demography* 14(4):581-590.
Wolf, A.P.
1986   The preeminent role of government intervention in China's family revolution. *Population and Development Review* 12(1):101-116.
Wolpin, K.I.
1984   An estimable dynamic stochastic model of fertility and child mortality. *Journal of Political Economy* 92(5):852-874.

World Bank
  1995   *World Development Report, 1995: Workers in an Integrating World.* New York: Oxford
         University Press for the World Bank.
Yamada, T.
  1985   Casual relationships between infant mortality and fertility in developed and less devel-
         oped countries. *Southern Economic Journal* 52(2):364-370.
Zeng Yi, Tu Ping, Gu Baochang, Xu Yi, Li Bohua, and Li Yongping
  1993   Causes and implications of the recent increase in the reported sex ratio at birth in China.
         Population and Development Review 19(2):283-302.

2

Effect of a Child's Death on Birth Spacing: A Cross-National Analysis

Laurence M. Grummer-Strawn, Paul W. Stupp, and Zuguo Mei

INTRODUCTION

Our purpose in this chapter is to examine the potential pathways through which infant and child mortality can affect the interval between births. Specifically, we examine the extent to which the death of a child tends to shorten the time until the birth of the next child. To the extent that the shortening of the birth interval is attributable to direct physiological mechanisms (i.e., premature return of menses due to breastfeeding cessation), the linkage between mortality decline and fertility decline can be considered directly causal. On the other hand, if the linkage between child death and birth interval is related more to maternal behavior, such as cessation of contraceptive use, then the linkage depends on the widespread use of contraceptives. By teasing out the mechanisms for the linkage, we will better understand the future course of fertility and mortality in developing countries.

The analysis uses data from phases 1 and 2 of the Demographic and Health Surveys (DHS), which collect an extensive set of fertility-related variables for women of reproductive age and for live births that occurred in the 5 years before the date of interview. We first present evidence of the magnitude of the effects on the birth interval for a variety of countries and then address the mechanisms through which these effects may operate.

PATHWAYS OF INFLUENCE

The effects of infant and child mortality on the intervals between births probably act through both physiological mechanisms and volitional behaviors as noted by Preston (1978). Most prominent among the physiological mechanisms is lactational amenorrhea, by which breastfeeding inhibits the return of ovulation after a birth. If a child dies, the mother will stop breastfeeding (except perhaps in the case of a multiple birth), and she will become susceptible to pregnancy more quickly than if the child had survived. This effect is expected to be most pronounced in societies such as those in sub-Saharan Africa in which breastfeeding is nearly universal and is performed for an extended time. Studies in the early 1980s showed that the anovulatory effect of breastfeeding is related to its frequency, intensity, and duration (Konner and Worthman, 1980; McNeilly et al., 1980; Howie et al., 1982). For this analysis, duration of breastfeeding was the only variable for which data were collected for all births during a 5-year period.

To explore the role of lactational amenorrhea in spacing of births, we used data from the DHSs to examine the effect of death of a child on the length of time until return of menses and until the next live birth. We treat time to return of menses, which is among the data collected in the DHS, as a proxy for time to return of ovulation, which is not collected in the DHS.

Beyond its effect in delaying the return of ovulation, breastfeeding may also reduce the probability of conception among ovulating, sexually active women. We investigated the effect of the premature truncation of breastfeeding on the interval from return of menses and resumption of sexual relations to a subsequent pregnancy.

The DHS do not collect information on pregnancies that do not result in a live birth (i.e., spontaneous abortions and stillbirths). This restriction prevents us from considering another potential physiological mechanism by which the death of a child could lengthen the interval to the subsequent birth. If infant mortality is correlated with fetal mortality in the same woman it could lengthen the subsequent interval due to fetal losses. This effect related to maternal health or genetic endowment appears realistic, especially in the case of neonatal mortality, and could be substantial for a subset of women. Unfortunately, we cannot use DHS data to measure this effect.

The primary behavioral pathways through which death of a child can affect the interval before a subsequent pregnancy involve sexual activity and contraceptive use. If a society observes a norm of traditional sexual abstinence for a period after a birth, then the death of a child may reduce that period. The DHS contain data on duration of postpartum abstinence and thus make it possible to investigate directly whether the death of a child affects this component of the birth interval.

Once a woman has resumed sexual relations and is ovulating after a birth, the behavioral factors affecting the time to conception are frequency of sexual intercourse and contraceptive use. We do not have good measures of either of these variables during the pertinent periods for all of the surveys used in this analysis. We presume, however, that the shortening of this portion of the interval, once we control for breastfeeding status, must be related to one or both of these factors.

We predict that the effect of the death of a child during this period of susceptibility to pregnancy will be more pronounced in countries with more frequent contraceptive use. Unfortunately, the DHS do not generally provide appropriate data on changes in contraceptive use throughout the intervals of interest, so it was not possible to examine the effect of contraceptive use. Use of a contraceptive calendar would be appropriate for this purpose, but only in high prevalence countries DHS included a contraceptive use calendar.

Frequency of sexual relations is another factor that may be related to the effect of death of an infant on the length of the susceptible period. A couple could respond to a child's death by increasing the frequency of sexual activity in an effort to replace a dead child. Unfortunately, this hypothesis could not be tested because DHS do not provide data on coital frequency during each period of the interval.

Induced abortion is another factor we could not address. This is probably an important factor only in very low fertility settings where child mortality is more rare. Such countries have generally been excluded from the DHS program.

INTERVENING VARIABLES

It is well documented that the length of the birth interval affects child mortality and that shorter previous intervals are associated with higher infant and child mortality rates (Sullivan et al., 1994). Some of the association between a child's death and a short subsequent birth interval could therefore be confounded by the association between short previous intervals and a subsequent child death. If some women are more prone to shorter intervals than average, because of differentials in fecundity, sexual activity, or contraceptive use, then child mortality may be a spurious factor. It is therefore important that we control for the length of the previous interval in studying the association between child mortality and the length of subsequent intervals.

Similarly, child mortality may be higher if there is a shorter subsequent interval. For a short subsequent interval to affect a child's death, the death should take place after the conception of the child who is born subsequently. Similarly, for a death to affect the length of the subsequent interval it should logically occur before the conception leading to the birth that closes the interval. To avoid the possibility of reverse causality, we took great care in the modeling to limit the effect of the death to the period before the conception leading to the subsequent live birth.

Other factors that may simultaneously affect both child survival and birth interval are maternal age and education, birth order, sex of the child, whether the child was wanted, socioeconomic status of the household, and whether the woman resides in an urban or rural community. Among these factors, sex of the child, whether the child was wanted, and maternal age tend to mask the association between death and short birth intervals. If the child is female, she is less likely to die and the birth interval is likely to be shorter because of the desire to have another birth following the birth of a girl (assuming preference for a son). Similarly, infants who are unwanted experience higher mortality, and subsequent birth intervals are likely to be longer. Children born to older mothers are at greater risk of death, but their birth is often followed by longer birth intervals because of the mother's reduced fecundity. Other factors may tend to generate the expected association between death of a child and length of the birth interval. If maternal education or socioeconomic status is higher, if birth order is lower, or place of residence is urban, infant mortality is likely to be lower and birth interval longer. Data on these variables are available in the DHS and are thus included in the multivariate analyses.

This list of intervening factors is by no means comprehensive. Other characteristics of the mother or child might be correlated with both interval length and the survival of the child. For example, mothers with a strong desire to have healthy children may opt for longer birth intervals (knowing that they are safer for the child) but also invest more resources in nutrition and medical care for the child. The continued presence of a male partner in the household certainly affects the probability of closing the birth interval, but also influences socioeconomic well-being of the household and allocation of resources within the household. Other characteristics that affect birth intervals but that are not necessarily correlated with child mortality, such as the woman's underlying fecundability, can bias estimation of the parameter estimates as well (Heckman and Singer, 1982, 1984). This problem of unobserved heterogeneity has been addressed by a variety of complex statistical procedures (Trussell and Richards, 1985; Trussell and Rodriguez, 1990; Guo and Rodriguez, 1992). Unfortunately, we were unable to find a suitable method that accounts for left- and right-censoring, time-varying covariates and time-varying effects in a manner that could be applied easily to 45 surveys. Our hope is that the variables controlled in the analysis are reasonable proxies for the unobserved characteristics, such that the degree of bias is minimized.

DATA AND METHODS

For this analysis, we used data from the DHS phases 1 and 2 (Lapham and Westoff, 1986). All data sets available at the time this study was started were included. Recoded data sets for 46 surveys were provided by Macro International, Inc. (Calverton, Maryland). Conducted in developing countries in the late 1980s and early 1990s, DHS were based on household interviews of women of reproductive age (age 15-49). Standard core questionnaires were used, encompassing topics on family planning, fertility, child mortality, and maternal and child health. Additional questions and slight modifications were implemented in each country. Results are comparable across countries because the DHS use standard questionnaire modules and standardized sampling procedures, field-work, and data processing.

The core questionnaire included data on the timing of a woman's live births, the survival status for these births, and the interval to death of a child, where applicable. For births occurring in the 5 years before the survey, data were obtained on the duration of breastfeeding, amenorrhea, and sexual abstinence.[1] Our analysis is restricted to births in the previous 5 years because a major aim is to examine the mechanisms through which the death of a child affects the subsequent birth interval, specifically the premature truncation of breastfeeding leading to earlier return of menses and resumption of sexual activity. Countries included in the analysis are listed in Table 2-1 and the number of births for each country is shown.

Outcome Measures

Interval Between Births

We examined the relationship between the birth interval and the death of the child that started the interval. Several problems are apparent. First, many of the birth intervals (a majority in many countries) are open intervals, that is, last births. For these births, the time to the next birth is censored; thus, we had to use life table techniques in the data analyses. Second, because a short subsequent birth interval can contribute to the premature death of the index child (Hobcraft et al., 1985), we must account for the possibility of reverse causality by ensuring that the death occurs before the conception of the child whose birth closes the birth interval. Thus, death must be accounted for as a time-varying variable.

To handle these problems, we have chosen to model birth intervals by using proportional hazards models; the baseline hazards are modeled with a piecewise exponential (Trussell and Guinnane, 1993). This model is specified as

$$\lambda(t \mid X) = \lambda_0(t) \exp(X\beta),$$

---

[1]Data on the duration of breastfeeding, postpartum amenorrhea, and postpartum abstinence are based on the mother's retrospective reports. It is well known that the quality of retrospectively reported data on duration is rather poor. Durations are frequently reported as multiples of 3 or 6 months and thus do not reflect accurate recollection of the events. To test whether this rounding or "heaping" problem affected our results, we tested models in which we excluded women who reported amenorrhea or breastfeeding durations of 3, 6, 9, 12, 15, 18, 24, 30, or 36 months. In all cases, the differences were so small that the results described here are not substantively changed.

Data quality could be related to the main variable of interest here (child death). Interviewers may be reluctant to ask about dead children because of cultural norms. Mothers may inaccurately report breastfeeding the dead child out of a feeling of guilt.

TABLE 2-1 Sample Sizes and Years of Surveys Included in Analysis

Region and Country	Survey	Year	Number of Births in Previous 5 Years
Africa			
Botswana	DHS1	1988	3,086
Burkina Faso	DHS2	1992	5,828
Burundi	DHS1	1987	3,811
Cameroon	DHS2	1991	3,350
Egypt	DHS1	1988	8,647
Ghana	DHS1	1988	4,136
Kenya	DHS1	1988-1989	6,980
Liberia	DHS1	1986	5,299
Madagascar	DHS2	1992	5,273
Malawi	DHS2	1992	4,495
Mali	DHS1	1987	3,358
Morocco	DHS1	1987	6,102
Morocco	DHS2	1992	5,197
Namibia	DHS2	1992	3,916
Niger	DHS2	1992	6,899
Nigeria	DHS2	1990	7,902
Ondo State, Nigeria	DHS1	1986-1987	3,280
Rwanda	DHS2	1992	5,510
Senegal	DHS1	1986	4,287
Senegal	DHS2	1992-1993	5,645
Sudan	DHS1	1989-1990	6,644
Togo	DHS1	1988	3,134
Tunisia	DHS1	1988	4,477
Uganda	DHS1	1988-1989	4,959
Zambia	DHS2	1992	6,299
Zimbabwe	DHS1	1988-1989	3,358
Asia			
Indonesia	DHS1	1987	8,140
Indonesia	DHS2	1991	15,708
Pakistan	DHS2	1990-1991	6,428
Sri Lanka	DHS1	1987	4,010
Thailand	DHS1	1987	3,627
Latin America			
Bolivia	DHS1	1989	5,814
Brazil	DHS1	1986	3,573
Brazil	DHS2	1991	3,159
Colombia	DHS1	1986	2,715
Colombia	DHS2	1990	3,751
Dominican Republic	DHS1	1986	4,767
Dominican Republic	DHS2	1991	4,164
Ecuador	DHS1	1987	3,051
El Salvador	DHS1	1985	3,339
Guatemala	DHS2	1987	4,627
Mexico	DHS1	1987	5,327
Paraguay	DHS2	1990	4,246
Peru	DHS1	1986	3,131
Peru	DHS2	1991-1992	9,362
Trinidad and Tobago	DHS1	1987	1,946

where λ is the hazard of the birth interval being closed by a subsequent live birth at time t, λ_0 is the baseline hazard, and X is a set of covariates. The baseline hazard is a step function, with steps defined for age groups 9-17, 18-23, 24-29, 30-35, 36-41, and 42-59 months. The hazard of closing the birth interval is assumed to be zero in the first 9 months of a child's life, allowing for a 9-month gestation for a subsequent birth. Therefore, all exposure and events in these first 9 months are ignored. We excluded intervals in which the date of either the index birth or the subsequent birth was imputed and intervals that began with a multiple birth.

We began with model 1 in which the only covariate is whether the index child was alive 10 months ago. In this way, the risk of a conception occurring after the index child had died was compared with the risk of conception while the child was living. Whether the index child is dead was treated as a time-varying covariate, with a lag of 10 months (assuming a gestation of 9 months). Thus, for example, death of the index child at the age of 6 months can only affect the birth of the next child at durations of 16 months and greater.

In model 2 of the birth interval we introduced controls for place of residence (urban or rural), an index of the socioeconomic status of the household, the mother's highest level of completed education (none, primary, or secondary), the mother's age at the time of the index birth, the sex of the child, parity, length of the previous birth interval, and whether the child was wanted at that time, at a later time, or not at all. The index of socioeconomic status was a continuous covariate based on a count of the number of goods and services available in the household from among the following: automobile, motorcycle, bicycle, refrigerator, television, radio, and electricity. The mother's age was modeled with a linear and quadratic term to account for nonlinearity in the declining fecundity with age. We considered parity and previous birth interval jointly by using a categorical variable with categories of first-births, parity of two to five with an interval less than 24 months, parity of two to five with an interval of at least 24 months, parity of six or more with an interval less than 24 months, and parity of six or more with an interval of at least 24 months. As noted, some of these factors tend to mask the association between death and short birth intervals, but others tend to generate such an association. Therefore, we had no prior expectation as to whether the effect of the index child's death would be stronger or weaker after adjustment for these factors.

In model 3, we added the effect of breastfeeding on closure of the birth interval. Breastfeeding was modeled in the same way as was the index child's death, that is, as a time-varying covariate with a 10-month lag. Although a woman can continue breastfeeding during pregnancy, we focused only on breastfeeding before the time of conception to avoid any possibility of reverse causality that occurs if a woman stops breastfeeding because she is pregnant. The addition of a breastfeeding dummy variable to the model along with child death had the effect of creating three possible statuses of the index child 10 months earlier:

dead, weaned but alive, and still breastfed. The parameter on the variable for death of the index child thus measured the effect of that event relative to the effect of survival of the index child who was weaned. Because we expected that a major mechanism for the association between death of the index child and a shorter subsequent birth interval was the premature truncation of breastfeeding, we anticipated a large reduction in the effect of a child's death. In fact, if breastfeeding were the only mechanism for the prolongation of the birth interval, as might be the case in countries where contraceptives are seldom used, then we would expect that the effect of child death might be reduced to zero.

Interval from Birth to Menses

To better understand the mechanisms through which the death of a child might affect the subsequent birth interval, it is useful to consider the various components of the birth interval. Two events must take place before the conception of the subsequent birth. The couple must resume sexual relations and the woman must begin ovulating again. Either event could occur first. Thus, the birth interval can be thought of in three distinct parts: insusceptible period (amenorrheic or abstinent), susceptible period, and gestation. Because data on gestational age are not available in the DHS, the part of the interval related to gestation was not examined separately.

Components of the Birth Interval

Return of Menses

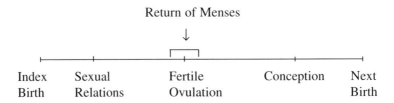

| Index | Sexual | Fertile | Conception | Next |
| Birth | Relations | Ovulation | | Birth |

The timing of ovulation is not directly observable; thus, no data are available on ovulation. However, data on the timing of first menses after each birth were obtained from the DHS. Menses can occur several months before ovulation, with the first few cycles being anovulatory, or ovulation can precede menses. Nevertheless, the return of menses is considered to be a good proxy for ovulation. For this reason, we modeled the effect of a child's death on the resumption of menses. A series of models was estimated, as were the full models for the birth interval, by adding control variables and breastfeeding in turn. The piecewise hazards were modeled with steps placed at 0-2, 3-5, 6-8, 9-11, 12-14, 15-17, 18-23, and 24-35 months. The amount of exposure and the number of events beyond 36 months are so low that it was deemed imprudent to fit the model beyond 36 months.

In many cases a woman reported that her menses never returned between one birth and the next. In such cases, the return of menses was assumed to have occurred 9 months before the birth. This treatment is consistent with our assumption that menses is a proxy for ovulation. In other cases a woman reported that menses returned, but the duration of amenorrhea exceeded the current age of the child (for open intervals) or exceeded the interval from birth to the next conception (for closed intervals). We dropped these cases from the analysis of the duration of amenorrhea.

It was expected that the death of the index child would shorten the time from birth to return of menses (increase the risks) but that this effect would work exclusively through the truncation of breastfeeding. Once breastfeeding was accounted for, the effect was expected to be zero.

Interval from Birth to Sexual Relations

We estimated a set of models exactly parallel to those for postpartum amenorrhea using the timing of the resumption of sexual relations as the outcome. The baseline hazard was estimated in the same way, and the same set of models was estimated. Whereas postpartum amenorrhea is related to breastfeeding through biological mechanisms, postpartum abstinence is related to breastfeeding only through social norms and cultural taboos. Thus, the degree to which death of a child affects the duration of postpartum abstinence and the degree to which this effect is explained by breastfeeding were expected to vary from country to country.

Duration of Susceptibility to Pregnancy

A series of models was also estimated on the second part of the birth interval, that is, after both menses and resumption of sexual relations had taken place. The models were specified in the same way as the models on the full birth interval, but all exposure during the periods of postpartum amenorrhea and postpartum abstinence was excluded. Births were excluded for which return of menses or resumption of sexual relations was reported in the same month as the conception because they would contribute no exposure. In these models, exposure and the occurrence of subsequent births are classified by time since the index birth rather than by time since the start of susceptibility to pregnancy. We estimated alternative formulations of the model by using time since menses or time since relations, but results did not change substantively.

The effect of the death of a child on this portion of the interval could be explained partially by breastfeeding because breastfeeding reduces the probability of conception even for ovulating women. After adjustment for breastfeeding, the effect was expected to be small in countries where contraceptive use was infrequent because women have few means to control their fertility in response to the death of a child.

Results

Interval Between Births

The first hazards model estimated (model 1) considered the time to the next live birth, including only covariates of age and the survival status of the index child. The coefficients of this model can be used to calculate a survival curve. The point at which this curve reaches 50 percent represents the median duration of the birth interval corresponding to the estimated model. In Figure 2-1a, the estimated median duration of the birth interval for intervals after the birth of a child who survives 5 years is compared with the estimated median birth interval after the birth of a child who dies in the neonatal period. This comparison is shown for each of the countries[2] for which data were analyzed. It thus gives a sense of the amount of reduction in the median birth interval that can be associated with child mortality, without taking other factors into consideration.

The results have been grouped by three regions: Africa, Asia, and Latin America. For each region the data have been arranged in order from the country with the longest median duration to the country with the shortest median duration. Median birth intervals after the birth of children who are still living appear to be shorter in Africa than in Asia or Latin America. However, birth intervals after a child has died are generally similar across the three regions.

Table 2-2 gives the ratio of the estimated median interval for subsequent births of children who survive to the median interval for births of children who die. This ratio varies between 1.21 and 3.15, indicating that the increase in birth interval associated with eliminating an early infant death is 21 to 215 percent. The average reduction in the median interval is 60 percent for the 46 DHS used for this analysis.

Figure 2-2 shows a plot of the estimated coefficient of the variable *DIED* for all three models of the log of the hazard of closing the birth interval (conception resulting in live birth). Because explanatory covariates are added to the models in turn (confounders, then breastfeeding), the coefficients on *DIED* show the degree to which the effect of *DIED*, independent of covariates, continues to be a predictor of interval length. In this way, we try to assess how much of the effect of the child's death can be explained away by controlling for other factors that we also expect to affect birth interval length.

---

[2]Several of the countries analyzed here were actually surveyed twice. In the ensing presentation of results we refer to "countries" as a matter of convenience, although the data points of interest in fact represent countries at a point in time.

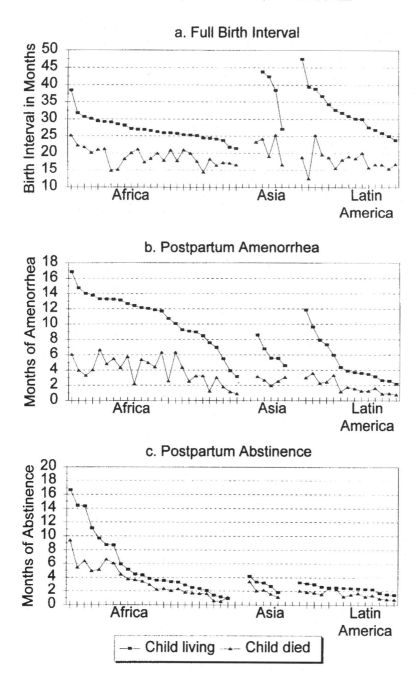

FIGURE 2-1 Predicted length of interval by survival status of the index child.

TABLE 2-2 Ratio of Predicted Median Interval Length Assuming the Child
Survived to the Predicted Median Interval Length Assuming the Child Died

Region and Country	Survey	Birth Interval	Time to Menses	Time to First Coitus
Africa				
Botswana	DHS1	1.53	2.61	1.43
Burkina Faso	DHS2	1.43	2.76	2.65
Burundi	DHS1	1.42	2.78	1.28
Cameroon	DHS2	1.44	2.78	1.28
Egypt	DHS1	1.88	3.05	1.43
Ghana	DHS1	1.40	2.21	1.32
Kenya	DHS1	1.37	2.12	1.30
Liberia	DHS1	1.45	n.a.	n.a.
Madagascar	DHS2	1.46	2.68	1.21
Malawi	DHS2	1.28	1.85	n.a.
Mali	DHS1	1.24	2.00	1.62
Morocco	DHS1	1.54	6.19	n.a.
Morocco	DHS2	1.96	3.49	2.33
Namibia	DHS2	1.41	2.32	1.33
Niger	DHS2	1.33	3.04	1.57
Nigeria	DHS2	1.43	2.26	1.89
Ondo State, Nigeria	DHS1	1.28	1.59	1.77
Rwanda	DHS2	1.53	4.23	0.84
Senegal	DHS1	1.31	3.70	1.63
Senegal	DHS2	1.35	3.41	1.51
Sudan	DHS1	1.27	5.68	1.41
Togo	DHS1	1.38	2.41	2.25
Tunisia	DHS1	1.69	3.39	2.29
Uganda	DHS1	1.26	3.58	1.46
Zambia	DHS2	1.21	2.42	1.35
Zimbabwe	DHS1	1.49	4.18	1.25
Average		1.44	2.95	1.44
Asia				
Indonesia	DHS1	1.81	2.71	1.64
Indonesia	DHS2	2.22	2.53	1.72
Pakistan	DHS2	1.63	2.84	1.60
Sri Lanka	DHS1	1.52	2.18	1.23
Thailand	DHS1	n.a.	1.50	1.50
Average		1.79	2.35	1.54
Latin America				
Bolivia	DHS1	1.55	2.68	1.59
Brazil	DHS1	1.87	2.97	1.85
Brazil	DHS2	1.83	2.84	1.80
Colombia	DHS1	1.54	2.78	1.05
Colombia	DHS2	2.52	1.96	1.13
Dominican Republic	DHS1	1.60	2.21	1.86
Dominican Republic	DHS2	1.74	2.86	1.63
Ecuador	DHS1	1.62	1.80	1.97

TABLE 2-2 (*continued*)

Region and Country	Survey	Birth Interval	Time to Menses	Time to First Coitus
El Salvador	DHS1	1.50	n.a.	n.a.
Guatemala	DHS1	1.41	3.97	1.67
Mexico	DHS1	1.75	2.39	1.58
Paraguay	DHS1	1.62	3.79	1.82
Peru	DHS1	1.62	3.01	1.69
Peru	DHS2	2.09	3.50	1.72
Trinidad and Tobago	DHS1	3.15	2.74	1.41
Average		1.83	2.63	1.52

NOTE: n.a., data not available.

The results for all 46 surveys are shown by region, arranged in the figure in order from the country with the largest crude effect of *DIED* (no other covariates) to the country with the smallest crude *DIED* effect. This is the same model that was used to generate the median durations shown in Figure 2-1A. The coefficients of the crude *DIED* effect tend to lie in a range between 0.4 and 1.0 in all three regions, which corresponds to relative risks between 1.5 and 2.7. Morocco (DHS2) and Trinidad and Tobago are outliers with relative risks greater than 3.0.

Model 2, labeled "with confounders," adds to the crude model the set of variables thought to be associated with both infant mortality and birth interval. These variables are mother's age, mother's education, birth order and previous interval, wantedness, socioeconomic status, residence, and sex of the child. Because some of these variables were expected to mask a real association between death and the birth interval, but others were expected to artificially create an association, we had no prior expectations about what the net effect of these variables taken as a group would be on the coefficient of *DIED*. As shown in Figure 2-2, the net effect of these variables on this coefficient is virtually nil.

In Table 2-3, we examine the degree to which the effect of child death is "explained" by each model. In the table, we compute the percentage of reduction in excess risk associated with death of a child, where excess risk is the estimated relative risk minus 1. The next to the last column of Table 2-3 shows the percentage of reduction in the excess relative risk in moving from the crude model (model 1) to the model with confounders (model 2). For example, in model 1 for Botswana the risk of closing the birth interval when the child has died is 1.89 times the risk when the index child is still alive. This relative risk has been reduced to 1.86 in model 2 where confounders were introduced. The excess relative risk is reduced by 2.9 percent, which was calculated as 100 x (1.89 – 1.86)/(1.89 – 1.0). By introducing the confounders, we have moved 2.9 percent

Parameter Estimate   Relative Risk

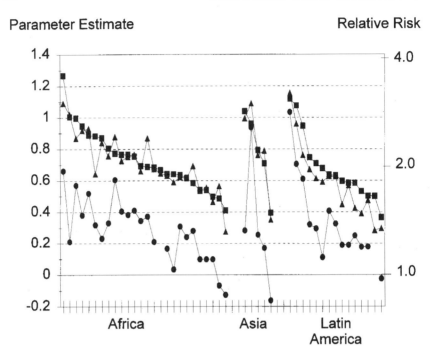

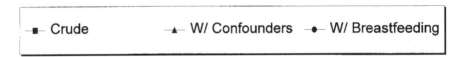

FIGURE 2-2 Effect of child death on rate of closing the birth interval.

of the way from the relative risk of 1.89 for the crude effect to a complete explanation of the effect of death of a child, for which the relative risk is 1.0 (i.e., a model in which there is no excess risk of closing the interval when the child has died).

With some exceptions, introducing the confounding variables did not reduce excess risk. In some cases the percentage of the reduction was negative, indicating that the set of confounding variables as a whole was masking an association between child death and the birth interval.

Model 3, labeled "with breastfeeding" in Figure 2-2, introduces an additional variable to model 2. This new variable, *BF*, is modeled in the same way as *DIED* (*BF* is a time-varying covariate that is set to true if the index child was still being breastfed 10 months before the hazard of closing the interval is being estimated).

Again, the 10-month lag is introduced to allow for the 9-month delay from conception to birth. By introducing the *BF* parameter, we change the interpretation of the parameter for *DIED*. In models 1 and 2, the comparison group for the relative risk for this variable was all children who are still alive. In model 3, the comparison group for both variables is living children who have been weaned.

Figure 2-2 shows that the relative risk of closing the birth interval when the child is dead at a given age, compared with being weaned at that age, was considerably less for all countries than when the comparison group included breastfed children. This finding gives strong evidence that much of the excess risk of a shorter birth interval after death of a child is explained by the physiological effects of breastfeeding. The relative risks of closing the interval when the child has died, as opposed to when the child has been weaned, generally are 1.1 to 1.5. Many of these effects are no longer statistically significant (Table 2-3). There are, however, notable exceptions in which the effect of child death remains high despite adjustments for the breastfeeding status of living children. These exceptions include Morocco (DHS2) with a relative risk or 1.94, Thailand with 2.55, Peru (DHS2) with 2.03, and Trinidad and Tobago (DHS1) with 2.81.

As shown in the comparison of model 3 with model 1 in Table 2-3 (last column), introducing an adjustment to control for breastfeeding generally produces a large percentage of reduction in the excess risk of child mortality on the hazard of closing the birth interval. In 14 of the 25 surveys analyzed for 22 African countries, controlling for breastfeeding status explains 65 percent or more of the excess risk of child death seen in the initial crude model. The same is true for 4 of the 5 surveys analyzed for 4 countries in Asia and for 8 of the 14 surveys analyzed in 11 countries in Latin America. Latin America seems to stand out as the region where the initially large effect of child death cannot be so consistently explained by premature weaning.

The statistical models used here examine the effect of a child's survival status at a point in time on the risk of an event occurring at the next point in time. These models cannot address the question of whether it matters when the death occurred. We might want to know whether the effect of death of a child is immediate, that is, whether it affects events in the next 1 or 2 months and whether the effect persists several months after the child has died. To address this question, we selected a subset of five African countries. In these countries, we estimated an alternative formulation of the *DIED* variable in which we considered the time since death.

We considered if the risk of closing the interval is affected by whether the index child had died within specific intervals of time before the duration for which the risk is being estimated. Intervals used for this analysis were 10-12, 13-18, 19-24, 25-30, and more than 30 months. In all previous models presented we only consider whether or not the index child was dead in the month before the duration for which the risk is estimated. As with the crude models discussed above, the comparison group for these models was living children. The lagged

TABLE 2–3 Effect of Child Death on the Rate of Closing the Birth Interval in Hazards Models

Region and Country	Survey	Relative Risk			Reduction in Excess Risk (%)	
		Model 1 (crude)	Model 2 (with confounders)	Model 3 (with breastfeeding)	Model 2 versus Model 1	Model 3 versus Model 1
Africa						
Botswana	DHS1	1.89*	1.86*	1.36*	2.9	59.5
Burkina Faso	DHS2	2.57*	2.50*	1.46*	4.5	70.6
Burundi	DHS1	2.39*	2.32*	1.26*	5.3	81.2
Cameroon	DHS2	2.17*	2.41*	1.83*	-20.5	28.8
Egypt	DHS1	2.70*	2.38*	1.77*	18.8	54.9
Ghana	DHS1	2.12*	2.15*	1.51*	-2.3	55.0
Kenya	DHS1	1.85*	1.85*	1.27*	0.2	68.2
Liberia	DHS1	1.95*	1.91*	n.a.*	4.3	n.a.
Madagascar	DHS2	2.15*	2.07*	1.50*	7.4	56.6
Malawi	DHS2	1.71*	1.71*	1.10*	1.0	85.5
Mali	DHS1	1.63*	1.76*	0.93*	-21.6	110.4
Morocco	DHS1	2.15*	2.12*	1.47*	2.5	59.6
Morocco	DHS2	3.55*	2.98*	1.94*	22.4	63.2
Namibia	DHS2	1.79*	2.00*	1.32*	-26.3	59.3
Niger	DHS2	1.90*	1.88*	1.18*	2.3	80.0
Nigeria	DHS2	2.00*	1.94*	1.41*	6.5	58.8
Ondo State, Nigeria	DHS1	1.99*	2.39*	1.45*	-39.9	54.5
Rwanda	DHS2	2.73*	2.77*	1.24*	-2.7	86.4
Senegal	DHS1	1.90*	1.80*	1.03*	10.6	96.1
Senegal	DHS2	1.98*	1.96*	1.23*	2.2	76.3
Sudan	DHS1	1.51*	1.32*	0.88*	37.4	123.2

Togo	DHS1	2.43*	2.53*	1.68*	-7.1	52.5
Tunisia	DHS1	2.42*	1.90*	1.37*	36.5	73.7
Uganda	DHS1	1.71*	1.74*	1.10*	-3.9	85.4
Zambia	DHS2	1.64*	1.59*	1.10*	8.3	83.8
Zimbabwe	DHS1	2.24*	2.13*	1.39*	8.6	68.3
Asia						
Indonesia	DHS1	2.03*	2.20*	1.19*	-16.9	82.0
Indonesia	DHS2	2.82*	2.70*	1.32*	6.6	82.2
Pakistan	DHS2	2.21*	2.14*	1.29*	5.6	76.1
Sri Lanka	DHS1	1.48	1.42	0.85*	13.3	130.9
Thailand	DHS1	2.61*	2.97*	2.55*	-22.4	3.8
Latin America						
Bolivia	DHS1	2.11*	1.96*	1.38*	13.4	65.9
Brazil	DHS1	1.79*	1.53*	1.28*	33.2	64.4
Brazil	DHS2	1.70*	1.48*	1.19*	31.9	72.5
Colombia	DHS1	1.44	1.35	0.98*	21.4	105.4
Colombia	DHS2	2.57*	2.14*	1.84*	27.2	46.5
Dominican Republic	DHS1	1.65*	1.61*	1.19*	7.0	70.2
Dominican Republic	DHS2	2.03*	1.85*	1.34*	17.8	66.9
Ecuador	DHS1	1.81*	1.57*	1.21*	30.6	74.5
El Salvador	DHS1	1.65*	1.33*	n.a.*	49.4	n.a.
Guatemala	DHS1	1.97*	1.81*	1.12*	17.0	88.0
Mexico	DHS1	1.89*	1.87*	1.50*	2.1	43.7
Paraguay	DHS2	1.88*	1.87*	1.38*	1.5	56.6
Peru	DHS1	1.79*	1.77*	1.21*	3.6	73.9
Peru	DHS2	2.93*	2.61*	2.03*	16.7	46.9
Trinidad and Tobago	DHS1	3.06*	3.18*	2.81*	-5.6	12.1

NOTES: n.a., data not available. *Parameter coefficient is statistically significant at the 5 percent level.

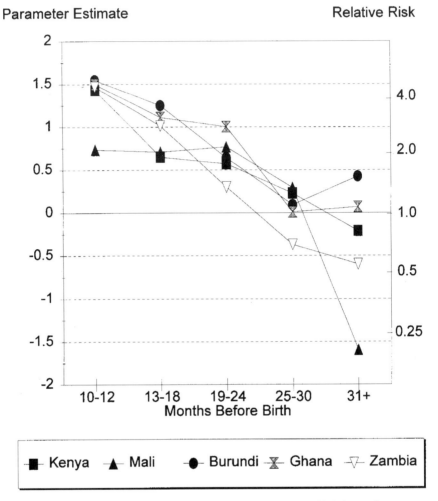

FIGURE 2-3 Lagged effect of child death on rate of closing the birth interval.

effects of a child death are shown in Figure 2-3. In all five countries, the effects
are greatest immediately after the death occurs and wane over time. If a birth has
not occurred within 2 years after the death, the death of the index child is irrelevant to the closure of the birth interval.

To address whether the observed effects are stronger if a child is older or
younger when it dies, we used the same five African countries to estimate models
in which the *DIED* variable was allowed to have time-varying effects. For the
full birth interval, effects of a child death are strongest for closing the birth
interval within 24 months (Figure 2-4). Effects fall off quickly beyond this point;

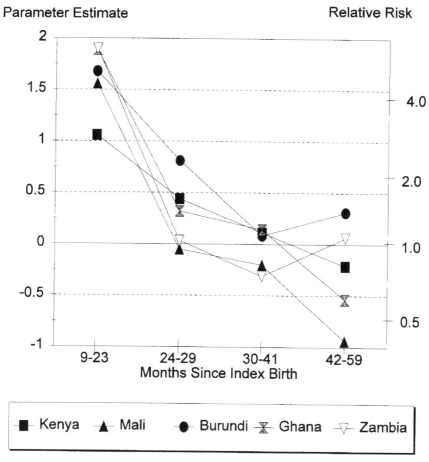

FIGURE 2-4 Age-dependent effect of child death on rate of closing the birth interval.

for intervals that are still open at 2.5 years postpartum (30 months), the occurrence of a child's death does not affect the propensity to close the interval.

Interval from Birth to Menses

The major physiological pathway through which the death of a child is
hypothesized to shorten the subsequent birth interval is by hastening the return of
menses and ovulation because the mother is not breastfeeding. In Figure 2-1b,
the predicted duration of postpartum amenorrhea after the birth of a child who
survives until menses returns is compared with the duration after the death of a
neonate for the full set of countries in the DHS. Figure 2-1b indicates the

magnitude of the overall crude effect of an early infant death on the duration of postpartum amenorrhea. As in Figure 2-1a, the intervals were calculated from the coefficients of a hazards model of time to resumption of menses in which the only covariates are age and whether the child is dead at the beginning of each month.

Africa stands out as having considerably longer median durations of postpartum amenorrhea, both when the index child who started the interval dies and when the child survives until return of menses (Figure 2-1b). The percent increase in the median duration of amenorrhea associated with the child's survival is considerably greater than was the case for the effect on the overall birth interval (see Table 2-2). The percent increase in the time until return of menses when the child survives over when the child dies is 50-468 percent and usually is 100-250 percent.

Analogous to the models of the hazard of conception resulting in a live birth, three separate models have been estimated for the hazard of return of menses. Figure 2-5 shows the estimated coefficient of *DIED* for each of the three models for all of the countries. As before, the countries are ordered, within regions, by the size of the *DIED* coefficient estimated in model 1.

As expected, the relative risks for the duration of amenorrhea in mothers of children who died compared with that in mothers of those who lived are highest in Africa (range, 2.07 to 5.14), lowest in Asia (range, 1.58 to 2.69), and intermediate in Latin America (range, 1.95 to 4.65).

As in the models for overall birth interval, there was little change in the estimated coefficients of *DIED* when the confounder variables were added for model 2. In Latin America there was a tendency for the addition of the confounding variables in model 2 to increase the effect of *DIED* over the effect seen in the crude model. This increase indicates that, as a whole, the confounders actually mask an association between death of a child and return of menses in women in Latin America.

In model 3 of the hazard of the return of menses, the addition of the variable on breastfeeding status considerably reduced the effect of *DIED* for all but a few countries (Table 2-4). But surprisingly, the risk of return of menses after a death, relative to the risk after weaning a living child (Table 2-4, model 3), remains high, especially in Africa where it is greater than 2.0 for 16 of the 25 countries. Also, the percent reduction in the excess risk of *DIED* that was achieved by adding the variable for breastfeeding (Table 2-4, model 3 versus model 1) is not as great as the reduction in the analogous model estimated for the birth interval (Table 2-3, model 2 versus model 1). The percent reduction in excess risk for Africa and Asia rarely exceeded 60 percent, whereas the percent reduction was greater than 60 percent for all but three countries in Latin America.

As with the full birth interval, we examined the data from the five African countries to determine the lagged effect of a child's death on the risk of menses

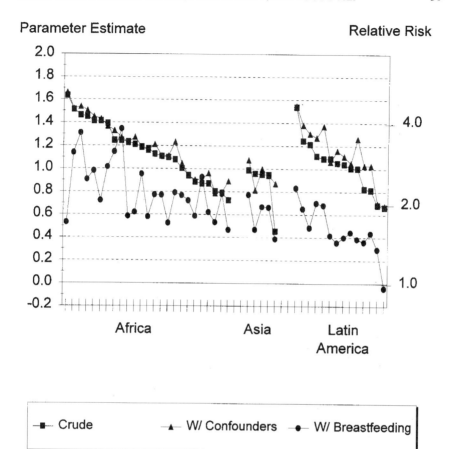

FIGURE 2-5 Effect of child death on rate of resuming menses postpartum.

returning (Figure 2-6). We considered whether the death took place 1, 2-3, 4-5, 6-7, or more than 7 months previously. These intervals are shorter than those for the full birth interval because the duration of amenorrhea is so much shorter than the birth interval and there are more events on which the hazards can be estimated. Again, risks are estimated relative to intervals in which the index child was still alive. The largest effect of death of a child on return of menses occurs immediately after the death (Figure 2-6). Effects wane with time and are negligible beyond 7 months after the death.

We also considered age dependencies in the effect of a child's death on return of menses for these five countries. The effect was essentially confined to the first year of life (Figure 2-7). Except in Burundi, effects were minimal in the second year. In the third year of life (24-35 months), the parameter estimates

TABLE 2-4 Effect of Child Death on the Rate of Resuming Menses Following a Birth in Hazards Models

Region and Country	Survey	Relative Risk			Reduction in Excess Risk (%)	
		Model 1 (crude)	Model 2 (with confounders)	Model 3 (with breastfeeding)	Model 2 versus Model 1	Model 3 versus Model 1
Africa						
Botswana	DHS1	3.47*	3.56*	3.85*	-3.7	-15.1
Burkina Faso	DHS2	3.23*	3.20*	1.79*	1.8	64.7
Burundi	DHS1	3.43*	3.41*	1.80*	1.2	67.2
Cameroon	DHS2	2.94*	3.43*	2.21*	-25.1	37.8
Egypt	DHS1	2.43*	2.47*	1.80*	-3.2	43.9
Ghana	DHS1	3.29*	3.28*	2.59*	0.5	30.4
Kenya	DHS1	2.57	2.56*	2.06*	1.0	32.6
Madagascar	DHS2	4.26*	4.51*	2.48*	-7.4	54.7
Malawi	DHS2	3.36*	3.58*	1.86*	-9.0	63.4
Mali	DHS1	3.03*	3.04*	2.16*	-0.7	42.8
Morocco	DHS1	2.39*	2.62*	1.86*	-16.6	37.7
Morocco	DHS2	2.21*	2.21*	2.19*	-0.7	1.7
Namibia	DHS2	2.39*	2.48*	2.53*	-6.6	-10.1
Niger	DHS2	3.09*	3.36*	2.17*	-12.9	44.1
Nigeria	DHS2	2.24*	2.20*	1.71*	3.3	43.0
Ondo State, Nigeria	DHS1	2.07*	2.44*	1.60*	-35.1	44.2
Rwanda	DHS2	4.54*	4.58*	3.12*	-1.1	40.0
Senegal	DHS1	4.31*	4.66*	3.71*	-10.5	18.2
Senegal	DHS2	5.14*	5.29*	1.70*	-3.6	83.0
Sudan	DHS1	4.11*	4.27*	2.68*	-5.1	46.1

Togo	DHS1	3.47*	3.78*	3.15*	−12.4	13.0
Tunisia	DHS1	3.00*	3.04*	1.69*	−2.0	65.4
Uganda	DHS1	4.11*	4.18*	2.06*	−2.3	65.8
Zambia	DHS2	2.73*	2.85*	2.16*	−6.6	33.2
Zimbabwe	DHS1	4.03*	3.93*	2.76*	3.4	41.8
Asia						
Indonesia	DHS1	2.69*	2.94*	2.17*	−14.8	30.6
Indonesia	DHS2	2.59*	2.72*	1.95*	−7.8	40.3
Pakistan	DHS2	2.61*	2.26*	1.60*	22.1	62.8
Sri Lanka	DHS1	2.59*	2.57*	1.94*	1.3	40.7
Thailand	DHS1	1.58*	2.39*	1.47	−141.5	17.9
Latin America						
Bolivia	DHS1	3.05*	3.57*	2.02*	−25.5	50.3
Brazil	DHS1	2.97*	2.90*	1.52*	3.6	73.6
Brazil	DHS2	2.84*	3.04*	1.49*	−11.2	73.2
Colombia	DHS1	2.73*	3.54*	1.47*	−46.4	72.7
Colombia	DHS2	1.95*	1.97*	0.96	−2.7	104.3
Dominican Republic	DHS1	2.28*	2.80*	1.43*	−40.6	66.3
Dominican Republic	DHS2	2.86*	3.19*	1.43*	−17.4	77.0
Ecuador	DHS1	1.99*	2.01*	1.35*	−2.5	65.0
Guatemala	DHS1	4.65*	4.69*	2.30*	−1.3	64.3
Mexico	DHS1	2.26*	2.80*	1.55*	−42.4	56.5
Paraguay	DHS2	2.97*	3.93*	1.98*	−48.6	50.4
Peru	DHS1	3.47*	3.98*	1.92*	−20.5	62.7
Peru	DHS2	3.36*	3.69*	1.63*	−13.9	73.5
Trinidad and Tobago	DHS1	2.74*	2.87*	1.56*	−7.6	67.5

*Parameter coefficient is statistically significant at the 5 percent level.

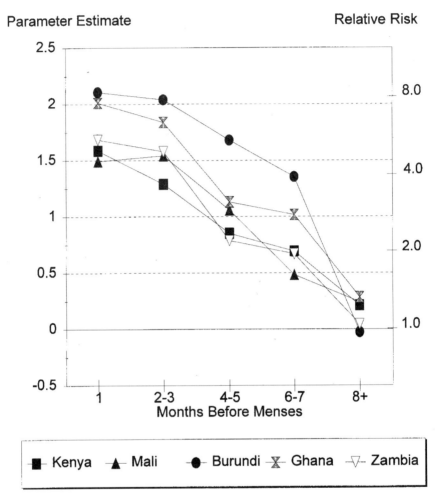

FIGURE 2-6 Lagged effect of child death on rate of menses returning postpartum.

vary considerably across the countries, most likely because of the small amount of exposure in this group.

Interval from Birth to Sexual Relations

A behavioral pathway through which a child's death may shorten the subsequent birth interval is by shortening the period of postpartum abstinence. In Figure 2-1c, the estimated duration of postpartum abstinence after the birth of a child who survives until sexual relations are resumed is compared with the duration after the death of a neonate. The death of a child consistently results in a shorter duration of abstinence in all countries.

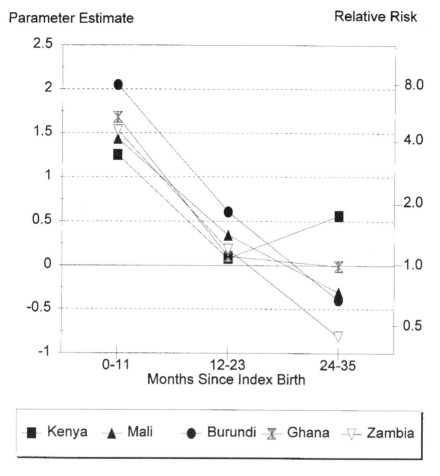

FIGURE 2-7 Age-dependent effect of child death on rate of menses returning postpartum.

Table 2-2 (column 3) gives the ratio of the estimated median duration of postpartum abstinence for births of infants who were still alive, to the duration following births of infants who died as neonates. Except in Rwanda, where the relationship is oddly reversed, the ratios are 1.05 to 2.65. This variation indicates that the lengthened abstinence associated with eliminating an early infant death is 5-165 percent. The relative effect of a child's death is not as great as that for postpartum amenorrhea or for the overall birth interval. On average, across the 46 surveys, child survival increased the birth interval by 60 percent, postpartum amenorrhea by 178 percent, and postpartum abstinence by 47 percent.

Again, three separate models were estimated for the hazard of resuming sexual relations. Figure 2-8 shows that the effect of *DIED* estimated in the crude model is virtually unchanged by the addition of either the confounding variables or the variable for breastfeeding status. We conclude that the effect of a child's death on increasing the risk of resuming sexual relations is direct and does not appear to operate through breastfeeding.

However, there does appear to be a group of African countries for which an addition of the breastfeeding status variable actually increases the effect of *DIED* over that in the initial crude model. In Table 2-5 (model 3 versus model 1), the percentage of reduction in the excess risk is negative for most African countries. This finding is puzzling and requires further investigation.

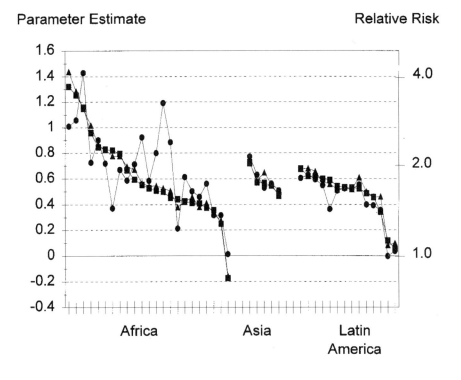

FIGURE 2-8 Effect of child death on rate of resuming sexual relations.

Interval from Menses and Sexual Relations to Birth

For the first set of models for the entire birth interval, some countries showed a general excess effect of a child's death on the risk of conception resulting in a live birth, even in comparison to the effect of a living child who was weaned (model 3 in Figure 2-2 and Table 2-3). This finding was more likely in Latin America than in either Africa or Asia. We decided to estimate an analogous series of three models of the risk of conception resulting in a live birth. In these models, all the exposure before resumption of menses and sexual relations has been excluded. In this way, we eliminated postpartum amenorrhea and abstinence from being explanatory mechanisms for the effect of *DIED*.

Figure 2-9 and Table 2-6 show the results of these three models. The results of the first model show that, with just the crude effect of *DIED*, for all the countries there is an excess risk for death of a child when conception of a subsequent child results in a live birth. This excess risk exists even when postpartum abstinence and amenorrhea are removed as possible mechanisms. In Africa, the crude relative risk associated with a child's death is greater than 1.5 in only 8 of the 23 surveys analyzed in 21 countries, whereas it is greater than 1.5 in 3 of the 5 surveys analyzed in 4 Asian countries and in 8 of the 14 surveys analyzed in 10 Latin American countries. We can thus see that in Africa much of the effect of *DIED* is operating through postpartum amenorrhea and abstinence, as expected. Even within Africa an effect larger than 1.5 is primarily limited to two regions: North Africa (Morocco, Egypt, and Tunisia) and East Africa (Burundi, Rwanda, and Zimbabwe).

As before, a second set of models was estimated in which the confounding variables were added to the first model. This generally had little effect on the coefficients for the effect of *DIED* in Africa and Asia, but did substantially reduce the effect in most Latin American countries. In Table 2-6, the addition of the confounding variables in Latin America generally explained 30-60 percent of the excess risk of conception resulting in a live birth, which is associated with death of a child in the first model.

When a control for breastfeeding status was added to the model, the effect of *DIED* was essentially eliminated for most countries in Africa and Asia. In Africa, the effect of *DIED* is insignificant in all countries except Morocco; in Asia, only Thailand has a relative risk (2.31) greater than 1.17 (Table 2-6). In Latin America, five countries continue to show a significant effect of a child's death, but there is a substantial reduction relative to the crude model. This effect of breastfeeding is not acting through lactational amenorrhea because menses has already returned for these women.

We examined interactions of the effect of *DIED* with the sex of the child, birth order, previous birth interval, and whether the child was wanted at that time. We hypothesized that the effect of death of a child would be greatest if the child were male, were of a low parity (especially first), or were wanted at that time.

TABLE 2–5 Effect of Child Death on the Rate of Resuming Sexual Relations Following a Birth in Hazards Model

Region and Country	Survey	Relative Risk			Reduction in Excess Risk (%)	
		Model 1 (crude)	Model 2 (with confounders)	Model 3 (with breastfeeding)	Model 2 versus Model 1	Model 3 versus Model 1
Africa						
Botswana	DHS1	3.19*	3.15*	4.18*	1.7	−45.0
Burkina Faso	DHS2	2.28*	2.17*	1.45*	8.1	64.9
Burundi	DHS1	1.28*	1.32*	1.37	−13.1	−33.1
Cameroon	DHS2	2.61*	2.77*	2.07*	−10.3	33.7
Egypt	DHS1	1.43*	1.39*	1.37*	9.7	12.2
Ghana	DHS2	1.95*	2.00*	1.80*	−5.9	15.7
Kenya	DHS1	1.69*	1.72*	1.79*	−3.7	−14.3
Madagascar	DHS2	2.33*	2.37*	2.47*	−3.1	−10.4
Mali	DHS1	1.51*	1.58*	1.65*	−13.6	−28.4
Morocco	DHS2	1.81*	1.95*	2.04*	17.6	−28.0
Namibia	DHS2	2.21*	2.17*	1.95*	3.3	21.4
Niger	DHS2	1.57*	1.66*	2.43*	−14.1	−148.0
Nigeria	DHS2	1.55*	1.46*	1.24	16.6	57.0
Ondo State, Nigeria	DHS1	3.75*	4.21*	2.74*	−16.9	36.6
Rwanda	DHS2	0.84	0.86	1.01	10.3	107.9
Senegal	DHS1	1.53*	1.52*	1.85*	1.1	−59.9
Senegal	DHS2	1.66*	1.73*	2.23*	−10.1	−85.6
Sudan	DHS1	1.65*	1.69*	3.29*	−7.2	−254.5

Togo	DHS1	3.50*	3.61*	2.88*	-4.3	24.9
Tunisia	DHS1	2.29*	2.29*	2.05*	0.3	18.3
Uganda	DHS1	1.46*	1.51*	1.75*	-12.3	-65.0
Zambia	DHS2	1.74*	1.76*	2.52*	-3.2	-106.2
Zimbabwe	DHS1	1.50*	1.46*	1.58*	8.5	-15.5
Asia						
Indonesia	DHS1	1.77*	1.80*	1.88*	-3.3	-14.3
Indonesia	DHS2	1.72*	1.74*	1.75*	-1.7	-4.0
Pakistan	DHS2	2.07*	2.05*	2.17*	1.5	-9.0
Sri Lanka	DHS1	1.60*	1.59*	1.66*	1.6	-9.9
Thailand	DHS1	1.76	1.91*	1.70*	-19.7	8.7
Latin America						
Bolivia	DHS1	1.70*	1.68*	1.68*	3.6	3.1
Brazil	DHS1	1.85*	1.93*	1.81*	-8.6	5.2
Brazil	DHS2	1.80*	1.75*	1.44*	6.7	45.2
Colombia	DHS1	1.05	1.10	1.04	-87.7	33.2
Colombia	DHS2	1.13	1.09	1.00	31.1	101.7
Dominican Republic	DHS1	1.86*	1.97*	1.88*	-13.8	-2.7
Dominican Republic	DHS2	1.63*	1.65*	1.49*	-3.4	21.4
Ecuador	DHS1	1.97*	1.97*	1.83*	0.5	14.4
Guatemala	DHS2	1.71*	1.70*	1.69*	1.3	2.4
Mexico	DHS1	1.58*	1.58*	1.48*	0.5	17.4
Paraguay	DHS2	1.69*	1.84*	1.74*	-22.9	-8.3
Peru	DHS1	1.72*	1.67*	1.66*	6.2	8.3
Peru	DHS2	1.82*	1.78*	1.73*	4.8	11.1
Trinidad and Tobago	DHS1	1.41	1.59	1.43	-43.3	-4.5

*Parameter coefficient is statistically significant at the 5 percent level.

Parameter Estimate   Relative Risk

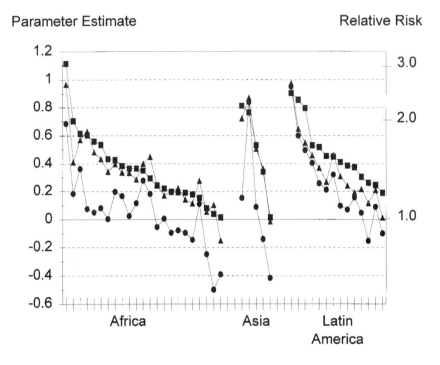

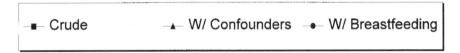

FIGURE 2-9 Effect of child death on rate of closing the birth interval after menses and sexual relations have resumed.

For none of these interactions did we find a consistent pattern of effect across the countries.

DISCUSSION

In this analysis, we have demonstrated that the death of a child has a substantial effect on the birth interval. We estimated that the median birth interval is 60 percent longer when a child lives than when it dies in early infancy. Preston (1978) estimated that the death of a child would shorten the average birth interval by 30 percent. However, the methods we used here are quite different from those Preston used. First, for our estimate, we use the median birth interval associated with the death of a child, rather than the overall mean birth interval, as the denominator. Second, the 1978 estimate does not account for the timing of the events of death of a child and the end of postpartum sterility and therefore allows for a potential reverse causality. If menses returns early while the child is still living, the subsequent interval to the next birth will likely be short, which may itself be a risk factor for infant death (Hobcraft et al., 1985). Furthermore, early weaning could lead to both the death of the child and the early return of menses. In our analysis, the survival status of the child is considered in the month prior to the month for which risks are being estimated, so reverse causality is not a problem. Third, our predicted birth intervals are based on creating a survival function in which the child's status is dead or living for all durations. Thus, the 60 percent estimate presented here is the reduction associated with elimination of all child death, not just infant death. Finally, whereas Preston's figure was based only on the mechanism of shortening the period of postpartum sterility, our estimate includes postpartum sterility as well as the interval when the woman is susceptible to pregnancy because of not using contraceptives and coital frequency.

Our analysis has demonstrated that a major portion of the effect of a child's death on shortening the subsequent birth interval operates through the premature truncation of breastfeeding. Overall, of the excess risk associated with an early infant death on closing the birth interval, 64 percent is explained by breastfeeding. This percentage is nearly identical in all three continents.

As expected, we found that the duration of amenorrhea is longest in the African countries. Death of a child has a substantial effect on the return of menses. Although premature weaning explains part of this effect, we were surprised to find a large effect remaining even after adjustment for breastfeeding.

The substantial effect of child death on the duration of postpartum abstinence was also surprising, as was the finding that the effect does not seem to operate through breastfeeding. We had expected that a major reason for prolonged periods of postpartum abstinence was a social taboo against intercourse during breastfeeding and a belief that intercourse would poison the milk (Aborampah, 1985). Instead, the norms for sexual activity appear to relate to the presence of the child, rather than to feeding patterns.

The duration of postpartum abstinence from sexual activity is generally not an important determinant of the length of birth interval because the period of abstinence is much shorter than the period of amenorrhea. With the exception of a few countries in Africa where the duration of abstinence is exceptionally long, the median duration of amenorrhea is longer than the duration of abstinence in every country. Particularly long durations of abstinence exist in the countries on the Gulf of Guinea: Ondo State, Burkina Faso, Togo, Ghana, Cameroon, and Nigeria. Notably, the effect of a child's death is far greater in Togo and Ondo State than in any other countries, and a large portion of the effect is explained by breastfeeding.

The effect of a child's death continues to operate even after menses and

TABLE 2–6 Effect of Child Death on the Rate of Closing the Birth Interval in Hazards Model in which Menses and Sexual Relations Have Resumed

Region and Country	Survey	Relative Risk			Reduction in Excess Risk (%)	
		Model 1 (crude)	Model 2 (with confounders)	Model 3 (with breastfeeding)	Model 2 versus Model 1	Model 3 versus Model 1
Africa						
Botswana	DHS1	1.25	1.19	1.01	24.0	97.7
Burkina Faso	DHS2	1.71*	1.54*	1.09	23.1	87.9
Burundi	DHS1	1.75*	1.62*	1.05	17.1	93.0
Cameroon	DHS2	1.42*	1.49*	1.32	-17.5	23.2
Egypt	DHS1	1.85*	1.77*	1.44	9.3	48.1
Ghana	DHS1	1.53*	1.49*	1.22	8.4	58.8
Kenya	DHS1	1.27*	1.27*	0.95	0.0	118.9
Madagascar	DHS2	1.44*	1.33*	1.12	24.8	72.0
Mali	DHS1	1.04	1.11	0.61	-168.9	1072.1
Morocco	DHS2	3.05*	2.63*	1.98*	20.5	51.9
Namibia	DHS2	1.34*	1.57*	1.20	-66.5	41.2
Niger	DHS2	1.44*	1.40*	1.03	10.3	93.8
Ondo State, Nigeria	DHS1	1.17	1.32*	1.12	-91.1	28.7
Rwanda	DHS2	1.83*	1.88*	1.08	-5.9	90.4
Senegal	DHS1	1.21*	1.15	0.91	28.2	142.7
Senegal	DHS2	1.08	1.06	0.78	32.0	360.6
Sudan	DHS1	1.01	0.86	0.68	1100.7	2449.8

Togo	DHS1	1.22	1.22	0.91	-2.9	142.0
Tunisia	DHS1	2.02*	1.51*	1.20	50.1	80.2
Uganda	DHS1	1.21*	1.25*	0.93	-18.3	135.2
Zambia	DHS2	1.19*	1.12*	0.87	36.9	169.1
Zimbabwe	DHS1	1.54*	1.41*	1.00	24.8	99.2
Asia						
Indonesia	DHS1	1.41*	1.44*	0.87*	-8.2	131.8
Indonesia	DHS2	2.26*	2.06*	1.17*	15.8	86.7
Pakistan	DHS2	1.70*	1.66*	1.09	6.2	86.7
Sri Lanka	DHS1	1.01	0.99	0.66*	204.0	2607.9
Thailand	DHS1	2.15*	2.39*	2.31*	-21.3	-14.5
Latin America						
Bolivia	DHS1	1.47*	1.27*	1.07	41.6	84.6
Brazil	DHS1	1.57*	1.31*	1.24	46.3	58.6
Brazil	DHS2	1.45*	1.21	1.17	52.8	62.2
Colombia	DHS1	1.36	1.24	1.05	32.2	86.6
Colombia	DHS2	2.35*	1.91*	1.82*	32.5	39.3
Dominican Republic	DHS1	1.28*	1.23	1.10	17.0	66.0
Dominican Republic	DHS2	1.68*	1.45*	1.30	34.1	56.5
Ecuador	DHS1	1.21	1.01	0.90	94.0	145.9
Guatemala	DHS1	1.30*	1.12	0.86	58.7	147.3
Mexico	DHS1	1.70*	1.58*	1.50*	16.4	28.6
Paraguay	DHS2	1.57*	1.59*	1.38*	-3.3	33.0
Peru	DHS1	1.51*	1.36*	1.10	29.0	79.9
Peru	DHS2	2.21*	1.73*	1.64*	39.7	47.0
Trinidad and Tobago	DHS1	2.47*	2.65*	2.59*	-12.7	-8.3

*Parameter coefficient is statistically significant at the 5 percent level.

sexual relations have resumed. Part of the effect operates through the truncation of breastfeeding when the child dies. It is not clear whether direct physiological mechanisms are at work here (such as anovulatory cycles after return of menses or reduced fecundity) or whether indirect effects of the breastfeeding experience are more important (such as fatigue and nighttime feedings which reduce coital frequency). But whatever the reason, breastfeeding does seem to confer a protective effect against closing the birth interval, even after return of menses and sexual relations.

Breastfeeding explains most of the susceptible period *DIED* effect in Africa—after controlling for breastfeeding, the effect of *DIED* is insignificant in every country in this region except Morocco (DHS2). This finding is not surprising since contraceptive use is generally low in Africa. The effect of child death is virtually explained away by breastfeeding because women have few mechanisms to increase their fertility, such as stopping contraception after the death of a child. On the other hand, the effect is largely explained by confounders in much of Latin America. One hypothesis for this finding is that, in Latin America, the confounders (especially mother's education, residence, socioeconomic status, and parity) are acting as proxies for the propensity to use contraceptives. As expected, the effect of a child's death on the length of the susceptible period appears to operate primarily through breastfeeding and contraception.

We were surprised to find that the effect of *DIED* did not depend on whether the child was wanted. We would have expected a much stronger effect of the child's death if the child had been wanted, in that there would be a desire to replace the lost child. It is unclear whether this result reflects the difficulties mothers have in describing a child (even one who has died) as unwanted or whether the wantedness of a previous child is simply not a good predictor of subsequent behavior.

ACKNOWLEDGMENT

We thank Bridgette James for help in obtaining the Demographic and Health Survey data sets and Sandy Jewell and Ellen Borland for their assistance in managing the original data sets.

REFERENCES

Aborampah, O.M.
    1985   Determinants of breast-feeding and postpartum abstinence: Analysis of a sample of Yoruba women, Western Nigeria. *Journal of Biosocial Science* 17(4):461-469.
Guo, G., and G. Rodriguez
    1992   Estimating a multivariate proportional hazards model for clustered data using the EM algorithm, with an application to child survival in Guatemala. *Journal of the American Statistical Association* 87:969-976.

Heckman, J., and B. Singer
  1982 Population heterogeneity in demographic models. Pp. 567-599 in K. Land and A. Rogers, eds., *Multidimensional Mathematical Demography*. New York: Academic Press.
  1984 A method for minimizing the impact of distributional assumptions in econometric models for duration data. *Econometrica* 52(2):271-320.
Hobcraft, J.N., J.W. McDonald, and S.O. Rutstein
  1985 Demographic determinants of infant and early child mortality: A comparative analysis. *Population Studies* 39(3):363-385.
Howie, P.W., A.S. McNeilly, M.J. Houston, A. Cook, and H. Boyle
  1982 Fertility after childbirth: Infant feeding patterns, basal PRL levels and postpartum ovulation. *Clinical Endocrinology* 17(4):323-332.
Konner, M., and C. Worthman
  1980 Nursing frequency, gonadal function, and birth spacing among !Kung hunter-gatherers. *Science* 207:788-791.
Lapham, R.J., and C.F. Westoff
  1986 Demographic and Health Surveys: Population and health information for the late 1980s. *Population Index* 52:28-34.
McNeilly, A.S., P.W. Howie, and M.J. Houston
  1980 Relationship of feeding patterns, prolactin and resumption of ovulation postpartum. Pp. 102-116 in G.I. Zatuchni, M.H. Labbok, and J.J. Sciarra, eds., *Research Frontiers in Fertility Regulation*. New York: Harper & Row.
Preston, S.H., ed.
  1978 *The Effects of Infant and Child Mortality on Fertility*. New York: Academic Press.
Sullivan, J., S. Rutstein, and G. Bicego
  1994 Infant and Child Mortality. Demographic and Health Surveys Comparative Studies no. 15. Columbia, Md.: Macro International, Inc.
Trussell J., and T. Guinnane
  1993 Techniques of event history analysis. Pp. 181-205 in D. Reher and R. Schofield, eds., *Old and New Methods in Historical Demography*. Oxford, England: Clarendon Press.
Trussell, J., and T. Richards
  1985 Correcting for unmeasured heterogeneity in hazard models using the Heckman-Singer procedure. Pp. 242-276 in N. Tuma, ed., *Sociological Methodology*. San Francisco, Calif.: Jossey-Bass.
Trussell, J., and G. Rodriguez
  1990 Heterogeneity in demographic research. Pp. 111-132 in J. Adams, D. Lam, A. Hermalin, P. Smouse, eds., *Convergent Issues in Genetics and Demography*. Oxford, England: Oxford University Press.

3

The Impact of Infant and Child Mortality Risk on Fertility

Kenneth I. Wolpin

INTRODUCTION

The relationship between the infant and child mortality environment and human fertility has been of considerable interest to social scientists primarily for two reasons: (1) The fertility and mortality processes are the driving forces governing population change, so an understanding of the way they are linked is crucial for the design of policies that attempt to influence the course of population change. (2) The "demographic transition," the change from a high fertility-high infant and child mortality environment to a low fertility-low mortality environment, which has occurred in all developed countries, has been conjectured to result from the fertility response to the improved survival chances of offspring.

Fundamental to either of these motivations is an understanding of the micro foundations of fertility behavior in environments where there is significant infant and child mortality risk. My purpose in this chapter is to clarify and summarize the current state of knowledge. To that end, I survey and critically assess three decades of research that has sought to understand and quantify the impact of infant and child mortality risk on childbearing behavior. To do so requires the explication of theory, estimation methodology, and empirical findings.

I begin by posing the basic empirical (and policy relevant) question: "What would happen to a woman's fertility (children born and their timing and spacing) if there was a once-and-for-all change in infant or child mortality risk?" Alternative behavioral formulations, encompassing static and dynamic decision-theoretic models found in the literature, answer that question and are reviewed. An illustrative three-period decision model, in which actual infant and child deaths are revealed sequentially and behavior is both anticipatory and adaptive, is developed in some detail, and the empirical counterparts for theoretical constructs derived from that model are developed and related to those found in the literature. Specifically, I demonstrate how replacement and hoarding "strategies," which are prominent hypotheses about reproductive behavior in this setting, fit explicitly into the dynamic model and how these concepts are related to the question posed above.

I review a number of empirical methods for estimating the quantitative effect of infant and child mortality risk on fertility, connecting them explicitly to the theoretical framework. I pay particular attention to the relationship between what researchers have estimated and the basic behavioral question. Finally, I present and discuss an overview of empirical results.

THEORY

Static Lifetime Formulations

The earliest formal theoretical models were static and lifetime (i.e., the family attempts to satisfy some lifetime fertility goal decided at the start of its "life"). The "target fertility" model is the simplest variety of such models.[1] Suppose a couple desired to have three surviving children. If the mortality risk were zero, they could accomplish their goal by having three births; if instead they knew that one of every two children would die, then they would need six births. Thus, it appeared straightforward that fertility would be an increasing function of mortality risk. Also, quite obviously, the number of surviving children would be invariant to the fraction of children who survive because the number of births is exactly compensatory.[2] The target fertility model provides the intuitive basis for the concept of "hoarding," that is, of having more births than otherwise would be optimal if mortality risk were zero.

The target fertility model ignores the fact that children are economic goods, that is, that they are costly. A number of authors have introduced a budget constraint into the optimization problem (O'Hara, 1975; Ben-Porath, 1976). Although most formulations included additional decision variables, usually following the quality-quantity trade-off literature (Becker and Lewis, 1973; Rosenzweig and Wolpin, 1980), the essential features of the mortality-fertility link can be

---

[1]The theoretical notion of a target level of fertility, leading to a positive association between fertility and infant and child mortality, was conceptualized at least as early as 1861 (see the quotation from J.E. Wappaus in Knodel, 1978).

[2]More formally, if the utility function is $U(N)$ and achieves a maximum at $N = N^*$ (the "target" fertility level) where N, the number of surviving children, is equal to sB, the (actual) survival rate (s) times the number of births (B), then by maximizing utility and performing the comparative statics, it can be shown that $dB/ds = -B/s < 0$ (sB is constant).

demonstrated in a simpler framework in which the family maximizes a lifetime utility function only over the number of surviving children and a composite consumption good, subject to a lifetime budget constraint.[3] In this model, as in the target model, there is no uncertainty; parents know exactly how many children will survive for any number of births.

In this model it is easily shown that an increase in the survival rate will reduce the number of births, as in the target model, only if fertility has an inelastic demand with respect to its price (i.e, to the cost of bearing and rearing a child).[4] Thus, it could be optimal to have fewer births at a positive mortality rate than at a zero mortality rate (the opposite of hoarding).[5] This result can arise because births per se are costly. At the higher mortality rate, although the number of surviving children is lower for the same number of births, increasing the number of surviving children by having additional births is costly. Depending on the properties of the utility function, the optimal response may be to reduce births. Therefore, the hoarding-type implication of the target fertility model is not robust to the addition of a resource cost to bearing a child.

These models have several shortcomings. First, although the family might be assumed to know the survival risk their children face, they cannot know with certainty the survival fraction (realized survival rate) (i.e., exactly how many children will die for any given number of births). Furthermore, if the number of surviving children is a random variable, these formulations are inconsistent with expected utility analysis unless utility is linear. Second, fertility is clearly discrete. The number of children can take only integer values. Third, fertility decision making would seem a priori to be best described as a sequential optimization problem in which one child is born at a time and in which there is, therefore, time to respond to realized deaths (Ben-Porath, 1976; Knodel, 1978; O'Hara, 1975; Williams, 1977)).

Sah (1991) considered the case of an expected utility maximizing family choosing the number of discrete births to have. He showed that if there is no *ex ante* birth cost (a cost that is incurred regardless of whether or not the child

---

[3]If X is a composite consumption good, Y is wealth, and c the fixed cost of bearing a child, the problem is to choose the number of births B that will maximize $U(sB, X)$ subject to $Y = cB + X$.

[4]The optimal number of births is found by setting the marginal rate of substitution between the consumption good and the number of surviving births, U_1/U_2, equal to the "real" price of a surviving birth, c/s. An increase in the survival rate reduces this price. The elasticity of fertility with respect to the survival rate, d ln B/d ln s, is equal to negative one plus the elasticity of fertility with respect to its cost, $-(1 + d \ln B/d \ln c)$.

[5]However, although the number of births may rise or fall as the survival fraction increases, the number of surviving children must increase. The elasticity of the number of surviving children (sB) with respect to s equals minus the elasticity of births with respect to c. Strictly speaking, the result follows if children are not Giffen goods. The target fertility result will arise only if the elasticity of fertility with respect to c is zero (fertility is perfectly inelastic with respect to c).

survives), then the number of births must be a nonincreasing function of the survival risk (as is true of the previous model). Consider the case in which the choice is between having two, one, or no children. In that case, the difference in expected utilities associated with having one versus no child is the survival risk s times the difference in utilities (i.e., $s[U(1) - U(0)]$. Similarly, the difference in expected utilities between having two children versus having one child is $s^2\{[U(2) - U(1)] - [U(1) - U(0)]\} + s[U(1) - U(0)]$. Now suppose that for a given s, it is optimal to have one child but not two, a result that requires satiation at one surviving offspring $[U(2) - U(1) < 0]$. Clearly, at a higher s, it will be optimal to have at least one child. However, at the higher value of s it will still not be optimal to have a second child, and indeed the difference in expected utilities between having two and having one cannot increase. As Sah demonstrates, the argument generalizes beyond a feasible set of two children to any discrete number of children.

This result, that increasing the mortality risk of children cannot reduce fertility (except in the neighborhood of certain mortality, $s = 0$), is the obvious analog to the target fertility result. However, unlike the target fertility model, it does not imply that the number of surviving children will be invariant to the survival rate. The reason is due to the discreteness (and the uncertainty). An example may be helpful. Suppose that $U(1) - U(0) = 2$ and $U(2) - U(1) = -1$. Now, assuming s is nonzero, it will always be optimal to have at least one child, $s[U(1) - U(0)] = s > 0$. However, in this example, for any survival rate less than two-thirds, it will be optimal to have two children. At a survival rate just below two-thirds, the expected number of surviving children is close to 1.33, whereas at a survival rate just above two-thirds, the expected number of surviving children is close to 0.67. There is, thus, a decline in the expected number of surviving children as the survival rate increases in the neighborhood of two-thirds. However, the relationship is not monotonic; the higher the survival rate within the zero to two-thirds range, and again within the two-thirds to unity range, the more surviving children there will be on average because the number of births is constant within each range.

The example also illustrates hoarding behavior. Because utility is actually lower when there are two surviving children as opposed to one, if the survival rate were unity (zero mortality risk) only one child would be optimal. However, when survival rates are low enough, below two-thirds in the example, the couple will bear two children because there is a significant chance that they will wind up with none who survive to adulthood. Indeed, at survival rates above one-half (but below two-thirds), on average the couple will have more than one surviving birth, exceeding the optimal number of births with certain survival. The key to this result, as will be apparent in the dynamic framework considered below, is that the family's fertility cannot react to actual infant and child deaths.

Sah (1991) demonstrates, however, that adding a cost of childbearing, as before, leads to ambiguity in the effect of the survival rate on fertility. He develops two sets of sufficient conditions for fertility (in the general case of any finite number of children) to decline with the survival rate (for hoarding to be optimal) that depend on properties of the utility function: that the utility function is sufficiently concave (in discrete numbers of children), or that for any degree of concavity the marginal utility of the last optimally chosen birth be nonpositive, that is, that the marginal utility of the last child be nonpositive if all of the optimally chosen children were to survive. Obviously, this second condition will fail to hold if there is no target fertility level, that is, if children always have positive marginal utility. Sah shows that these conditions are weaker than those that would be required if fertility were treated as a continuous choice within the same expected utility framework, and it is in that sense that discreteness reduces ambiguity.

Sequential Decision Making

In formulating the theoretical linkages between infant and child mortality and fertility, the early contributors to this area of research clearly had in mind sequential decision-making models under uncertainty. No biological or economic constraints would force couples to commit to a particular level of fertility that is invariant to actual mortality experience. However, as in other areas of economics, the formalization of such dynamic models of behavior, particularly in the context of estimation, awaited further development.[6] To illustrate the informal argumentation of that time, consider the following discussion by Ben-Porath (1976:S164):

> Let us distinguish between two types of reaction to child mortality: "hoarding" and "replacement." Hoarding would be the response of fertility to expected mortality of offspring; replacement would be the response to experienced mortality. . . . If children die very young and the mother can have another child, the same life cycle can be approximated by replacement. Where the age profile of deaths is such that replacement can reconstitute the family life cycle, replacement is superior to hoarding as a reaction, since the latter involves deviations from what would be the optimum family life cycle in the absence of mortality. If preferences are such that people have a rigid target of a minimum number of survivors at a given phase in the life cycle, hoarding involves a large number of births and the existence of more children than necessary who have to be supported in other phases of the life cycle. . . .
>
> The superiority of replacement is clear, but of course it is not always possible. The risks of mortality are often quite significant beyond infancy. Parents

---

[6]Not all researchers believed that it was necessary to specify the optimization problem formally, however. In describing fertility strategy, Preston (1978:10) states, "These are obviously simplifications of what could be exceedingly complex 'inventory control' problems. But it is probably reasonable to apply no more sophisticated reasoning to the problem than parents themselves would."

may be afraid of a possible loss of fecundity or some health hazard that will make late replacement impossible or undesirable. The reaction to mortality which is expected to come at a late phase of either the children's or the parents' life cycle may be partly in the form of hoarding.

It is obvious from Ben-Porath's remarks that he viewed the replacement decision as a sequential process made in an environment of uncertain mortality and that the hoarding of births is a form of insurance that depends on forward-looking behavior. Furthermore, Ben-Porath postulated that the essential features of the environment that lead to hoarding behavior as an optimal response are those that make replacement impossible, namely that children may die beyond the period of infancy and that the fertile period is finite (and possibly uncertain).

Although several sequential decision-making models of fertility are discussed in the literature, which include nonnegligible infant mortality risk (Wolpin, 1984; Sah, 1991; Mira, 1995), none explicitly model sequential fertility behavior when mortality past infancy is significant (probably because of its intractability in a many-period setting). However the essential behavioral implications of sequential decision making and the intuition for them can be demonstrated in a sequential decision-making model with only three periods. Moreover, a three-period formulation is sufficient to illustrate and operationalize replacement and hoarding concepts.

Suppose that births are biologically feasible in the first two periods of a family's life cycle, but that the woman is infertile in the third (Figures 3-1 and 3-2 provide a graphical representation of the structure of the model). Each offspring may die in either of the first two periods of life, as an infant or as a child, with probabilities given by p_1 (the infant mortality rate) and p_2 (the child mortality rate, conditional on first-period survival). Within periods, deaths occur subsequent to the decision about births. Thus, an offspring born in the first period of the family's life cycle may die in its infancy (its first period of life) before the second-period fertility decision is made. However, that same offspring, having survived infancy, may instead die in its childhood (its second period of life) after the second-period fertility decision is made. Such a death cannot be replaced by a birth in the third period because the woman will be infertile. For the same reason, a birth in the second period is not replaceable even if its death occurs in that period (as an infant). It is assumed for simplicity that the survival probability to the adult period of life, conditional on surviving the first two nonadult periods, is unity. The family is assumed, for ease of exposition, to derive utility from only those offspring who survive to adulthood.[7] This corresponds to the notion that children are investment goods as in the old age security hypothesis (e.g., Willis, 1980) that offspring provide benefits only as adults.

---

[7]One can think of the third period of the couple's life as longer than a single period of life so that a birth in the second period that survives its infancy (in the couple's second period) and its childhood (the couple's third period) (i.e., $d_2^0 = d_3^1 = 0$) will survive to adulthood while the couple is still alive.

PERIOD 1

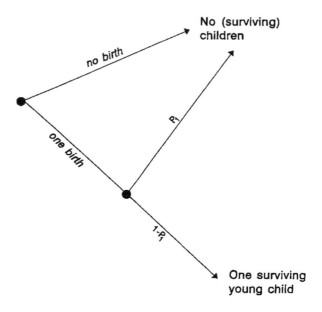

FIGURE 3-1 Decision tree: Period 1.

Formally, let $n_j = 1$ indicate a birth at the beginning of period $j = 1, 2$ of the family's life cycle and zero otherwise. Likewise, let $d_j^k = 1$ indicate the death of an offspring of age k, $k = 0, 1$ at the beginning of period j, zero otherwise, given that a birth occurred at the beginning of period $j - k$. By convention, an infant is age 0 (in its first period of life) and a child is age 1 (in its second period of life). Thus, letting N_{j-1} be the number of surviving offspring at the beginning of period $j = 1, 2, 3, 4$ of the family's life cycle,

$$N_0 = 0, \tag{1}$$
$$N_1 = n_1(1 - d_1^0) = M_1^0,$$
$$N_2 = M_1^0(1 - d_2^1) + n_2(1 - d_2^0) = M_2^1 + M_2^0,$$
$$N_3 = M_2^1 + M_2^0(1 - d_3^1) = M_3^2 + M_3^1.$$

where $M_j^k = \{0,1\}$ indicates the existence of an offspring of age $k = 0, 1, 2$ at the end of period j (and beginning of $j + 1$). Further, let c be the fixed exogenous cost of a birth and Y the income per period. Finally, utility in period 1 is just period 1

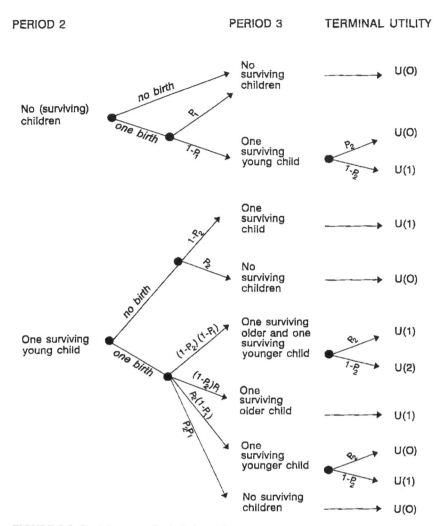

FIGURE 3-2 Decision tree: Periods 2 and 3.

consumption, $Y - cn_1$, utility in period 2 is that period's consumption, $Y - cn_2$, and period 3 utility is consumption in that period plus the utility from the number of surviving children in that period, $Y + U(N_3)$.[8] Lifetime utility is not discounted and income is normalized to zero for convenience.[9]

---

[8]Note that the couple does not care about the age distribution of children.

[9]One can normalize income at zero without loss of generality because utility is linear in consumption.

Because the decision horizon is finite, the problem of optimally choosing a sequence of births so as to maximize lifetime utility is most easily solved backwards. Define $V_t^n(N_{t-1})$ to be the expected lifetime utility at time t if fertility decision $n_t = 1$ or 0 is made at the beginning of period t, given that there are N_{t-1} surviving offspring at the end of period $t - 1$. Furthermore, define $V_t(N_{t-1}) = \max[V_t^1(N_{t-1}), V_t^0(N_{t-1})]$ to be the maximal expected lifetime utility at period t for given surviving offspring at the end of period $t - 1$. Because no decision is made at the beginning of period 3, consider the lifetime expected utility functions at period 2 conditional on the number of surviving children, namely

$$V_2^0(0) = U(0), \tag{2}$$

$$V_2^1(0) = (1 - p_1)(1 - p_2)U(1) + [(1 - p_1)p_2 + p_1]U(0) - c,$$

$$V_2^0(1) = (1 - p_2)U(1) + p_2 U(0),$$

$$V_2^1(1) = (1 - p_2)^2(1 - p_1)U(2) + (1 - p_2)[2p_2(1 - p_1) + p_1]U(1)$$
$$+ p_2[p_2(1 - p_1) + p_1]U(0) - c.$$

For either of the two states, $N_1 = 0$ or 1, the decision of whether or not to have a birth is based on a comparison of the expected lifetime utilities of the two alternatives. If the family has no surviving offspring at the beginning of period 2, either because there was no child born in period 1 or because the infant did not survive to period 2, then from equation (2), the family will choose to have a birth in period 2 if and only if $V_2^1(0) > V_2^0(0)$, or $(1 - p_1)(1 - p_2)[U(1) - U(0)] - c > 0$. If there is a surviving offspring at the beginning of period 2, then the condition for choosing to have a birth is that $V_2^1(1) > V_2^0(1)$ or $(1 - p_1)(1 - p_2)\{(1 - p_2)[U(2) - U(1)] + p_2[U(1) - U(0)]\} - c > 0$. It is easily seen from these expressions that as long as the utility function exhibits diminishing marginal utility in the discrete stock of surviving offspring, that is, $U(2) - U(1) < U(1) - U(0)$, then for all values of p_1 and p_2, the difference between expected lifetime utilities associated with having and not having a birth in period 2 is greater when there is no surviving offspring at the beginning of period 2 ($N_1 = 0$) than when there is a surviving offspring ($N_1 = 1$) (i.e., the gain to have a birth in period 2 is larger if an offspring born in period 1 dies as an infant than if it survives to period 2). The extent to which the gain from a birth in period 2 is increased by the death of an infant born in period 1 $[V_2^1(0) - V_2^0(0)] - [V_2^1(1) - V_2^0(1)]$ is equal to $(1 - p_2)^2(1 - p_1)\{[U(1) - U(0)] - [U(2) - U(1)]\}$. This gain is clearly larger the more rapid the decline in the marginal utility of surviving offspring and the smaller the age-specific mortality probabilities. It is this gain that represents the motivation for "replacement" behavior.

To isolate the effect of the infant mortality risk on second-period fertility, suppose that the child mortality probability p_2 is zero. In this case, the birth decision in period 2 is governed by the sign of $(1 - p_1)[U(2) - U(1)] - c$ if there is a surviving first-period birth and by the sign of $(1 - p_1)[U(1) - U(0)] - c$ if there is not. Clearly, the family would not have a second birth as insurance against the child death of the firstborn (i.e., there would be no hoarding because such a death, given the survival of infancy, is impossible by assumption). However, the absence of such a hoarding motive does not imply that there is no effect of mortality risk on fertility.

An increase in infant mortality risk p_1 has two effects on fertility. First, because an offspring born in period 1 is more likely to die during infancy, the family is more likely to enter the second period without a surviving offspring ($N_1 = 0$). In this case, according to the previous analysis, the gain from a birth in period 2 would be larger. Second, the value of having a second-period birth is lower in the new mortality environment regardless of the existing stock of children (assuming nonsatiation). The effect of a (unit) change in the infant mortality probability on the gain from having a second-period birth is $- [U(N_1 + 1) - U(N_1)]$. For expositional purposes, call this the "direct" effect of mortality risk. If at an initial level of p_1 it were optimal for the household to have a second birth even if the first survived infancy, $(1 - p_1)[U(2) - U(1)] - c > 0$, then increasing infant mortality risk sufficiently would make it optimal to have a second birth only if the first died in infancy. Further increases in the infant mortality rate would eventually lead to optimally having zero births (at some level of p_1 $(1 - p_1)[U(1) - U(0)] - c < 0$). If having a second surviving child reduces utility (satiation), then a second birth would only be optimal if the first died during infancy.

To illustrate the effect on second-period fertility of increasing the probability of death in the second period of life, assume that the increase occurs from an initial state in which there is no mortality risk in either period of life, $p_1 = p_2 = 0$. It is useful to contrast that effect relative to the effect of increasing the first-period mortality risk from the same state. Furthermore, assume that in the zero mortality environment it is optimal to have only one surviving child (i.e., $[U(2) - U(1)] - c < 0$ and $[U(1) - U(0)] - c > 0$). Then, taking derivatives of the relevant expressions in equation (2) evaluated at zero mortality risk yields

$$\frac{d[V_2^1(1) - V_2^0(1)]}{dp_1}\bigg|_{p_1 = p_2 = 0} = -[U(2) - U(1)], \tag{3}$$

$$\frac{d[V_2^1(1) - V_2^0(1)]}{dp_2}\bigg|_{p_1 = p_2 = 0} = -[U(2) - U(1)] + \{[U(1) - U(0)] - [U(2) - U(1)]\}.$$

The effect of a change in the "infant" mortality rate is, as previously derived, the direct effect, which is negative if there is no satiation at one surviving offspring. The effect of a change in child mortality risk is the negative direct effect plus an additional non-negative term whose magnitude depends on the degree of concavity of the utility function. As with Sah's result, this positive offset arises because survival of the first offspring to adulthood is now uncertain and the decision about the second birth must be made before that realization. The hoarding effect generalizes to any levels of mortality risk in the sense that concavity is a necessary condition for its existence. Both replacement and hoarding behavior depend on the curvature of the utility function.

The analysis of the second-period decision, taking the first-period birth decision as given, does not provide a complete picture of the effect of infant and child mortality risk on the family's fertility profile. To see how the decision to have a birth in the first period varies with mortality risk, it is necessary to consider the relevant expected lifetime utilities in period 1, namely,

$$V_1^0 = \max[V_2^0(N_1 = 0), V_2^1(N_1 = 0)] = V_2(0), \qquad (4)$$

$$V_1^1 = (1 - p_1)\max[V_2^0(N_1 = 1), V_2^1(N_1 = 1)]$$
$$+ p_1 \max[V_2^0(N_1 = 0), V_2^1(N_1 = 0)] - c,$$
$$= (1 - p_1)V_2(1) + p_1 V_2(0) - c.$$

The value (expected lifetime utility) of forgoing a first-period birth is simply the maximum of the values attached to entering period 2 without a surviving offspring. The value attached to having a first-period birth depends on the probability that the infant will survive. If the offspring survives infancy, the family receives the maximum of the values associated with entering the second period with an offspring and choosing either to have or not to have a birth in that period [see equation (2)]. If the offspring does not survive, the family receives the maximum of the values associated with entering the second period without a surviving offspring [see equation (2)]. The couple has a birth in period 1 if $V_1^1 > V_1^0$.

To characterize the decision rules in period 1, consider the types of behavior that would be optimal in period 2 under each of the two regimes, having or not having a surviving offspring at the beginning of period 2. There are three scenarios to consider:

(1) It is optimal to have a birth in period 2 regardless of the value of $N_1[V_2^1(0) > V_2^0(0), V_2^1(1) > V_2^0(1)]$.

(2) It is optimal to have a birth in period 2 only if $N_1 = 0$ (i.e., if there are no surviving offspring $[V_2^1(0) > V_2^0(0), V_2^1(1) < V_2^0(1)]$).

(3) It is not optimal to have a birth in period 2 regardless of the value of N_1, $[V_2^1(0) < V_2^0(0), V_2^1(1) < V_2^0(1)]$.

Without providing the details, which are straightforward, the optimal behavior in period 1 is as follows:

(1) If it is optimal to have a birth in period 2 when there is already a surviving offspring, then it will be optimal to have a birth in period 1.
(2) If it is optimal to have a birth in period 2 only if there are no surviving offspring, then it will be optimal to have a birth in period 1.
(3) If it is not optimal to have a birth in period 2 regardless of whether there are surviving offspring, then it will not be optimal to have a birth in period 1.[10]

Together, these results imply that increasing infant mortality risk cannot increase fertility. At very low mortality risk, it will be optimal (also assuming that the birth cost is low enough) to have a second birth independent of whether there is a surviving first birth, implying that case (1) holds. As infant mortality risk increases, it will eventually become optimal to have a second birth only if there is not a surviving first birth, implying that case (2) holds. Finally, at some higher level of mortality risk, it will not be optimal to have a second-period birth regardless of whether there is a surviving first birth, implying that case (3) holds.

The effect of increasing child mortality risk is more complex. If we assume that infant mortality risk (when child mortality risk is zero) is such that case (2) holds, then increasing child mortality risk will at some point produce case (3) (having two children regardless of the mortality experience of the first child, i.e., hoarding behavior as in Sah). Further increases in child mortality risk will lead eventually to a decline in births back to case (2) and then to case (1).

Table 3-1 provides a numerical example. It presents two scenarios, one in which the infant mortality probability is varied, holding the child mortality probability fixed at zero, the other allowing for the opposite (although the infant mortality probability is positive). In both cases, the expected number of births and the expected number of survivors to adulthood are calculated as the relevant mortality risk is varied. In the example, the values of the utility differences $U(2) - U(1)$ and $U(1) - U(1)$ are fixed and exhibit concavity and nonsatiation, as is the cost of a birth, c.

With respect to p_1, the expected number of births is piecewise linear. Between $p_1 = 0$ and the value of p_1 given by the solution to $V_2^1(1) = V_2^0(1)$ (i.e., the

---

[10]These results are special to the assumption that offspring do not yield contemporaneous utility flows.

TABLE 3-1 Dependence of the Expected Number of Births and Surviving Children on Infant and Child Mortality Risk

Outcome	Risk							
	0.000	0.025	0.050	0.075	0.100	0.125	0.150	0.175
Infant mortality[a]								
Expected births	2.000	2.000	2.000	2.000	2.000	1.125	1.150	1.175
Expected survivors	2.000	1.950	1.900	1.850	1.800	0.984	0.978	0.969
Child mortality[b]								
Expected births	1.120	1.120	2.000	2.000	2.000	2.000	2.000	1.120
Expected survivors	0.986	0.961	1.672	1.628	1.584	0.154	1.496	0.813

NOTES: $U(2) - U(1) = 0.8$, $U(1) - U(0) = 1.8$, and $c = 0.71$.
[a] $p_2 = 0$.
[b] $p_1 = 0.12$.

value of p_1 at which there is indifference between having a birth and not having a birth when there is a surviving offspring, 0.1125 in the example), the family will have a birth in both periods regardless of the survival outcome of the first birth (the expected number of births is two). Between the above solution and the value of p_1 that makes the family indifferent between having a birth or not when there is no surviving child, the value that solves $V_2^1(0) = V_2^0(0)$ (0.606 in the example), the family will have a birth in period 1, but only have a birth in period 2 if the first offspring dies. The expected number of births is $1 + p_1$ over this range. At higher levels of infant mortality (greater than 0.606), it will not be optimal to have any births (the expected number of births and survivors are zero). Thus, there is a positive relationship between the number of births and the infant mortality risk over a considerable range of values of the infant mortality rate (from 0.1125 to 0.606 in the example). But rather than indicating hoarding behavior, the positive relationship arises because over this range of increasing infant mortality risk it is optimal to replace infants who die. Notice, however, that the expected number of surviving children (as seen in Table 3-1) never declines (increases) with decreasing (increasing) infant mortality risk.

With respect to p_2, there may be as many as five possible piecewise linear segments of the expected birth function over the p_2 domain. In the first segment, beginning from zero (and ending at 0.044 in the example), it is optimal to have a birth in both periods only if the first offspring dies (the expected number of births is $1 + p_1$). The expected number of surviving children (to adulthood) declines in this segment. In the second segment, it is optimal to have a birth in both periods, and the utility gain from the second birth is an increasing function of p_2 (between $p_2 = 0.044$ and 0.10 in the example). The third segment repeats the second except that the gain is now declining in p_2 (between $p_2 = 0.10$ and 0.157 in the example). The fourth segment repeats the first with the expected number of births equal to $1 + p_1$ ($p_2 = 0.157$ to 0.552), while in the last segment the family has no births (between $p_2 = 0.552$ and 1.0). As seen in the table, expected births first increase and then decrease as the child mortality rate increases. Notice that the jump in fertility between the first and second segments (between p_2 equal to 0.025 and 0.05) is exactly the hoarding response. Moreover, it is accompanied by an increase in the expected number of surviving children. Thus, increased child survival induces, over this range, a decrease in the expected number of surviving children.

As Table 3-1 makes clear, knowledge of the values of utility differences and of the cost of a birth are sufficient for the calculation of fertility behavior under any hypothetical mortality environment. Thus, if the model provides an accurate representation, or at least approximation, of fertility behavior, it would provide a tool for assessing the effect of health-related policy interventions and thus of the experiment postulated at the beginning of this chapter. Of course, the three-period model is intended to be only illustrative. For example, in a model with a longer fertile period and in which there are non-negligible age-specific mortality risks over an extended range of childhood ages, there would be a considerably more complex fertility response to a change in the mortality environment.

ESTIMATION ISSUES

It is possible within this theoretical framework to describe all of the methods that demographers and economists have used to estimate the responsiveness of fertility to changes in mortality risk. In the three-period model, the family decides deterministically in each of the two fecund periods whether or not to have a birth. A population of homogeneous families with respect to preferences (the two utility differences) and constraints (the cost of childbearing and the infant and child mortality probabilities) will all act identically. Moreover, because knowledge of preferences and constraints by the researcher would imply perfect prediction of behavior by the model (assuming for this purpose that the model is literally true), there would be no statistical estimation problem. But suppose the population differs randomly in the cost of childbearing, c.[11] Furthermore, assume that different values of c for periods 1 and 2, c_1 and c_2, are drawn independently from the same distribution, $F(c;\Theta)$, at the beginning of their respective periods. Thus, the decision in period 1 is conditioned on knowledge of c_1 only.[12] Neither period birth cost is known to the researcher, so that, although each family's behavior is still deterministic (each family either decides to have a birth or not in each period), the researcher can determine behavior only probabilistically.

What can be learned from estimation obviously depends on the data that are available. In this regard, it is useful to divide the discussion of estimation issues into two cases corresponding to whether the population is homogeneous or heterogeneous with respect to mortality risk.

Population-Invariant Mortality Risk

Consider a sample of families for whom we observe fertility and infant and child mortality histories. By assumption, they have the same utility function, draw their period-specific birth costs from the same distribution, and face the same mortality schedule for their offspring. In the context of the three-period model, it is sufficient for our purpose that we have information on n_1, n_2, and N_1, that is, that we know about all births and at least whether the firstborn died in

---

[11]Alternatively, utility differences could have a random component.

[12]The assumption of imperfect foresight with respect to the future cost of childbearing is not consistent with the solution of the model presented for the first-period fertility decision. In deciding on first-period fertility, the family would have to take into account the possible future actions that would be optimal for all possible values of the randomly drawn second-period cost of childbearing. Changing the informational structure in this way simplifies the estimation problem and its exposition.

infancy. It is not necessary to know the mortality experience in period 2 because there can be no subsequent fertility response in period 3. In addition, let us suppose that the researcher also knows the mortality schedule faced by the sample, p_1 and p_2, and in addition, for identification purposes, knows the form and parameter values that describe the birth cost distribution $F(c; \Theta)$.[13]

Then the likelihood function for this sample is

$$L(\omega \mid \text{data}) = \prod_{i=1}^{I} \Pr(n_{1i}, n_{2i} \mid d_{1i}, p_1, p_2, F), \tag{5}$$

$$= \prod_{i=1}^{I} \Pr(n_{2i} \mid N_{1i}, p_1, p_2, F) \Pr(n_{1i} \mid p_1, p_2, F),$$

where ω consists of the two utility differences. There are I families in the sample, with the lack of an i subscript implying constancy in the population.

Now, the probability (from the researcher's perspective) that a randomly drawn family will be observed to have a birth in period 2 conditional on the two possible values of the beginning period stock of surviving offspring is

$$\Pr(n_2 = 1 \mid N_1 = 1) = \Pr\big(c_2 < (1 - p_2)(1 - p_1)\{(1 - p_2)[U(2) - U(1)] \tag{6}$$
$$+ p_2[U(1) - U(o)]\}\big),$$

$$\Pr(n_2 = 1 \mid N_1 = 0) = \Pr\big(c_2 < (1 - p_2)(1 - p_1)[U(1) - U(0)]\big).$$

Similarly, the probability of a first-period birth is given by

$$\Pr(n_1 = 1) = \Pr\big(c_1 < (1 - p_1)\{E_1[V_2(1)] - E_1[V_2(0)]\}\big), \tag{7}$$

where E_1 is the expectations operator given the information set at period 1 and is taken over the distribution of infant and child mortality and birth costs, and the value functions in the integral of equation (7) are given by equation (4). There are three sample proportions, corresponding to the theoretical probabilities in equations (6) and (7), from which the utility differences can be recovered.[14]

---

[13]This is a strong assumption. In the two-period decision context, where there are only two utility differences, adopting a specific functional form for the utility function would not reduce the number of parameters. For the longer-horizon model, that would realistically apply, the reader can think of placing parametric restrictions on the form of the utility function and on the distribution function for birth costs. Such assumptions would be sufficient for identification of the distribution function parameters.

[14]It might appear that we could have relaxed the assumption that all of the parameters of the birth cost distribution are known, given that there are more sample proportions than unknown parameters. However, this turns out not to be the case given the structure of the model. As an example, if F is assumed normal and we normalize the variance to unity, the mean of the cost distribution does not enter the decision rule in a way that allows it to be identified separately from the utility differences.

Given these estimates, the response of fertility behavior in the population to variations in mortality risk can be obtained by solving the behavioral optimization problem. More specifically, given the estimates of the utility differences, it is possible to forecast the impact of changing age-specific mortality risk on the expected number of births and surviving children exactly as in Table 3-1.

Notice that in this example there is no other way to estimate policy responses to mortality risk variation because mortality risk is assumed not to vary in the population. However, the sample proportions of births, the data analogs of equations (6) and (7) used in the structural estimation, obviously provide information about behavior. Indeed, taking the difference in the probabilities in equation (6) provides a natural way to define a measure of replacement behavior. Specifically, the definition of the replacement rate r is given by

$$r = \Pr(n_2 = 1 \mid n_1 = 1, d_1 = 1) - \Pr(n_2 = 1 \mid n_1 = 1, d_1 = 0), \qquad (8)$$

where the conditioning event in equation (8) is restricted to a first-period birth with and without its death. (This detail is unnecessary given the construction of the model, because the second-period birth probability is the same regardless of why the stock of children is zero.) Analogous to the three-period dynamic model, if there is diminishing marginal utility, then the probability of a birth is larger when there is no surviving offspring than when there is, and $r > 0$. According to equation (8), full replacement, $r = 1$, would require that the probability of having a second birth be unity when the first birth did not survive and zero otherwise. On the other hand, the replacement rate will be zero if the probability of a birth is independent of the number of surviving offspring, a result that requires [see equation (6)] that the marginal utility of surviving offspring be constant, $U(2) - U(1) = U(1) - U(0)$.

What do we learn from this transformation of the underlying probabilities (i.e., from calculating r)? Or alternatively, for what policy experiment would calculation of r be relevant? Implicit in the original policy experiment is the notion that the effect of the change in mortality risk of infants and children is known to families or becomes immediately obvious from its (population) impact (for example, as seems to have been the case when the polio vaccine was introduced in the United States).[15] However, suppose that, although effective, families did not alter their beliefs about mortality risks (or did so only very slowly, as might be the case with generalized improvements in nutrition). Then we would observe families responding only to the reduced number of infant deaths as they

---

[15]It should be noted that the behavioral formulation assumes that the policy is itself a surprise (i.e., that families attach a zero probability to its occurrence). Otherwise, in the dynamic model, one would have to allow for a distribution over future infant and child mortality risk (conditional on current information). Introducing additional parameters would require a reconsideration of identification.

are experienced and not to the decline in the infant and child mortality risk per se. In this case, the replacement rate would measure the full response to the program.

Now the replacement rate times the number of first-period infant deaths in a population yields the number of extra births that arise in that population because of the infant deaths. This result follows from the fact that the definition of r in equation (8) is equivalent to the expected number of births given a birth and infant death in the first period, $1 + \Pr(n_2 = 1 \mid n_1 = 1, d_1 = 1)$ minus the expected number of births given a birth and no infant death, $1 + \Pr(n_2 = 1 \mid n_1 = 1, d_1 = 0)$. So suppose, for example, that the government institutes a health program that will reduce the infant mortality risk by 0.05. Following its introduction, there will be a reduction in the number of first-period deaths of $0.05 \times \Pr(n_1 = 1) \times$ (number of families). If $r = 1$ at the preprogram, and perceived to be postprogram, mortality risk, then all of the second-period births that had resulted from the replacement of first-period deaths will not occur and the number of second-period births will thus decline by the same amount as the number of first-period deaths. Furthermore, the number of surviving children would be approximately unchanged. Alternatively, if $r = 0$ so that no first-period deaths were replaced, the number of second-period births will be unaffected by the reduction in the number of deaths, and the number of surviving children will increase by the number of averted deaths.

If the fertile stage is extended beyond two periods, the replacement rate would have to account for births, arising from a death, that occur in later periods.[16] If there are T fecund periods, then the replacement rate for the specific case of a birth in the first period and its subsequent infant death is given by

$$r = \sum_{j=2}^{T} [\Pr(n_j = 1 \mid n_1 = 1, d_1 = 1) - \Pr(n_j = 1 \mid n_1 = 1, d_1 = 0). \qquad (9)$$

Notice that to calculate equation (9) knowledge of the probabilities of all future birth sequences conditional on N_1 is required. In the T-period case, a replacement rate can be calculated at any period for any given birth and death sequence. For example, in a setting in which the entire birth and death sequence determined the decision rule, there would be, for example, a seven-period replacement rate given the death of a 3 year old in period 6, and it would be conditional on other births and deaths as of the end of period 6.[17] There is thus potentially a very large set of replacement rates, all of which are determined by the parameters of the underlying behavioral model.[18]

Although perhaps less transparent than was the case in the three-period

---

[16]Replacement births could be postponed in this model due to random fluctuations in birth costs. In richer models there could be additional reasons.

[17]Thus, replacement rates are not restricted to infant deaths.

[18]It is also possible for the replacement rate to be larger than one if children die at older ages. A death close to the end of the fertile period might induce hoarding behavior.

model, the expression for the replacement rate in equation (9) is equivalent to the difference in the expected number of births given the birth and death of a child in period 1 and the expected number of births given the birth and survival of a child in period 1. Therefore, equation (9) measures exactly the excess births that arise from an infant death. Analogous replacement rates would measure the excess births that would arise from the death of a child of any age given any birth and death history.

The value in estimating replacement effects for policy analysis rests on an assumption about the extent to which effective programs alter families' perceptions about mortality risk. Eventually, one would expect that the new mortality environment would become known, in which case replacement rates would provide an inaccurate picture of the fertility response. The value of structural estimation of the behavioral model does not depend on assumptions about learning, because identifying the fundamental parameters allows either policy experiment (or any combination) to be simulated (although predicting the effect of the change would depend on those assumptions).[19] For the rest of the discussion I will assume, as has the literature, that replacement rates correspond to experiments of interest.

Longitudinal or retrospective data on birth and death histories are not always available. Often, only information on total births and deaths is reported for a cross section of households (i.e., in the three-period model, $n_1 + n_2$ and d_1).[20] If mortality risk is the same for all families, it would seem natural to estimate a regression of the number of births on the actual number of infant and child deaths. Such a regression would determine the additional births that arise from one additional death (i.e., the replacement rate in equation (8) or equation (9) in the T-period case). Thus, for the regression

$$B_j = b_o + rD_j + v, \tag{10}$$

where B_j is the number of births in family j, D_j is the number of deaths, and v is a stochastic element, the regression coefficient r is the replacement rate in equation (8). In the three-period model, B can equal only 0, 1, or 2, whereas D can be only 0 or 1, and the only relevant deaths are those of infants. Again, second-period deaths are ignored because they cannot influence fertility.

From the birth probabilities given in equation (6), it is possible to derive the

---

[19]Here, mortality risk was assumed not to be changing over the family's decision period. If mortality risk was not constant, some assumption about how families forecast future mortality risk would have to be incorporated into the behavioral model.

[20]Additional information contained in d_1 results from the special nature of the three-period formulation, namely that with one total birth and one death, the timing of the birth is known. With a longer horizon, such inferences would be unavailable from total births and total deaths.

set of probabilities for numbers of births given any number of deaths (e.g., $\Pr(B = 0 \mid D = 0)$, $\Pr(B = 1 \mid D = 0)$, etc.), and, from these, the expected number of births for each number of deaths. With some tedious algebra, it can be shown that the ordinary least-squares regression estimator—the difference in the expected number of births given one death and the expected number of births given zero deaths—is

$$\hat{r} = E(B \mid D = 1) - E(B \mid D = 0) = \frac{g_1 + g_2 r}{g_1 + g_2}, \qquad (11)$$

where $g_1 = \Pr(n_1 = 0)$ and $g_2 = \Pr(d_1 = 1 \mid n_1 = 1)\Pr(n_1 = 1)$. It is easy to see from equation (11) that the ordinary least-squares regression coefficient of births on deaths in general will overstate the replacement effect.[21]

There have been several attempts to provide estimates of replacement effects that correct for the "spurious" correlation between births and deaths.[22] Olsen (1980) considers the following joint stochastic representation of total births and deaths:

$$B_j = \overline{B} + r(D_j - \overline{D}) + v_j, \qquad (12)$$
$$D_j = pB_j + \varepsilon_j,$$

where the overbars indicate means. Substituting the first equation in (12) into the second yields

$$D_j = p\overline{B} + \frac{pv_j}{1 - pr} + \frac{\varepsilon_j}{1 - pr}. \qquad (13)$$

As Olsen argues, because the number of deaths is not statistically independent of v_j, as seen in equation (13), the regression coefficient estimator of r from the B_j equation will be biased and inconsistent. Specifically, the probability limit of the regression estimator is

---

[21]Notice that the replacement rate can be estimated correctly by restricting the estimation sample to couples with at least one birth ($g_1 = 0$ in that subsample). However, this is an artifact of the three-period model. In general, the number of deaths must rise with the number of births for a constant mortality rate, and the resulting positive correlation between births and deaths is built into the estimated replacement effect.

[22]Notice that in the three-period model, knowledge of g_1, the proportion of families not having a child in period 1, and of g_2, the proportion of families who have both a birth in the first period and for whom the infant dies, is sufficient to solve equation (11) for the true replacement effect. Of course, if one had this information it would not be necessary to estimate the replacement effect from equation (11), as equation (6) could be computed directly as discussed above. The use of equation (11), as noted, is predicated on the lack of such event history data.

$$\mathrm{plim}(\hat{r}) = r + \frac{\mathrm{cov}(D_j, v_j)}{\mathrm{var}(D_j)} > r. \qquad (14)$$

The ordinary least-squares regression estimator overstates the true replacement rate because deaths and births are positively correlated independently of the existence of replacement; families with more births experience more deaths simply because their "sample" size is larger. Deriving expressions for the moments in equation (14) under the assumption that Dj and Bj are binomial random variables, Olsen further shows that

$$\mathrm{plim}(\hat{r}) = r + \{(1 - pr)[p + \frac{(1-p)\overline{B}}{\mathrm{var}(B)}]\}^{-1}. \qquad (15)$$

The probability limit of the ordinary least-squares estimator can deviate substantially from the true replacement rate. Assuming $r = 0$, Olsen reports that the ordinary least-squares regression estimate of r ranges between 0.9 and 1.7 for five different populations. But what is important is that equation (15) can be used to "correct" the replacement effect estimate using the observed mortality rate p (along with the mean and variance of births). Given the ordinary least-squares estimate ($\hat{r}$), the sample mortality rate (p), and the first two moments of the sample birth distribution [$\overline{B}$, var(B)], equation (15) can be explicitly solved for r.

Mauskopf and Wallace (1984) present a somewhat different procedure for estimating the replacement rate that solves explicitly for the death distribution that is consistent with replacement behavior.[23] To outline their method, define B^* to be the number of births that would occur if the family experienced no child deaths. In the three-period model, B^* is a well-defined entity obtained by solving the sequential model for n_1 and n_2 conditional on there being no deaths. Given that c varies randomly in the population, B^* is a random variable with expectation in the three-period model given by $1 \times \Pr(B = 1 \mid D = 0) + 2 \times \Pr(B = 2 \mid D = 0)$. In general, one can write $B^* = E(B^*) + u$, where $E(u) = 0$, $E(u^2) = \sigma^2$, and where $E(B^*)$ is determined by the exact optimizing model that is adopted.

Because replacement children can themselves die and be replaced, Mauskopf and Wallace (1984) conceptualize the process as sequential (although they conceive of the actual decision process as being static), consisting of separate rounds of deaths, replacement births, deaths of the replacement births, replacement births of the replacement birth deaths, etc. So in the first round, $d_0 = pB^* + \varepsilon_0 = pE(\mathrm{B}^*)$

---

[23]Mauskopf and Wallace (1984) argue that Olsen's correction is only strictly valid at a zero replacement rate. Olsen assumed that the distribution of deaths conditional on births was binomial (i.e., $E(D) = pB$). However, if deaths are in part replaced, the binomial assumption cannot be valid as the number of deaths will depend on the replacement rate and on the number of births that would occur if there were no deaths.

+ ω_0, where $\omega_0 = pu + \varepsilon_0$ and p is the (non-age-specific) mortality rate of children. First round deaths, d_0, conditional on B^*, are assumed to be binomially distributed. Assuming independence between u and ε_0, the variance of ω_0 is $\text{var}(\omega_0) = p^2\sigma^2 + p(1-p)E(B^*)$. First-round replacements are $r_0 = rd_0 + \eta_0 = rpE(B^*) + \xi_0$, where $\xi_0 = r\omega_0 + \eta_0$ and r is the replacement rate. The variance of ξ_0 given the independence between η_0 and the other stochastic elements is $\text{var}(\xi_0) = r^2 \text{var}(\omega_0) + r(1-r)pE(B^*)$. In general, in the ith round, $d_i = pE(r_{i-1}) + \omega_i$ and $r_i = rE(d_i) + \xi_i$. Summing over all rounds, $I = 0, 1, \ldots$, they derive the following expressions for the first two moments of total deaths and total births:

$$E(D) = \frac{pE(B^*)}{1-pr}, \tag{16}$$

$$E(B) = \frac{E(B^*)}{1-pr},$$

$$\text{var}(D) = \frac{[p^2\sigma^2 + pE(B^*)(1 + pr - p)]}{(1-pr)^2},$$

$$\text{var}(B) = \frac{[\sigma^2 + prE(B^*)]}{(1-pr)^2},$$

$$\text{cov}(D, B) = \frac{[p\sigma^2 + prE(B^*)]}{(1-pr)^2}.$$

These five equations have four unknowns, p, r, $E(B^*)$, and σ^2, satisfying the necessary condition for identification. Mauskopf and Wallace estimate the parameters by matching the theoretical moments to the observed moments in the data.

In the T-period model, the replacement rate estimated from the total birth and total death relationship using either Olsen's correction or the Mauskopf and Wallace method would be an "average" of replacement rates specific to the actual birth and death sequences in the sample. Such "average" replacement rates could be quite different for samples that differ, for example, only in the age distribution of the families (women), but with the same underlying infant mortality risk, preferences, and birth costs.

Population-Variant Mortality Risk

Observable Heterogeneity

Assume now that population variation in the mortality environment is observable to the researcher (e.g., geographic variation in mortality rates). Structural estimation could proceed with the pooled (over geographic areas) data if utility differences (the structural parameters) were cross-sectionally invariant or separately by geographic area if not.

A possible alternative estimation procedure is to approximate the decision rules of the optimization problem as a general function of the state variables. Birth probabilities could be approximated by

$$\Pr(n_2 = 1 \mid N_1) = \Pr[h_2(N_1, p_1, p_2, c_2) > 0], \qquad (17)$$
$$\Pr(n_1 = 1) = \Pr[h_1(p_1, p_2, c_1) > 0],$$

where, as before, the c's are random variables. Given distributional and functional form assumptions, the impact of a change in mortality risk can be calculated from the h functions estimated with likelihood function shown in equation (5). For example, linearizing the h function in its arguments and assuming normality of the cost distribution leads to a standard (bivariate) probit estimation problem.[24] Although the estimates could be used to assess the effect of policy interventions that reduce mortality risks, the ability to extrapolate from equation (17) so as to assess large policy changes would depend on the global properties of the approximation of the h function. And clearly this estimation method is unavailable without population variation in mortality risk.

Nonparametric estimation of replacement rates (equation (8) or (9)) could be obtained for each geographic area, recalling that replacement rates depend on the level of infant mortality risk. Because Olsen's correction factor (equation (15)) depends on the mortality rate, Olsen's analysis could be conducted within areas, recognizing as well the direct dependence of the replacement rate on mortality risk. Similarly, Mauskopf and Wallace's analysis could be conducted within geographic areas, obtaining separate location-specific estimates of replacement rates.

Unobservable Heterogeneity

In this case, families differ in their underlying mortality risk to an extent not fully observed by the researcher (see Rosenzweig and Schultz, 1983, or Olsen and Wolpin, 1983, for evidence of the existence of permanent unobserved heterogeneity in mortality risk). Structural estimation, using maximum likelihood as before, would require either that couple-specific mortality schedules be treated as estimable parameters or that they be assumed to have a known distribution whose parameters would be estimated. Suppose, for example, that $p_2 = 0$ (i.e., that there

---

[24]Because the second-period birth probability depends on the lagged dependent variable N_1, the two decision rules could be estimated separately only if c_1 and c_2 are drawn independently.

is no mortality risk beyond infancy). Then, because realized deaths provide information on family-specific mortality risk, the likelihood function would incorporate both fertility and mortality events, namely

$$L = \prod_{i=1}^{I} \Pr(n_{1i}, n_{2i}, d_{1i}^0, d_{2i}^0 \mid p_{1i}) \tag{18}$$

$$= \prod_{i=1}^{I} \Pr(d_{1i}^0, d_{2i}^0 \mid p_{1i}) \Pr(n_{2i} \mid N_{1i}, p_{1i}) \Pr(n_{1i} \mid p_{1i}),$$

where d_1^0 and d_2^0 indicate a death of a first- or second-period birth in infancy as in the prior notation, and where conditioning on p_{1i} indicates that the infant mortality rate is now family specific. It is important to note that, to implement the estimation procedure (maximize equation (18)), the optimization problem of the family would have to be solved for each family separately. If instead we had assumed a specific parametric distribution for p_1 or a nonparametric distribution having a fixed number of discrete values (a fixed number of family types), the likelihood function would contain an integration or discrete mixture over the possible values of p_1 that each family could be exposed to. The optimization problem would, in this case, have to be solved for each possible value of mortality risk. Notice that there are cross-equation restrictions implied by the behavioral model. Not only are birth probabilities in the two periods connected by the same fundamental parameters (the last two components of the likelihood function in the second line of equation (18)), but also those probabilities are functions of the mortality risk that also enters the determination of actual deaths in the first component of the likelihood function. Thus, the estimates of mortality risk would be influenced not only by observed mortality rates, but also by the fertility response to mortality risk.

Approximate decision rules (equation (17)) can be estimated using likelihood function (equation (18)). Heckman (1982) deals with this class of models in the multinomial probit case when there is also unobserved heterogeneity. Estimating approximate decision rules differs from structural estimation in that cross-equation restrictions are ignored. Estimation must take into account that the unobserved heterogeneity is correlated with the existing stock of children in each period of the family's life cycle (see, for example, Mroz and Weir, 1989). Subject to the usual caveat about the inconsistency of fixed-effects estimates in "short" panels, one would recover an (unbiased) estimate of each family's permanent mortality risk and also obtain an estimate of the effect of mortality risk on birth probabilities. However, this procedure is equivalent to a two-step procedure of estimating the family-specific mortality risk from realized family-specific mortality rates and "regressing" measures of fertility on them. Because the realized rates measure the true risk with error, these policy-relevant estimates would be biased downward. Replacement effects estimated from the effect of a death on birth probabilities or total births, holding the estimated mortality risk constant, would be upwardly biased (since deaths are positively correlated with the family's true mortality risk).

Replacement rates estimated nonparametrically using sample birth probabilities would not correspond to the replacement rate for any particular family. The replacement rate in equation (8) or (9) holds mortality risk constant, whereas the sample birth proportions reflect the unobserved variation in mortality risk. The number of excess births calculated this way would also not provide the correct population effect. That calculation would have to be performed for each family separately and then summed over families to obtain the correct estimate. Nonparametric replacement estimates based on birth and death histories can be used for policy analysis only if one can assume that mortality risk is homogeneous (or otherwise held constant).

Olsen suggests estimating the replacement effect from the regression (equation (10)) using realized sample (infant) mortality rates among families, reflecting in part variation in underlying mortality schedules and in part "luck," as an instrumental variable for total deaths (to correct for the spurious correlation between total births and total deaths). Although such a procedure would be valid in the case in which mortality risk was constant in the population (and also unnecessary), when mortality risk varies but is unobserved, regression equation (10) is misspecified; the dynamic model, for example, implies that the expected number of births will vary with the true infant mortality risk (recall the direct effect of mortality risk demonstrated in the three-period model). If it is not included as a regressor because it is unobserved, then it enters through the regression error, and the realized mortality rate, being correlated with it, cannot be a valid instrument for the number of deaths. It is important to stress that the problem with this procedure exists even if there is no child mortality risk; it has nothing to do with hoarding behavior. However, if there was significant child mortality and the risk varied in the population, child mortality rates would also not be a valid instrument for estimating replacement effects because they affect fertility independently (through the direct effect and the hoarding effect).

Both Olsen and Mauskopf and Wallace extended their methodologies to the case in which population heterogeneity in mortality risk is unobservable. It is sufficient to consider the Mauskopf and Wallace paper because the problem with the method, shared by both, is more easily demonstrated. Assume that child (but, not infant) mortality risk is zero. As Mauskopf and Wallace note, one can view the moment equations (16) as conditional on a particular value of p (p_1 under the above assumption). To obtain the unconditional (population) moments, Mauskopf and Wallace integrate the conditional moments over p, assuming that p comes from the two-parameter beta distribution. They then estimate the beta distribution parameters instead of p. However, this procedure is inconsistent with the dynamic model presented above; both the replacement rate (r) and $E(B^*)$, which appear in the moment equations, depend on p. Integrating over p requires that one solve for their optimal values as p changes. Ignoring this dependence leads, in principle, to incorrect estimates of the replacement effect.

Additional Mortality-Fertility Links

There are two biological links between mortality and fertility, recognized in the literature, that create special problems for the estimation and interpretation of empirical relationships (for more details see Wolpin, in press).

Breastfeeding There is a strong presumption that lactation reduces the propensity to conceive. Thus, in societies where breastfeeding is customarily practiced, the death of an infant may hasten the birth of another child. What may appear to be a behavioral replacement response may be due to the premature cessation of breastfeeding that accompanies the infant death (see, for example, Preston, 1978).

Endogenous Mortality Risk To the extent that the timing and spacing of children itself influences mortality risk and there is unobserved heterogeneity in mortality risk, estimating the effect of mortality risk on fertility is problematic. In addition to biological links, a further difficulty arises if mortality risk is unknown to the decision maker.

Learning Families may not know their own infant and child mortality risk. Deaths may provide useful information about that risk. Replacement effects, for example, will then reflect not only the direct effect of a death but also on its signal about the families' underlying propensity to experience deaths (see Mira, 1995).

A BRIEF SURVEY OF EMPIRICAL RESULTS

This section presents results of representative studies that have had as their main goal either the estimation of replacement effects or the effect of mortality risk on fertility. Estimates of replacement provide information about the effect of a hypothetical policy intervention that reduces mortality risk but for which the change in mortality risk is not perceived by families. Studies that estimate the effect of mortality risk on fertility provide information about the effect of an intervention when the change in mortality risk it induces is known to families.

Replacement Effects

Estimates Based on Birth and Death History Data

The definition of replacement given in equation (8) or (9) has rarely been adopted as the statistical measure in practice when complete fertility and mortality histories have been available. Rather, two other measures, having their roots in the demographic literature, have been more prominent: the parity progression ratio and the mean closed interval to the next birth. They are both easily defined in terms of birth probabilities. If we let L equal the duration to the next birth, then conditional on the first-period state, the probability that $L = t$ is

$$\Pr(L = t \mid n_1, d_1) = \Pr(n_{t+1} = 1, n_t = 0, ..., n_2 = 0 \mid n_1, d_1). \tag{19}$$

These probabilities define the duration density function, say $g(L)$. There is actually a different density for each period and a different longest duration. If there is a longest feasible duration, L^*, then for $g(L)$ to be a proper density it must include the probability of having no more children, for example,

$$g(\infty) = 1 - \sum_{t=1}^{L^*} \Pr(L = t \mid n_1, d_1). \tag{20}$$

(In the three-period model, $L = 1$ is the only feasible duration.) The parity progression ratio (PPR) is simply the probability that the couple will have (at least) one more birth, the next parity. A measure of replacement behavior is the difference between the PPR when there is a death and the PPR when there is not, that is, in the case in which there is a birth in period 1 (as in equation (6)):

$$\Delta\text{PPR} = G(L^* \mid n_1 = 1, d_1 = 1) - G(L^* \mid n_1 = 1, d_1 = 0), \tag{21}$$

where G is the cumulative duration distribution function. PPRs can be calculated analogously for any birth and death history and are usually calculated by conditioning on a particular parity (rather than on age). Conditioning on parity rather than age leads to a different quantitative measure for replacement because it combines the different age-specific responses (i.e., experiencing one infant death out of three births will induce a different replacement response depending on the number of periods left until the end of the fecund horizon). However, calculating the excess number of births due to a reduction in the mortality risk for a population with homogeneous mortality risk would be identical using PPRs to that calculated from equation (8) or (9). For a population with heterogeneous mortality risk, the excess birth calculation using PPRs would be incorrect, as was the case with using equation (8) or (9).

The other prominent measure of replacement behavior, based on birth and death histories, found in the literature is the differenced mean closed interval (DMCI). The DMCI is the difference in mean birth durations, conditional on having an additional birth before the end of the fecund stage, under alternative mortality experiences. The DMCI is given by

$$\text{DMCI} = E(L \mid n_1 = 1, d_1 = 1, L \le L^*) - E(L \mid n_1 = 1, d_1 = 0, L \le L^*) \quad (22)$$

$$= \sum_{t=1}^{L^*} \left[\frac{tg(t \mid n_1 = 1, d_1 = 1)}{G(L^* \mid n_1 = 1, d_1 = 1)} - \frac{tg(t \mid n_1 = 1, d_1 = 0)}{G(L^* \mid n_1 = 1, d_1 = 0)} \right].$$

Because the DMCI is conditional on having a birth subsequent to the death, its relationship to the other replacement measures is not straightforward. For example, in the last fertile period the expected duration to the next birth, conditional on there being a birth, must be one period independent of the prior mortality experience; thus, in this case the DMCI will be zero even though the probability of an additional birth would be responsive to the mortality history (r in equation (8) is not zero). The DMCI should be more closely related to the other replacement measures in populations of younger families and higher fertility. This measure is clearly the most problematic in calculating excess births.

Knodel (1978) uses reconstituted birth and death information from three German villages for women who married between 1840 and 1890 and whose marriages were intact at age 45. Mean closed intervals and PPRs for the three villages are shown in Table 3-2. All of the villages have high fertility rates; total fertility is over 6. The women in the village of Mömmlingen are known to have breastfed their children over extended periods, whereas in Schönberg and Anhausen breastfeeding was rarely practiced at all. This fact is consistent with the longer average birth interval in Mömmlingen, although the prolongation of postpartum sterility due to lactation may not be the only factor.

The differences between the mean closed intervals for women who did and did not experience child deaths are clearly largest in Mömmlingen, the village where breastfeeding was normally practiced. For example, over all birth intervals, the mean closed interval was more than 10 months shorter if a woman residing in Mömmlingen had experienced at least one death, but only two months shorter for women in Schönberg and less than one month shorter for women in Anhausen. The differences in PPRs by infant mortality experience, however, seem to be largest in Anhausen and are therefore more suggestive of replacement behavior. But PPRs do not uniformly rise with additional deaths; indeed, the likelihood of a women moving from a third to a fourth birth declines with the number of infant deaths. One possible explanation of this phenomenon would be that women with more deaths learn that they have a higher infant mortality rate, which reduces subsequent fertility (the direct effect). In an attempt to net out the lactation effect of an infant death, Knodel looks at the effect of the death of the firstborn on the mean closed interval between the second and third births. The differences are now largest in Anhausen, 5.8 months, and smallest in Schönberg, 2.8 months.

Vallin and Lery (1978) use a subsample of 92,000 French women who were born between 1892 and 1916 and were surveyed in 1962. As reported in

TABLE 3-2 Parity Progression Ratios and Mean Closed Intervals Based on Nineteenth Century Bavarian Village Data

Outcome	Mean Closed Intervals (months)		
	Mömmlingen	Schönberg	Anhausen
All birth intervals			
No infant deaths	30.0	22.0	19.9
One or more infant deaths	19.4	20.0	19.2
Second to third child			
First child survives	29.0	23.9	23.4
First child dies	25.4	21.1	17.6

	Parity Progression Ratios (percent)		
	Mömmlingen	Schönberg	Anhausen
Second to third child			
No infant deaths	96.3	97.4	84.0
One or more infant deaths	100.0	97.6	90.5
Third to fourth child			
No infant deaths	93.0	93.1	81.3
One infant death	94.5	87.9	92.9
Two or more infant deaths	85.7	76.5	90.0

SOURCE: Knodel (1978).

Table 3-3, for all levels of completed family size and regardless of the birth order of the infant death, retrospectively obtained mean closed intervals are about one year less when an infant death is experienced. PPRs differ by about 16 percentage points for the movement between first and second births when the firstborn did or did not die, by approximately the same amount for the movement between second and third births given that the secondborn did or did not die, and by about 10 percentage points for higher parities. As was the case for the German historical data, the later French data reveal similarly higher fertility subsequent to an infant death. Numerous other studies report mean closed intervals and PPRs by mortality experience. Most use cross-sectional data where birth and death information is collected retrospectively. Some report estimates based on regressions that hold individual characteristics constant (e.g., Ben-Porath) and in that sense are not completely nonparametric. The general findings in the literature are qualitatively the same as for the two papers discussed above, namely that the evidence is consistent with the existence of replacement behavior.

TABLE 3-3 Parity Progression Ratios and Mean Closed
Intervals Based on 1962 French Survey of Family Structure

Parity	Mean Closed Intervals	
	No Infant Death	Infant Death
Total fertility		
Two	4.14	3.17
Three		
First birth	3.35	2.43
Second birth	4.19	3.39
Four		
First birth	2.77	2.16
Second birth	3.43	2.48
Third birth	4.06	3.26
	Parity Progression Ratios (n to $n + 1$)	
	No Infant Death (birth n)	Infant Death (birth n)
First to second child	68.5	84.7
Second to third child	57.6	72.8
Third to fourth child	56.4	67.4
Fourth to fifth child	57.3	67.9
Fifth to sixth child	59.2	69.2

SOURCE: Vallin and Lery (1978).

Estimates Based on Total Births and Deaths

Tables 3-4 and 3-5 report estimates of replacement effects based on the use of total births and total deaths. Table 3-4 shows replacement effects obtained by Olsen and Table 3-5 those by Mauskopf and Wallace. Olsen uses data from the 1973 Columbia Census Public Use Sample and reports his results for different age and residential location groups. Only the oldest age group, women who were age 45-49 in 1973, are shown. The uncorrected estimates, that is, the regression coefficient on total deaths, imply a replacement rate of over one for both urban and rural women, regardless of whether controls are added. The corrected estimate that assumes a homogeneous mortality rate in the population is negative, implying that there are actually fewer births when there is an infant or child death. This result is consistent with the negative "direct" effect of higher infant mortality. The replacement effect obtained under the assumption that the mortality rate varies in the population (independently from births) yields point estimates of around 0.2.[25] Olsen also estimates a replacement effect when the mortality

---

[25]The independence assumption is inconsistent with optimizing behavior.

TABLE 3-4 Replacement Effects from Total Births Regressors: Olsen Method

Regressors	Urban, Age 45-49			Rural, Age 45-49		
		Corrected			Corrected	
	Uncorrected	Fixed Mortality Rate	Random Mortality Rate	Uncorrected	Fixed Mortality Rate	Random Mortality Rate
Death only	-1.27	-0.54	0.21	1.06	-0.53	0.19
Deaths, education of wife and husband, regional dummies	1.21	-0.49	0.20	1.04	-0.51	0.20

SOURCE: Olsen (1980).

TABLE 3-5 Replacement Effects from Total Births Regressors: Mauss-hopf and Wallace Method

| Mortality Rate | All Women | Years of Education | | |
		None	1-4	5+
Fixed	0.601	0.348	0.592	0.964
	$(0.03)^a$	(0.04)	(0.06)	(0.13)
Random	0.593	0.437	0.613	0.978
	(0.04)	(0.04)	(0.05)	(0.08)

[a]Standard errors in parentheses.

SOURCE: Mausshopf and Wallace (1984).

rate is correlated with births. Those estimates vary between 0.13 and 0.22 depending on the joint distributional assumption for the mortality rate and total fertility.[26]

The estimates based on the method developed by Mauskopf and Wallace are presented in Table 3-5. Mauskopf and Wallace use data from the 1970 Brazilian census, restricting attention to women who were between 40 and 50 years old at the time of the survey. The replacement rate, assuming the mortality risk to be fixed in the population, was estimated to be 0.6 for the total sample. It was 0.35 for those with zero schooling, 0.6 for women with 1-4 years of schooling, and almost unity for women with 5 or more years of schooling. Allowing the mortality rate to differ in the population, using the method described above, only changed the estimate significantly for the lowest education group.

Approximate Decision Rules

Mroz and Weir (1989) developed a discrete-time statistical representation of the timing of births that can be viewed as an approximation to the decision rules that arise from a dynamic sequential utility maximizing model. Three stochastic processes are specified as (1) the process generating the probability of resuming ovulation after a birth, (2) the process generating the probability of conception,

---

[26]Olsen (1983) adds an estimate of innate mortality risk to the regression of total births and total deaths in combination with his correction method as an attempt to separate replacement and hoarding behavior. However, the effect of early age mortality risk on fertility cannot be called a hoarding response, as hoarding would not exist in an environment without significant mortality risk among older children. Controlling for innate infant frailty, however, would provide an estimate of the replacement rate that is uncontaminated by unobserved mortality risk. Olsen estimates a replacement rate of 0.17 using this method.

and (3) the process generating the onset of secondary sterility. The waiting time to a birth is the convolution of the waiting time to the resumption of ovulation and the waiting time to a conception, conditional on the resumption of ovulation and conditional on not becoming infecund. The probability of observing a woman with a particular sequence of births up to any given age is specified in terms of these three stochastic processes. Mroz and Weir allow for unobserved heterogeneity in each of the three waiting times; women may differ biologically in the postanovulatory and fecund processes, and they may differ biologically and behaviorally in the conception process. However, there is neither observed nor unobserved heterogeneity in mortality risk (cross sectionally or temporally).

Monthly probabilities are modeled as logistic functions. The fecund hazard at any month depends on duration since the start of the interval, age, age at marriage, parity attained by that month (dummy variables for each attained parity), dummy variables for whether the particular month is the first month of risk of conception in the interval, a dummy for the first month of marriage, and the number of surviving children during that month. Heterogeneity shifts the monthly probability proportionately and is assumed to take on a small number of discrete values (Heckman and Singer, 1984). Identification in this model is achieved by a combination of functional form assumptions, assumptions about biological processes (for example, exactly 9 months gestation) and a clever use of data (using the timing of an infant death to tie down the beginning of the fecund period given the cessation of breastfeeding). The reader is referred to their paper for the exact details.

The model is estimated using reconstituted data between 1740 and 1819 from 39 French villages based on birth and death histories for women who were married at age 20-24. The results provide evidence on the importance of unobserved heterogeneity (in the fertility process) in the estimation of replacement effects. Mroz and Weir report that simulations conducted prior to estimation, omitting controls for unobserved heterogeneity in the fecund hazard rate and recognizing that they accounted for the cessation of lactation due to an infant death, resulted in the probability of a birth increasing in the number of surviving children (conditional on parity, age, duration, and age at marriage). Controlling for heterogeneity in estimation, however, resulted in a negative effect as is consistent with a behavioral replacement effect. Quantitatively, Mroz and Weir found that births increase by 13 percent due to the cessation of lactation alone following an infant's death and by 17 percent overall. Given an average of about seven births, the absolute behavioral replacement effect is 0.28. Mroz and Weir essentially assume that mortality risk does not vary in the population (given covariates).

The Impact of Infant and Child Mortality Risk on Fertility

Structural Estimation

Wolpin (1984) illustrates structural estimation. The model has the following characteristics: (1) Per-period utility is quadratic in the number of surviving children in that period and in a composite consumption good, (2) fertility control is costless and perfect, (3) there is a fixed cost of bearing a child and a cost of maintaining a child in its first period of life (if it survives infancy), (4) children can die in only their first period of life subject to an exogenous time-varying (and perfectly forecasted) infant mortality rate, (5) the household has stochastic income and consumption net of the cost of children that is equal to income in each period, and (6) the household's marginal utility of surviving children varies stochastically over time according to a known (to the household) probability distribution. Given this framework, the household chooses in each period whether or not to have a child.[27]

For the purpose of estimation, Wolpin assumes that the time-varying preference parameter is drawn independently over both time and across households from a normal distribution. The mortality rate faced by the household is assumed known to the researcher, measured by the state-level mortality rate in each period, and the researcher is assumed to forecast future mortality rates exactly as the household is assumed to do, namely based on the extrapolated trend in the mortality rate at the state level. Future income is forecasted from the time series of observed household income, again under the assumption that the household uses the same forecasting method.

The data are drawn from the 1976 Malaysian Family Life Survey that contains a retrospective life history on marriages, births, child deaths, household income, etc., of each woman in the sample. Wolpin used a subsample of 188 Malay women who were over age 30 in 1976, currently married, and married only once. The period length was chosen to be 18 months, the initial period was set at age 15 (or age of marriage if it occurred first), and the final decision period was assumed to terminate at age 45. Thus, there were 20 decision periods. In the implementation, the cost of a birth is allowed to be age varying as a way of capturing age variation in fecundity and in marriage rates. In addition, the woman's schooling is allowed to affect the marginal utility of surviving children.

Parameter estimates are obtained by maximum likelihood. As already alluded to, the procedure involves solving the dynamic programming problem for each household (given their income and mortality risk profiles) and calculating

---

[27]Mira (1995) recently extended that model to the case in which families learn about the innate mortality risk they face through their realized mortality experience.

the probability of the observed birth sequence. Because the woman's fertility is observed from what is assumed to be an exogenous initial decision period (either age 15 or age at marriage, whichever occurs first), the likelihood function is conditioned on the initial zero stock of children, which is the same for all women. The birth probability sequences that form the likelihood function can be written as products of single-period birth probabilities conditional on that period's stock of surviving children, the output of the dynamic programming solution.

Given the parameter estimates, the replacement effect is calculated in each period and for each number of surviving children for a representative couple. The replacement effect is estimated to be small, ranging between 0.01 and 0.015 additional children ever born per additional infant death. The reason for the negligible replacement effect is that the actual fertility behavior is best fit in the context of this optimization model with utility parameters that imply essentially a constant marginal utility of children. Wolpin also calculated that an increase in the infant mortality risk by 0.05 would lead to a reduction in the number of births by about 25 percent. (Note that this effect includes the potential replacement of the increased number of infant deaths, which is in this case negligible given the very small estimated replacement effects.) Thus, the impact of a policy that altered infant mortality risk would depend quite heavily on how quickly that policy change was perceived to have been effective.[28]

Nonstructural Estimation

A number of studies have attempted to estimate the effect of mortality risk on fertility using nonstructural estimation methods. As already discussed, obtaining correct estimates is particularly challenging if there is unobserved mortality risk variation, and more so when mortality risk is endogenous, as when fertility spacing affects mortality risk as discussed above. Mortality risk can also be endogenous if it is affected by behaviors that are subject to choice and if, in addition, there is population heterogeneity in preferences. Several studies, having recognized this problem, have attempted to estimate the effect of innate family-specific mortality risk on fertility. To do so requires that one estimate the production function for child survival, accounting for all behavioral and biological determinants.[29] Although the credibility of the estimates of the fertility-frailty relationship depends in part on the way frailty estimates are obtained, let

---

[28]Interestingly, direct evidence about hoarding comes from my 1984 study, although I failed to recognize it at the time. Given the finding there that the marginal utility of surviving children is essentially constant, which led to the negligible estimated replacement rates, the potential hoarding response, if child mortality were significant in that environment, would also be negligible since hoarding also depends on concavity as shown in equation (3).

[29]See Wolpin (in press) for a discussion of the methods used to estimate the survival technology as well as empirical findings.

us consider the findings of studies that estimate its effect on fertility behavior assuming the frailty estimates to be credible.

Rosenzweig and Schultz (1983), using data from the 1967, 1968, and 1969 National Natality Followback Surveys (U.S. Department of Health, Education and Welfare), find that the expected number of children ever born per woman would be 0.17 greater for an infant mortality risk of 0.1 as opposed to zero. Given that in their sample the infant mortality rate is less than 3 percent, this experiment may be within sample variation. At the sample average of 2.5 births per woman, an additional 0.25 deaths per woman leads to 0.17 more births and therefore to 0.08 fewer surviving children. Such a finding, it should be noted, must arise from replacement behavior to be consistent with the dynamic model presented above; in that model an increase in infant mortality risk cannot increase births for the same number of infant deaths.

Olsen and Wolpin (1983), also using the 1976 Malaysian Family Life Survey, estimate that a couple faced with a 1 percent higher monthly probability of death within the first 24 months of life will have their first birth approximately 2 weeks earlier. This effect is rather small given that the average interval between births is 30 months. Although seemingly inconsistent with the simple three-period model, that model is not rich enough to capture more complicated behaviors that might explain this result. For example, it is possible that greater mortality risk induces an earlier first birth so as to increase the time over which to respond to actual mortality.

CONCLUSIONS

The original question posed in the introduction to this chapter was intended to focus attention on the micro foundations of fertility behavior as a necessary prerequisite to informed population policies. It is fair to ask whether after several decades of empirical research we can confidently report to policy makers the quantitative estimates of the effects of changing infant and child mortality risk on fertility at the individual level. The answer, in my view, is unfortunately no. That assessment does not rest simply on the fact that estimates vary widely or that the empirical approaches are methodologically flawed. Rather it rests more fundamentally on the fact that we do not have a deep enough understanding of behavior to know how to generalize our results beyond the setting within which we obtain estimates. To ultimately accomplish that goal requires that we establish tighter links between theory (behavioral decision rules) and empirical methods (what is estimated).

ACKNOWLEDGMENTS

Support from National Science Foundation grant SES-9109607 is gratefully acknowledged. This chapter is in part a summarization and condensation of the paper "Determinants and Consequences of the Mortality and Health of Infants and Children," which will appear in the *Handbook of Population and Family Economics*, M. Rosenzweig and O. Stark, eds. I have received useful comments from Barney Cohen, Mark Montgomery, and several anonymous reviewers.

REFERENCES

Becker, G.G., and H.G. Lewis
   1973   On the interaction between the quantity and quality of children. *Journal of Political Economy* 81:S279-S288.
Ben-Porath, Y.
   1976   Fertility response to child mortality: Micro data from Israel. *Journal of Political Economy* 84(2):S163-S178.
Heckman, J.J.
   1982   Statistical models for discrete panel data. Pp 114-178 in C. Manski and D. McFadden, eds., *Structural Analysis of Discrete Data with Econometric Applications*. Cambridge, Mass.: MIT Press.
Heckman, J.J., and B. Singer
   1984   A method for minimizing the distributional assumptions in econometric models of duration data. *Econometrica* 52(2):271-320.
Knodel, J.
   1978   European populations in the past: Family-level relations. Pp. 21-45 in S.H. Preston, ed., *The Effects of Infant and Child Mortality on Fertility*. New York: Academic Press.
Mauskopf, J., and T.D. Wallace
   1984   Fertility and replacement: Some alternative stochastic models and results for Brazil. *Demography* 21(4):519-536.
Mira, P.
   1995   Uncertain Child Mortality, Learning, and Life Cycle Fertility. Unpublished Ph.D. dissertation, University of Minnesota, Minneapolis.
Mroz, T.A., and D. Weir
   1989   Structural change in life cycle fertility during the fertility transition: France before and after the revolution of 1789. *Population Studies* 44:61-87.
O'Hara, D.J.
   1975   Microeconomic aspects of the demographic transition. *Journal of Political Economy* 83:1203-1216.
Olsen, R.J.
   1980   Estimating the effect of child mortality on the number of births. *Demography* 17(4):429-443.
   1983   Mortality rates, mortality events, and the number of births. *American Economic Review* 73:29-32.
Olsen, R.J., and K.I. Wolpin
   1983   The impact of exogenous child mortality on fertility: A waiting time regression with exogenous regressors. *Econometrica* 51(3):731-749.
Preston, S.H.
   1978   Introduction. Pp 1-18 in S.H. Preston, ed., *The Effects of Infant and Child Mortality on Fertility*. New York: Academic Press.
Rosenzweig, M.R., and T.P. Schultz
   1983   Consumer demand and household production: The relationship between fertility and child mortality. *American Economic Review* 73:38-42.

Rosenzweig, M.R., and K.I. Wolpin
    1980   Testing the quantity-quality model of fertility: Results from a natural experiment using
            twins. *Econometrica* 48:227-240.
Sah, R.K.
    1991   The effects of child mortality changes on fertility choice and parental welfare. *Journal of
            Political Economy* 99(3):582-606.
Vallin, J., and A. Lery
    1978   Estimating the increase in fertility consecutive to the death of a young child. Pp 69-90 in
            S.H. Preston, ed., *The Effect of Infant and Child Mortality on Fertility.* New York:
            Academic Press.
Williams, A.D.
    1977   Measuring the impact of child mortality on fertility: A methodological note. *Demogra-
            phy* 14(4):581-590.
Willis, R.J.
    1980   The old age security hypothesis and population growth. Pp. 43-68 in T. Burch, ed.,
            Demographic Behavior: Interdisciplinary Perspectives on Decision Making. Boulder,
            Colo.: Westview Press.
Wolpin, K.I.
    1984   An estimable dynamic stochastic model of fertility and child mortality. *Journal of Politi-
            cal Economy* 92(5):852-874.
    In   Determinants and consequences of the mortality and health of infants and children. In M.
    press   Rosenzweig and O. Stark, eds., *Handbook of Population and Family Economics.*
            Amsterdam, Netherlands: North-Holland.

4

Learning and Lags in Mortality Perceptions

Mark R. Montgomery

Each culture has experts, people of unusual acumen or specialized knowledge, who detect covariations and report them to the culture at large.

Nisbett and Ross (1980:111).

Every demographer can sketch in two curves the broad outlines of the demographic transition. One curve depicts high and then falling mortality; the other shows how fertility, also high at the outset, follows a similar downward course after a lag. Fertility change depends on many factors other than mortality per se, but it is reasonable to believe that, as survival prospects improve, the need for high fertility must be reduced.

Although much empirical research supports the view that mortality decline is a causal factor in fertility decline (Schultz, 1981; Wolpin, in this volume), the literature also contains puzzling cases in which considerable mortality decline fails to evoke any response in fertility, as well as examples in which the usual sequence is reversed, with fertility decline preceding the decline in mortality (Matthiessen and McCann, 1978). In spite of the fundamental role assigned to mortality change, no theory has yet been formulated to explain the lag in fertility responses or to show why long lags are to be expected in some circumstances and rapid response in others.

In assembling the elements of such a theory, it is worthwhile to pose to ourselves this question: How, in fact, do people learn that mortality has declined? Imagine oneself semiliterate, situated in a rural area of a developing country, and isolated to a great degree from the media and from the formal health-care system. Suppose that even in such an environment, a decline in child mortality is under way. Are the improvements in child survival simply self-evident? Is it a trivial matter to learn the facts? How would one know of mortality decline without having been informed of the facts by health personnel or by those who are better educated?

These questions came to mind in the course of a series of focus groups that Olukunle Adegbola and I conducted in Lagos, Nigeria, in 1989. Lagos is of course at the opposite end of the spectrum from the situation just described: It is perhaps Africa's largest urban community, saturated by information from radio, television, and newspapers, with a population that contains numerous health personnel and a mixture of the well-educated and the thoroughly uneducated. Without really expecting much from the question, we asked our focus group participants in Lagos whether they thought children were more likely to survive these days than a generation ago. We were somewhat taken aback by the range and variety of their replies. No consensus existed about mortality decline. The better-educated expressed confidence that a decline was under way and pointed to the many medicines and modern treatments that were unknown in their fathers' time. Some of the less-educated, by contrast, exhibited confusion about the direction of change, some arguing that children were more likely to die now than in the past, while others cited improvements in health care. Several participants observed that currently in Lagos, one sees many more funerals than used to be the case; to them, this was evidence of rising mortality. They were clearly thinking of the numerator of a mortality rate, rather than of the rate itself.

Evidently, it is not a simple matter to deduce mortality decline from observation alone. It may be that few people think naturally in terms of rates or probabilities, and that some training is required to appreciate the distinction between the number of deaths and the death rate. Perhaps educated Nigerians know of mortality decline because they have learned about it in school or because they are more attentive to information presented in the media or by health personnel. In addition, the mortality decline in Nigeria may have been uneven (Hill, 1993), with a clearer downward trend for socioeconomically advantaged groups and a slower change, perhaps too subtle to reach the threshold of perception (McKenzie 1994), among groups that are less well-off.

The aim of this chapter is to explore such issues with the aid of formal models of learning and decision making under uncertainty. I draw on a diverse literature that includes studies in economics, demography, and social and cognitive psychology. The chapter is frankly speculative. I know of only three empirical studies that have directly measured mortality perceptions in developing countries: Pebley et al. (1979) for Guatemala, Heer and Wu (1978) for Taiwan and urban Morocco, and Cleland et al. (1992) for five Central and West African countries. The Pebley et al. study focused on perceived child survival probabilities in four villages in the Institute of Central America and Panama (INCAP) study of Guatemala. Likewise, Heer and Wu (1978) considered child mortality perceptions in two Taiwanese townships and for Morocco they gathered data on perceptions of change. Cleland et al. explored the perceived threat of AIDS to adult survival and behavior. In developed country settings, recent work by Hurd and McGarry (1995) for the United States is concerned with the perceptions of mature and elderly men and women of old age survival prospects. In view of the prominent causal role thought to be played by child mortality decline in fertility transitions, it is surprising that the empirical literature on perceptions of survival remains so thin.

The chapter is organized as follows. In the first section I consider a model of Bayesian learning about child survival in which individual perceptions are determined by a prior distribution that summarizes initial subjective beliefs about mortality probabilities, these beliefs then being updated by reference to a sample of information on mortality experience, yielding a posterior distribution that summarizes how beliefs change in the light of experience. Bayesian learning supplies a natural benchmark for learning models, in that the approach assumes that individuals process information in an optimal fashion, acting much as statisticians do. In view of the difficulties that individuals may face in thinking in probabilistic terms, however, to assume Bayesian learning may well be inappropriate. An extensive literature in both psychology and economics, which makes use of experimental evidence on judgment and belief updating, provides strikingly little support for the Bayesian model. It seems that individual reasoning about uncertainty can and often does depart systematically from Bayesian predictions. In the second section some of the major findings from this experimental literature are reported, and I speculate about their implications for mortality perceptions. In the final section I present conclusions and offer suggestions for a demographic research agenda.

BAYESIAN LEARNING ABOUT CHILD SURVIVAL

The Bayesian approach to learning is perhaps viewed most usefully as an optimal benchmark, providing a standard against which less precisely formulated models can be judged. I focus on a type of learning that might be termed social learning (Montgomery and Casterline, 1996), whereby individuals gather information about child survival prospects by observing the experiences of their peers. Each family is assumed to be linked by way of its social networks to a sample of other families that provides N observations on child survival in each year. The true child survival probability will change from one year to the next, following an upward trend, and each year the family's beliefs about survival will be updated in a Bayesian fashion, taking into account that year's sample of size N.

To draw out the implications of survival probabilities for fertility, I rely on a simple utility maximization model (details are reported in the Appendix) that is an idealized representation of fertility decision making. Parents are assumed to choose the number of births they bear, denoted by B, so as to maximize an expected utility function $U(S)$, where $S \leq B$ is the number of surviving children. I explore a specification in which U is a quadratic function of S, that is,

$$U(S) = aS - bS^2,$$

with parameters $a, b > 0$. In this specification there is an ideal number[1] of surviving children S^* that corresponds to the maximum of $U(S)$. Because child survival is uncertain, parents are not assured of having S^* children and will adjust their fertility B to protect themselves against the possibility of child loss. The number of surviving children S is assumed to be binomially distributed given the number of births B and the child survival probability θ. In developing the examples below, I take θ to be the probability of surviving to age 5, that is, as the complement of the child mortality probability.[2]

Known Survival Probabilities

To begin, suppose that the survival probability θ is known with certainty. Figures 4-1 and 4-2 illustrate the optimal fertility distributions for a range of values of the survival probability θ. In developing these figures, I assumed that the desired number of surviving children is four[3] and that θ lies in the range that has been characteristic of the postwar experience in West Africa. To motivate the example, I take from Hill (1993:Table 5.2) a time series of child mortality estimates for Ghana, a West African country whose mortality decline is well documented. In the immediate postwar period (circa 1948) the probability of child mortality was about 0.301 in Ghana. A period of mortality decline then set in, bringing child mortality to a level of 0.199 by 1967. In the 1970s and 1980s little further improvement took place, and by 1985 Ghanaian child mortality had fallen only to 0.163. Figure 4-1 presents illustrative fertility estimates derived from θ values that range from 0.699, a number that corresponds to the immediate postwar years, to a maximum of 0.95, the latter being some 10 points above what Ghana had achieved as of the mid-1980s.

As can be seen in Figure 4-1, improvement in child survival brings about a reduction in mean desired fertility. The mean value of fertility declines from 5.5 to 4.2 over the range for θ, a difference of slightly more than one child. The net reproduction rate, however, remains essentially constant, this being a common

---

[1]For simplicity, I choose parameter values to ensure that there is only one maximum of $U(S)$, associated with an integer value for S.

[2]Alternatively, one could consider survival to adulthood rather than to age 5. In most developing country settings in which mortality rates are very low between age 5 and adulthood, there would be little empirical difference between the two survival probabilities. Where perceptions are concerned, however, the death an older child or young adult might exert a powerful influence out of proportion to its empirical likelihood.

[3]The optimal number of surviving children is produced by making assumptions on the ratio of utility parameters a and b such that $4 = a/(2b)$ or $a = 8b$. We can then consider different values for b. The greater the value for b, the sharper the fall off in utility as the number of surviving children deviates from four.

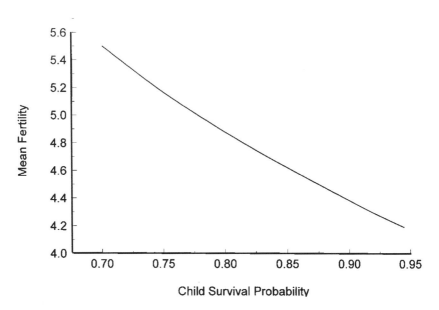

FIGURE 4-1 Mean fertility by child survival probability.

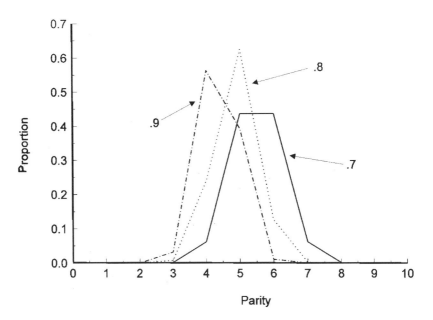

FIGURE 4-2 Distributions of fertility given different survival values.

feature of models that take births themselves to be costless (see the Appendix). The effects of child survival are perhaps clearer in Figure 4-2, which shows the distribution of desired fertility for several θ values.

Uncertain Survival Probabilities

Having sketched the main features of the case in which θ is known, I now ask how fertility decisions might differ if the survival probability θ is an unknown quantity about which individuals have more or less certain prior beliefs. Two questions must be addressed. First, how does one represent such prior beliefs? Second, how does experience cause these beliefs to be revised?

As they enter adulthood, most women and men in developing countries will have had some exposure, whether direct or indirect, to the risks of child mortality. Many will have experienced the death of a sibling, an event that must leave a deep and vivid impression, and the experiences of relatives might figure in as well.[4] Those who have attended school would have acquired some general information about health and survival, which could also shape initial perceptions of risk. But for many young adults, childbearing and the risks of child death are matters that belong to a stage of life that they have not yet entered and about which they know little. We would therefore expect perceptions of the survival probability θ to be hazy and subject to considerable uncertainty.

Imagine two young Ghanaian adults who begin their family building in 1948. In each year, they will have access, through social networks of relatives, friends, and peers, to a sample of N observations on child survival. Each year the family assesses the information contained in this sample and revises its subjective beliefs about θ accordingly. The size N of this sample will depend on the extent of social networks in general, the level of fertility in the population, and the degree of privacy that shrouds matters of birth and death. For example, it may be that the educated have access to larger social networks than do the less educated and so possess a larger sample of information. For simplicity, however, I take N to be a constant and set $N = 10$ for purposes of illustration.

Returning to the household's fertility choice, the problem is to choose the number of births B that maximizes

$$E \, U(S) = E \, (aS - bS^2).$$

As noted in the Appendix, if the value of the survival probability θ were known, this problem could be restated as

---

[4]As John Casterline (personal communication, 1996) notes, this supposition forms the basis of the sisterhood method for estimating adult mortality.

$$\max_{B} B(a - b)\, \theta - bB(B - 1)\theta^2.$$

With θ unknown, however, the values of θ and θ^2 must be replaced in the expression by their subjective expected values, $E(\theta)$ and $E(\theta^2)$, which in turn depend on prior beliefs and the available sample of child survival observations.

Illustrative Results

If we take the Ghanaian experience as a guide, Figure 4-3 shows the sequence over time of the actual survival probability as compared with the evolution of subjective beliefs about survivorship. Figure 4-3 shows the subjective mean $E(\theta)$ and the 25th and 75th percentiles of the subjective distribution. It illustrates the evolution of perceptions for a family beginning in 1948 with a prior distribution whose mean is identical to the true survival probability (0.699), but with considerable uncertainty about θ, as evident in the 25th to 75th percentile range that stretches from 0.57 to 0.86. In 1948 and in each year thereafter, the family updates its beliefs on the basis of ten new observations, each such sample being drawn from a binomial distribution characterized by that year's (true) survival probability. The learning shown here is therefore cumulative; that is, beliefs in 1980 are influenced to some degree by the initial prior distribution in 1948 as well as by the intervening sequence of social network samples.

As can be seen in the figure, although the uncertainty evident in the initial

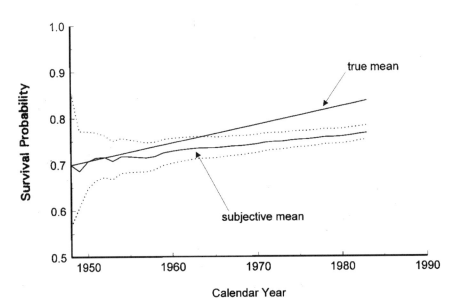

FIGURE 4-3 Actual trend versus subjective distribution.

prior distribution is quickly reduced, and even though the initial subjective mean and the true mean were selected to exactly coincide, the family's perception of child survival fails to keep pace with the empirical realities. There is an upward trend in the subjective mean, to be sure, but the year-to-year gain is smaller than the true improvement in survivorship. By the early 1960s even the 75th percentile of the subjective θ distribution has fallen below the true value for θ, and by the end of the period the gap between the subjective mean and the true θ value has grown to some eight percentage points.

One might ask whether larger social networks, which contain more annual observations on children's deaths and survival, would bring the subjective mean into line with the true survival probability. A change in the sample size N does have some effect, but the gap shown in Figure 4-3 persists even if N is doubled to 20 annual observations.

The persistent lag in expectations, as compared with the true level of child survival, is the product of two factors. The first is that the true values for θ follow a trend, whereas in the simple Bayesian model outlined above, beliefs are updated without there being a recognition that a trend in survivorship exists. If a more complex Bayesian model were employed (see Zellner and Rossi, 1984; Koop and Poirier, 1993; Poirier, 1994) in which both level and trend components for θ were updated from sample experience, the subjective values would adhere more closely to the actual trend. Such Bayesian trend models require greater sophistication on the part of decision makers, who must now make mental comparisons of their social network samples over time.

The second factor is that even with relatively small social network samples (recall that $N = 10$), only a few rounds of experience are required to substantially reduce subjective uncertainty about θ. As the distribution of beliefs becomes ever more concentrated about the subjective mean, upward revision of that mean is made ever more grudgingly. With time and experience, individuals become more and more set in their beliefs and begin to resist new evidence of improvements in survival.

Implications for Fertility

How much difference does learning and uncertainty make to fertility decisions? One way to assess the net effect of learning is to compare the mean level of desired fertility with the survival probability θ set equal to its true end-of-period value (see Figure 4-3) to the mean fertility level produced by the subjective distribution of θ for that year. The difference in fertility is on the order of 0.6 children. In other words, an objectively correct evaluation of survival prospects would be predicted to lead to 0.6 fewer desired births than in the case in which subjective mortality impressions are employed.

The projected difference of 0.6 desired births is in no way an empirical finding, being simply the outcome of a particular model and set of assumptions.

The model itself could be elaborated in any number of dimensions, for example by incorporating both trend and level components in learning and by adding a dynamic structure that would permit child replacement effects to be analyzed. These are worthwhile extensions; they will inevitably lead to a more sophisticated Bayesian model. Before we undertake to construct such an elaborate model, we should assess the experimental evidence on learning to determine whether any support exists for the type of optimal learning being considered here.

DEPARTURES FROM BAYESIAN LEARNING

Camerer (1995) has thoroughly reviewed the literature in cognitive psychology, social psychology, and economics and found evidence that indicates a departure from Bayesian learning in two principal areas: Individuals employ learning strategies that are cognitively much simpler than the Bayesian rules; and in some circumstances, individuals consistently make fundamental mistakes in probabilistic reasoning, tending to assign too much weight to certain types of evidence and not enough to others.

Nonexperimental economists have been inclined to dismiss such findings, arguing that, as individuals gather experience and are repeatedly subjected to the discipline of the market or other social institutions, their judgments will come to resemble optimal Bayesian judgments. Such conditions are unlikely to obtain in respect to mortality perceptions and fertility decision making. In developing transitional societies, individuals are often called upon to make decisions in novel situations and in environments that are in flux, where the old rules no longer quite apply but new rules and institutions have not yet evolved to take their place. Mistakes and misperceptions are to be expected as individuals traverse such new terrain.

To begin, it should come as no surprise that individuals prefer to use simple rules of thumb in making their judgments and updating beliefs, rather than to engage in complex Bayesian calculations. Such common decision rules usually involve a simple averaging of prior beliefs and new sample evidence (Lopes, 1985, 1987; McKenzie, 1994). This need not in itself put the Bayesian perspective in doubt, as one could argue that individuals often behave as if they were Bayesians. In the case of updating in mortality perceptions, the main features of Figure 4-3 above would probably not change greatly if individuals simply split the difference between their prior beliefs and the latest sample evidence.

However, there is considerable doubt that individuals consistently behave as if they were Bayesians. As Camerer (1995) and Conlisk (1996) demonstrate, when economic experiments are designed to reward optimal decisions and punish mistakes in judgment, as a market would, these incentives do not consistently lead participants to adopt Bayesian decision rules. A new area of research in economics, exemplified by El-Gamal and Grether (1995) and Cox et al. (1995), attempts to discover by statistical means the types of learning rules participants employ in experimental games. Bayesian decision making emerges as one in the set of rules employed, but other rules are equally prominent and substantial heterogeneity in learning evidently exists. Although this literature casts doubt on Bayesian learning, it has not yet succeeded in identifying a compelling and dominant alternative. Rather, it seems that the type of non-Bayesian reasoning that individuals employ is situation-specific, depending in a complicated fashion on the nature of the problem.

Where mortality perceptions are concerned, the experimental literature suggests that, on the whole, perceptions may be even more resistant to change than was illustrated in the simple Bayesian model above. Not every aspect of the literature supports such a conclusion, but the bulk of the evidence does.

It may be useful to preface the following discussion by reference to recent findings on the neurological basis of human learning and memory. The experiments of Knowlton et al. (1996), and the insightful comments on them by Robbins (1996), provide evidence that memory and learning in tasks related to probability classification involve a different section of the brain than do other tasks involving recognition and recall. (Their probabilistic experiments had to do with a weather forecasting game in which an arrangement of four cards imperfectly predicted the weather.) Moreover, as Knowlton et al. (1996:1400) observes, "the probabilistic structure of the task appears to defeat the normal tendency to try to memorize a solution, and individuals can learn without being aware of the information they have acquired." Because child survival and death are likewise imperfectly predictable chance events, one wonders whether humans process information about them in ways that are fundamentally distinct from other types of learning. Might individuals over time come to appreciate trends and covariations in child survival without ever being able to say quite why they know what they do? The anomalies in probabilistic learning to be discussed below may well have common neurological roots.

Null Events

Where mortality is concerned, the definition of an event is itself worth considering. A statistician would note both the occurrence of a child death and the occurrence of a child survival; both are "events." But for the lay person, only the former may be noteworthy. There is no news in a child's survival; nothing has happened; it is a "null event." It may therefore be difficult for the lay person to give recollections of child survival their fully appropriate subjective weight. The experimental literature (Estes, 1976) contains numerous examples in which subjects demonstrate their difficulty in retaining information about such null events. If an event X is always described in an experiment as being "not Y," this trivial semantic difference appears to have real implications for recall.

Use of Base Rates

It is often observed in experimental contexts that when presented with a statistical portrait of a population, termed by psychologists a "base rate," and a sample of evidence from that population, individuals tend to give too much emphasis to the sample evidence and not enough to the base rate. For example, when told that these days, 90 percent of children survive to adulthood, and when given a small sample in which only six children in a group of ten survived, individuals might tend to give the sample evidence too much weight in their thinking (Grether, 1980). When asked to compare two situations having different base rates, such as two different mortality levels, individuals will often ignore these base rates entirely in favor of sample evidence, unless their attention is specifically directed to the difference in the base rates (Bar-Hillel, 1980; Bar-Hillel and Fischhoff, 1981; Argote et al., 1986). It seems that the base rates are somehow viewed as rather abstract and pallid by comparison with the vividness and individuality of sample data (Bar-Hillel, 1980). Perhaps for a developing country villager, general media presentations on the likelihood of child survival, or similar presentations by health personnel, lack the immediacy and persuasive power inherent in a tiny sample of recent village experience. One source of data is "merely statistical," whereas the other commands attention and demands interpretation.

As Nisbett and Ross (1980:57) remind us, this bias in favor of sample evidence is reinforced by many folk sayings. Statements such as "Seeing is believing," or "You can prove anything with statistics," which stress the reliability of one's own experience, are not counterbalanced by other maxims that warn against the danger of inferring too much from a small sample. The experimental evidence (see Nisbett and Ross, 1980:56-60; Tversky and Kahneman, 1974) shows that people prefer to rely on sample evidence even when they are made aware that such evidence has very little diagnostic content.

Strength Versus Weight

Griffin and Tversky (1992) argue that in making judgments about the likelihood of an event, people focus first on the apparent "strength" of an effect (such as the size of a sample mean) and then make an adjustment, but typically an insufficient adjustment, for the "weight" of the sample evidence (the sample size or the standard error of the sample mean). To put this differently, ". . . people are highly sensitive to variations in the extremeness of evidence and not sufficiently sensitive to variations in its credence or predictive validity. . ." (Griffin and Tversky, 1992:413). This bias might cause certain unusual events, such as a case in which a single family in a rural village lost all of its children, to acquire a disproportionate influence in mortality perceptions.

Negative Events

A considerable literature in psychology testifies to the disproportionate influence wielded by negative events and information in the formation of impressions (Fiske 1993; Taylor 1991; Pratto and John, 1991; Skowronski and Carlston, 1989; Slovic, 1987). Taylor (1991) notes that the presentation of negative information often evokes physiological arousal, and that such physiological responses are not seen in the case of positive information. Taylor questions whether tests on positive information are sufficient to support this conclusion; her view is that the evidence is suggestive but not definitive. In addition, it seems that negative information often commands attention, occupying cognitive resources to a greater degree than would equally extreme but positive information.[5]

The possible evolutionary basis of all this has been discussed by Taylor (1991) and Pratto and John (1991), who note that an asymmetry in response to negative and positive information may have played an adaptive role over human history. By concentrating attention and mobilizing its physical and cognitive resources, the human organism would have prepared itself for rapid, effective response to external threat. One might think that this "mobilization" phase would also make it easier to recall memories of negative events.

Taylor argues, however, that humans in fact find it more difficult to recall negative events. Following the receipt and the intense cognitive processing of negative information, a "minimization" phase evidently sets in, during which humans make concentrated efforts to explain, explain away, mute, or otherwise suppress the negative event in question. Taylor cites a number of studies that suggest that memories of positive events are both richer and more accessible. As she writes, "The relative inaccessibility of negative events in memory would seem to create an evolutionary lacuna in the form of an inability to learn from past mistakes" (Taylor, 1991:78). Yet the minimization phase might also have an evolutionary basis, according to Taylor, in that, "from the standpoint of long-term adaptation, focus on negative events and the resulting negative mood state could be maladaptive for the organism. . . [being associated with] depression, . . . , lowered motivation, reduced creativity, and an overall reduced level of well-being" (Taylor, 1991:78).

---

[5]The experiments of Pratto and John (1991) are especially interesting in this regard. Their subjects were asked to name colors presented rapidly on a screen; within each color slide was inscribed an adjective chosen from a set ranging from extremely undesirable to extremely desirable. Pratto and John found that when negative adjectives were presented, subjects consistently took longer to name the color than in the case of neutral or positive adjectives. Evidently the need to attend to the negative adjectives interfered with the task at hand—to name the color—whereas positive adjectives did not bring about interference.

Assessment of the Probability of Negative Events

Slovic (1987; also see Savage, 1993) reports that assessments of "riskiness" are dominated by two factors: the degree to which event probabilities are unknown (such as might be the case with new technologies or with events whose consequences are manifested only with delay), and the dread with which an event is regarded, where dread is determined by the catastrophic nature of the event and the degree to which its incidence or consequences are preventable or controllable by individual actions, skill, and diligence. The suggestion in this work is that people may sometimes confound the probability of an event's occurrence with its consequences given that it does occur. Thus, when one family loses all of its children, the catastrophic nature of the event may convince others that mortality rates are higher than they truly are.

Order Effects

In the psychological literature on belief updating, there is considerable interest in the effects on perceptions or judgments of the order in which information is received (for a review, see Hogarth and Einhorn, 1992). The major concepts are those of primacy, which has to do with the disproportionate influence exerted by the first elements in a sequence of data, and recency, which refers to a similarly disproportionate effect for the most recent observations in that sequence. With regard to primacy, the first items of information may establish for an individual a mental representation of the situation, and later information may be interpreted in the light of this initial framework or context. Primacy can be thought of in terms of the enduring impact of first impressions. However, when the information sequence is long, or when each event in the sequence is complex and subject to differing interpretations, recent events may tend to loom larger in perceptions. In some traditional cultures, for example, each child death is viewed as the product of unique material and spiritual circumstances whose precise meaning requires careful consideration (Caldwell et al., 1983). The need to attend to these recent events may cloud the recollection of deaths in an earlier period. It is not yet clear under what conditions primacy or recency exerts the dominant influence on beliefs, although some authors (Nisbett and Ross, 1980) make a strong case for primacy effects. There is a link to the psychological literature on the phenomenon known as anchoring, whereby initial estimates of probabilities are resistant to revision (Tversky and Kahneman, 1974).

Order effects may be of particular interest in relation to mortality trends. One's first impressions of mortality risks may be formed during childhood, adolescence, or the early adult years. Even in the face of a strong downward trend in mortality, these initial impressions—themselves shaped in an era of higher mortality—may prove difficult to set aside. (They may be reinforced by the testimony of family elders who witnessed eras of even higher mortality.) Recency effects, by contrast, would highlight events nearer to the present, a period in which mortality risks are lower. Thus, a dominance of recency effects would seem to draw additional attention to low-mortality eras, and might thereby tend to accentuate the effects of mortality decline on fertility.

Although the concepts of primacy and recency have to do with the time ordering of events, they might be extended to refer to social ordering or social proximity (Barney Cohen, personal communication, 1996). If one's own niece or nephew dies, that event may be more socially salient than if another unrelated child in the village dies. In the social network that forms the sample of individual mortality experience, different subjective weights may be attached to the information derived from different network members.

Distinguishing Absolute from Relative Frequencies

A fundamental difficulty in the estimation of mortality risks is in separating conceptually the number of deaths from the number of persons exposed to the risk of death. Humans are evidently rather good at estimating probabilities when the number of trials is held constant, at least in simple experimental situations (Hogarth, 1975), but they experience considerable difficulty in gauging probabilities when the number of trials differs. Thus, it is hard for subjects to discriminate between low-probability events occurring in large samples and high-probability events in smaller samples (Estes, 1976). Yet it is precisely this difference that faces the lay person attempting to understand mortality trends. Downward mortality trends make lower mortality risks contemporaneous with larger population sizes and more rapid natural population growth. In urban areas, the confounding effect of in-migration adds to the difficulty of probability assessment.

Assessment of Covariation

Much of the discussion above has to do with the imperfections and limits of cognitive skills that might impede understanding of trends in mortality. The identification of trends is a special case of a more general task, that of understanding covariation and causation (McKenzie, 1994; Nisbett and Ross, 1980). As Nisbett and Ross (1980:102-103, 113-120) note, inference of causation depends on the factor of distinctiveness, that is, the degree to which an effect occurs primarily in the presence of one cause, and on consistency, or the likelihood that the effect will produce the outcome of interest.

These concepts may bear on the degree to which the presence of modern health personnel in a rural area contributes to a belief that mortality in that area has declined. An ill child may be treated in the health clinic and yet die, although the child was more likely to live than if treated by the local healer. Children treated by the healer often live, as do children treated at the clinic. Thus, modern health care is neither fully distinctive nor wholly consistent in its effect on child survival. Because of the probabilistic relationship of treatment to survival, in some circumstances individuals may not deduce survival improvement from the mere presence of the modern health care system.

In addition to the themes that have already been mentioned, the psychological literature on covariation assessment emphasizes the importance of preexisting beliefs and theories, which function as mental frameworks through which new evidence is interpreted. As Nisbett and Ross (1980:10) put it:

> If the layperson has a plausible theory that predicts covariation between two events, then a substantial degree of covariation will be perceived, even if it is present only to a small degree or even if it is totally absent. Conversely, even powerful empirical relationships are apt not to be detected or to be radically underestimated if the layperson is led not to expect such a covariation.

In traditional societies, death is often understood and explained in terms of a powerful and coherent mental framework, which supplies a theory and a context for each event. These frameworks are vividly illustrated in the work of Caldwell et al. (1983) in south India. In such settings, new ideas about mortality improvements and the role of modern medicines and health personnel must contend with older, well-established, internally consistent theories of the earthly and spiritual causes of death and traditional remedies for illness. The objective event or outcome—a death or a recovery from grave illness—can be interpreted in a variety of ways, and in transitional societies one would expect considerable disagreement about the causes of improvements. To quote again from Nisbett and Ross (1980:119):

> The lay scientist seems to search only until a plausible antecedent is discovered that can be linked to the outcome through some theory in the repertoire. Given the richness and diversity of that repertoire, such a search will generally be concluded easily and quickly. The subjective ease of explanation encourages confidence. . . [T]he possibilities for "alternative explanations" no less plausible than the first, are never allowed to shake the lay scientist's confidence.

If mortality decline is to be held credible, then the empirical facts suggestive of decline must be supported by a credible theory. If this is to happen, then older theories about cause and effect may have to give way or otherwise adjust, and one would expect the adherents of such theories to resist and offer counterexplanations for the observed changes (Nisbett and Ross, 1980:171). Such transition periods are no doubt lengthened by the general difficulties humans experience in detecting cause-and-effect relationships from their own empirical experience.

Individual Views and Group Judgments

Although one might imagine that group discussion might tend to eliminate the types of individual biases and departures from strict Bayesian rationality that have been described, this does not necessarily occur. Rather, groups are often more extreme in their judgments than individuals, sometimes (although not always) amplifying individual errors into an erroneous group consensus (Argote et al., 1986, 1990). Thus, groups as well as individuals may violate Bayes' rule.

Cultural Differences

A small literature explores cultural differences in how uncertainty itself is viewed and how degrees of uncertainty are expressed. This literature centers on the concept of probabilistic thinking, which Wright et al. (1978:285) define as "the tendency to adopt a probabilistic set, discrimination of uncertainty, and the ability to express the uncertainty meaningfully as a numerical probability." Reviews and experiments regarding probabilistic thinking are presented in Wright et al. (1978) and Kleinhesselink and Rosa (1991). The major conclusions appear to be as follows. In a study of factual knowledge about geography and other matters that included students from Hong Kong, Malaysia, Indonesia, and Great Britain, Wright et al. (1978) found that, as seems to be typical (Fischhoff et al., 1977), all students tended to be overconfident about their judgments in relation to true performance (that is, to be wrong too often when confident they are right). Given this, the Asian students tended to express their evaluations and degrees of confidence in absolute terms (e.g., 0 percent or 100 percent confidence in a judgment) more often than did the British students, who adopted gradations in language and used nuance to describe their confidence levels. These tendencies apparently could not be attributed to different levels of substantive knowledge (for similar findings see Wright and Phillips, 1980).

It may be, therefore, that the Asian students are less prone to think in probabilistic terms. An alternative explanation is that, however the Asian students may think, they are less likely to express themselves in terms of degrees of certainty. This literature hints that cultural differences may exist, but leaves uncertain their extent and depth.

Summary

If the literature described above can be taken as a guide, I would argue that on the whole, improvements in child mortality are likely to be perceived with a greater lag than suggested by optimal Bayesian calculations. There are clearly many subtleties here, and it may be that recency effects and different types of adaptive learning could reverse this conclusion. Nevertheless, it seems far from clear that when mortality improves, individuals will possess the cognitive equipment to correctly and rapidly perceive the trend.

CONCLUSIONS

My aim in this chapter has been to point to a gap in the theory of the demographic transition related to the factors that might induce lags or misperceptions of mortality change. If the wide-ranging literature cited above offers any basis for generalization, one might extract from it a few general themes.

Social Learning and the Demographic Transition

Economic development is associated with sweeping change in any number of social and economic arenas. Some of these changes require little effort to observe and interpret. Others, however, are difficult both to perceive and to understand. Among these society-wide changes, mortality is perhaps especially difficult in that some probabilistic thinking is required even to judge the direction of change. I have argued that individuals, if left to their own perceptual devices, are unlikely to infer that mortality prospects have improved; more precisely, they are unlikely to do so rapidly and without some interim period characterized by error, uncertainty, and debate.

Social learning may also be important in other arenas of behavior, particularly in cases in which individuals are considering the adoption of innovations. Elsewhere (Montgomery and Casterline, 1996) it has been argued that social learning is a fundamental element in the diffusion perspective on fertility transition. Diffusion models lay emphasis on factors affecting the demand for children, such as mortality, as well as those that affect the costs of fertility regulation. Some of the arguments made above with regard to mortality perceptions might also apply to learning about the properties of modern contraceptive methods or the risks and expected returns to be derived from educating children.

The role played by exogenous variability and the mediating functions of social institutions also deserve consideration. High-mortality environments are likely to be environments in which mortality is highly variable. High variance, in turn, must surely add to the difficulties that individuals face in learning about the central tendencies of their environments, that is, in extracting signal from noise. Stable social institutions can act as buffers against extreme risks, or may play an insurancelike function in spreading otherwise local risks over wider populations. When institutions play such roles, they act to dampen variance and may thereby facilitate individual learning.

Education and the Modern Health Sector

If mortality misperceptions are likely, it might now be asked how they come to be corrected. The argument developed above suggests a reconsideration of the special contribution of education and the provision of information. We do not yet understand how mortality perceptions are formed and whether they are influenced principally by direct experience, observed experience, or by the acquisition of learning in school, from the media, or from the health sector itself. Diffusion of information about mortality improvements—from those who were taught the facts to those who might otherwise not have perceived them—may be the fundamental source of changes in perceptions.

The roles that are played by national and international organizations charged with health interventions must surely be important. It is these agencies that communicate information about mortality and health change to the populations they serve. They can do so directly through presentations in the media and the discussions of health personnel. One wonders, in light of the discussion above, what factors determine the reception of these media messages. Are they typically judged persuasive, or abstract and irrelevant? The formal health organizations also communicate information indirectly by insertion of material related to health in national school curricula. LeVine et al. (1994) have argued that schooling itself equips individuals with the cognitive skills they need to translate the "decontextualized language" of the formal health sector into terms that are meaningful to individual experience and decisions.

Perhaps it is in the schoolroom that individuals learn to be attentive to information provided by government and the formal health sector. Of course, few students will emerge from school with an understanding of the germ theory of disease and the workings of modern medicines. Many will come to know that such knowledge exists and that it rests in the hands of modern health care personnel. They will also have been exposed to the knowledge that mortality is controllable, at least to a degree, and this in itself will tend to heighten attention to information about health (Simons, 1989).

The Western experience in such matters may be instructive. As Preston and Haines (1991) argue, citing Dye and Smith (1986), the nineteenth century experience in the United States was one of a gradually increased emphasis on the mother's role in protecting her children's health. There was an increasing faith in the controllability of mortality, although few effective means existed for prevention and even fewer for cure. Until the early twentieth century, the rising belief in controllability did little but increase anxiety and promote a sometimes frantic search for cures; when effective medicines finally emerged, however, the net effect was to improve child survivorship. Interestingly, in this era it was within the medical and public health professions that diffusion of information and the combat between traditional and modern health beliefs were important. Not until the second decade of the twentieth century did physicians fully relinquish nineteenth century beliefs in bodily imbalances, innate racial constitutions, and various miasmas as explanations for disease.

A Research Agenda

To know whether lags and learning are important in today's developing countries, there is no substitute for basic research aimed at eliciting perceptions of mortality levels, differentials, and change. This is a challenging area for research in that the populations whose perceptions are to be studied are not always fully literate and perhaps have a different vocabulary and understanding of uncertainty. In highly literate populations, several methods have been used successfully to elicit subjective probabilities (see Hurd and McGarry, 1995; Dominitz and Manski, 1994a,b; and Morgan and Henrion, 1990). The early study of Pebley et al. (1979) tested simple probability scales in Guatemala, evidently with good results. These methods might be adapted profitably for use in developing country settings in which mortality and fertility transitions are now under way.

APPENDIX

In the simple Bayesian fertility decision model, parents are assumed to choose the number of their births B to maximize the expected value of the utility function $U(S)$, where $U(S) = aS - bS^2$. The $U(S)$ function is symmetric, a specification that imposes equal penalties for falling short of the target S^* and exceeding it. This form of the utility function has been chosen principally for analytic convenience, and although I do not do so in what follows, other nonsymmetric specifications might also be considered.

Note that the number of births B does not enter $U(S)$ directly. The implicit assumption is that the costs of children—that is, the factors that cause $U(S)$ to slope downward beyond S^*—are largely the costs associated with surviving children. In high-mortality settings, where the probability of death after infancy is high, such an assumption is not entirely appropriate. An additional term involving B could be added to the specification above, yielding a more general expected utility function $U(S,B)$. This addition would certainly affect the fertility predictions derived from the model, but would not directly alter mortality perceptions and the process of learning. To simplify matters, therefore, I have not included B directly.

In keeping with Sah (1991), the number of surviving children S is assumed to be binomially distributed given the number of births B and the child survival probability θ. That is,

$$P(S = s \mid B, \theta) = \binom{B}{s} \theta^s (1 - \theta)^{B-s}.$$

The parameter θ represents the probability of surviving to age 5.

Known Survival Probabilities

To begin, suppose that the survival probability θ is known with certainty. In this case, parents confront the following maximization problem:

$$\max_{B} \sum_{s=0}^{B} U(s) \binom{B}{s} \theta^s (1-\theta)^{B-s}.$$

Although no analytic solution for B is available, the utility-maximizing B is easily found by numerical means for any given θ. Indeed, from the binomial assumption and the simple form adopted for $U(S)$, the problem reduces to finding the number of births B that maximizes

$$E[U(s) \mid B, \theta] = B(a-b)\theta - bB(B-1)\theta^2.$$

Without additional structure, the steps taken to this point would lead to a single utility-maximizing value B^* for fertility. It is perhaps more reasonable to allow for some heterogeneity in the population and to think of B^* as the most likely value for fertility. Heterogeneity is introduced by attaching "disturbance terms" ε_B specific to each level of fertility, giving

$$E[U(s) \mid B, \theta, \varepsilon_B] = B(a-b)\theta - bB(B-1)\theta^2 + \varepsilon_B.$$

Provided that the disturbance terms ε_B are mutually independent, extreme-value random variables, we are led to a distribution of the levels of optimal fertility of the form

$$\Pr(B \mid \theta) = \frac{\exp\left[B(a-b)\theta - bB(B-1)\theta^2\right]}{\sum_{j=0} \exp\left[j(a-b)\theta - bj(j-1)\theta^2\right]}.$$

The above is recognizable as the probability derived from a conditional-logit choice problem.

Subjective Beliefs

It is analytically convenient to summarize prior beliefs regarding θ by means of the beta distribution, whose density is

$$f(\theta \mid \alpha, \beta) = \frac{1}{\text{Be}(\alpha, \beta)} \theta^{\alpha-1} (1-\theta)^{\beta-1},$$

where $\text{Be}(a,b)$ is the beta function. This distribution is reasonably flexible and allows for a variety of representations of uncertainty (Lee, 1989; Pratt et al., 1995). The mean and variance of the beta distribution are

$$E(\theta) = \frac{\alpha}{\alpha + \beta},$$

$$\text{var}(\theta) = \frac{\alpha\beta}{(\alpha + \beta)^2 (\alpha + \beta + 1)} = \frac{E(\theta)\,[1 - E(\theta)]}{\alpha + \beta + 1}.$$

When $\alpha = \beta = 1$, the distribution of θ is uniform over the interval from 0 to 1; the case $\alpha = \beta = 2$ yields a symmetric distribution for θ about the value $\theta = 0.5$; and with $\alpha > \beta$, $\alpha > 2$ a skewed unimodal distribution emerges. I illustrate this last case in Figure 4A-1, for which α and β have been chosen so that the subjective mean of the survival probability $\theta = 0.699$, a value equal to Hill's initial estimated probability of child survival in postwar Ghana.

Social Learning

When beta-distributed prior beliefs about θ are updated by reference to a sample of N external observations on child survival, this sample being generated by the binomial distribution, the posterior distribution for θ is also a beta. In other words, the beta distribution is the conjugate prior for the binomial. We can see this as follows. Let $p_0(\theta)$ represent the prior distribution for θ and $p_1(\theta)$ represent the updated or posterior distribution. We then have

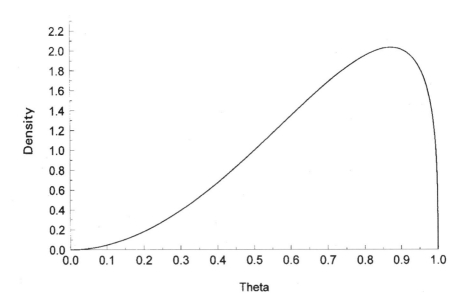

FIGURE 4A-1 The beta density (mean = 0.699).

$$p_1(\theta) = p_0(\theta) \binom{N}{s} \theta^s (1-\theta)^{N-s}$$

$$= \frac{1}{Be(\alpha,\beta)} \theta^{\alpha-1}(1-\theta)^{\beta-1} \binom{N}{s} \theta^s (1-\theta)^{N-s}$$

$$= \frac{1}{Be(\alpha+s,\beta+N-s)} \theta^{\alpha+s-1}(1-\theta)^{\beta+N-s-1},$$

so that the posterior distribution is a beta with parameters $\alpha_1 = \alpha + s$, $\beta_1 = \beta + N - s$.

Although flexible, the beta distribution is not an ideal choice for an application to child survival in that the distribution always assigns some subjective probability to values of θ near 1 and 0. This gives a potentially unrealistic representation of subjective beliefs, as few individuals believe either that all children will survive or that none will. However, by selecting values for α and β with some care, one can confine most of the subjective distribution for θ to a reasonable range.

Note that the principal advantage of the beta distribution is that, when it is combined with the binomial, the posterior distribution for θ has the same form as the prior distribution, both being betas. This is analytically convenient. By departing from the beta distribution one could represent subjective perceptions in a more reasonable way, perhaps by confining the perceived θ to a range, but this advantage would be offset by greater difficulty entailed in analytic comparisons when the prior and posterior differ in form.

Desired Fertility with θ Uncertain

Returning to the fertility choice facing households, the problem is to choose the number of births B that maximizes

$$E \, U(S) = E \, (aS - bS^2).$$

As noted above, if the value of the survival probability θ were known, this problem could be restated as

$$\max_B B(a - b) \, \theta - bB(B - 1)\theta^2 \, .$$

With θ unknown, however, the values of θ and θ^2 must be replaced in the expression by their subjective expectations, $E(\theta)$ and $E(\theta^2)$, which in turn depend on prior beliefs and the available sample of child survival observations. The utility maximization problem can be stated as

$$\max_{B} B(a-b)\,E(\theta) - bB(B-1)E(\theta)\left[E(\theta) + \frac{1-E(\theta)}{\alpha+\beta+1}\right],$$

where $E(\theta) = \alpha/(\alpha+\beta)$.

ACKNOWLEDGMENTS

This research was supported in part by a grant from the Rockefeller Foundation. I thank John Casterline, Barney Cohen, and two anonymous referees for their insightful comments.

REFERENCES

Argote, L., R. Devadas, and N. Melone
    1990   The base-rate fallacy: Contrasting processes and outcomes of group and individual judgment. *Organizational Behavior and Human Decision Processes* 46:296-310.
Argote, L., M. Seabright, and L. Dyer
    1986   Individual versus group use of base-rate and individuating information. *Organizational Behavior and Human Decision Processes* 38:65-75.
Bar-Hillel, M.
    1980   The base-rate fallacy in probability judgments. *Acta Psychologica* 44:211-233.
Bar-Hillel, M., and B. Fischhoff
    1981   When do base rates affect predictions? *Journal of Personality and Social Psychology* 41(4):671-680.
Caldwell, J., P. Reddy, and P. Caldwell
    1983   The social component of mortality decline: An investigation in South India using alternative methodologies. *Population Studies* 37(2):185-205.
Camerer, C.
    1995   Individual decision making. In J. Kagel and A. Roth, eds., *The Handbook of Experimental Economics*. Princeton, N.J.: Princeton University Press.
Cleland, J., M. Caraël, J.-C. Deheneffe, and B. Ferry
    1992   Sexual behavior in the face of risk: Preliminary results from first AIDS-related surveys. *Health Transition Review* 2(Suppl.):185-204.
Conlisk, J.
    1996   Why bounded rationality? *Journal of Economic Literature* 34:669-700.
Cox, J., J. Shachat, and M. Walker
    1995   An Experimental Test of Bayesian vs. Adaptive Learning in Normal Form Games. Unpublished manuscript, Department of Economics, University of Arizona, Tucson.
Dominitz, J., and C. Manski
    1994a   Eliciting Student Expectations of the Returns to Schooling. Unpublished manuscript, Institute for Social Research, University of Michigan, Ann Arbor.
    1994b   Using Expectations Data to Study Subjective Income Expectations. Unpublished manuscript, Institute for Social Research, University of Michigan, Ann Arbor.
Dye, N., and D. Smith
    1986   Mother love and infant death, 1750-1920. *Journal of American History* 73:329-353.

El-Gamal, M., and D. Grether
    1995   Are people Bayesian? Uncovering behavioral strategies. *Journal of the American Statistical Association* 90(432):1137-1145.

Estes, W.
    1976   The cognitive side of probability learning. *Psychological Review* 83(1):37-64.

Fischhoff, B., P. Slovic, and S. Lichtenstein
    1977   Knowing with certainty: The appropriateness of extreme confidence. *Journal of Experimental Psychology: Human Perception and Performance* 3(4):552-564.

Fiske, S.
    1993   Social cognition and social perception. *Annual Review of Psychology* 44:155-194.

Grether, D.
    1980   Bayes Rule as a descriptive model: The representativeness heuristic. *Quarterly Journal of Economics* 95:537-557.

Griffin, D., and A. Tversky
    1992   The weighing of evidence and the determinants of confidence. *Cognitive Psychology* 24:411-435.

Heer, D., and H.-Y. Wu
    1978   Effects in rural Taiwan and urban Morocco: Combining individual and aggregate data. Pp. 135-159 in S.H. Preston, ed., *The Effects of Infant and Child Mortality on Fertility.* New York: Academic Press.

Hill, A.
    1993   Trends in childhood mortality. Pp. 153-217 in K. Foote, K. Hill, and L. Martin, eds., *Demographic Change in Sub-Saharan Africa.* Washington, D.C.: National Academy Press.

Hogarth, R.
    1975   Cognitive processes and the assessment of subjective probability distributions. *Journal of the American Statistical Association* 70(350):271-289.

Hogarth, R., and H. Einhorn
    1992   Order effects in belief updating: The belief adjustment model. *Cognitive Psychology* 24:1-55.

Hurd, M., and K. McGarry
    1995   Evaluation of the subjective probabilities of survival in the Health and Retirement Study. *Journal of Human Resources* 30(Suppl.):S268-S292.

Kleinhesselink, R., and E. Rosa
    1991   Cognitive representation of risk perceptions: A comparison of Japan and the United States. *Journal of Cross-Cultural Psychology* 22(1):11-28.

Knowlton, B., J. Mangels, and L. Squire
    1996   A neostriatal habit learning system in humans. *Science* 273:1399-1402.

Koop, G., and D. Poirier
    1993   Bayesian analysis of logit models using natural conjugate priors. *Journal of Econometrics* 56(3):323-340.

Lee, P.
    1989   *Bayesian Statistics: An Introduction.* New York: Halsted Press.

LeVine, R.A., E. Dexter, P. Velasco, S. LeVine, A.R. Joshi, K.W. Stuebing, and F.M. Tapia-Uribe
    1994   Maternal literacy and health care in three countries: A preliminary report. *Health Transition Review* 4(2):186-191.

Lopes, L.
    1985   Averaging rules and adjustment processes in Bayesian inference. *Bulletin of the Psychonomic Society* 23(6):509-512.
    1987   Procedure debiasing. *Acta Psychologica* 64:167-185.

Matthiessen, P., and J. McCann
    1978   The role of mortality in the European fertility transition: Aggregate-level relations. Pp. 47-68 in S.H. Preston, ed., *The Effects of Infant and Child Mortality on Fertility*. New York: Academic Press.
McKenzie, C.
    1994   The accuracy of intuitive judgment strategies: Covariation assessment and Bayesian inference. *Cognitive Psychology* 26:209-239.
Montgomery, M., and J. Casterline
    1996   Social learning, social influence and new models of fertility. *Population and Development Review* 22(Suppl.):151-175.
Morgan, M., and M. Henrion
    1990   *Uncertainty: A Guide to Dealing with Uncertainty in Quantitative Risk and Policy Analysis*. New York: Cambridge University Press.
Nisbett, R., and L. Ross
    1980   *Human Inference: Strategies and Shortcomings of Human Judgment*. Englewood Cliffs, N.J.: Prentice-Hall.
Pebley, A., H. Delgado, and E. Brinemann
    1979   Fertility desires and child mortality experience among Guatemalan women. *Studies in Family Planning* 10(4):129-136.
Poirier, D.
    1994   Jeffreys' prior for logit models. *Journal of Econometrics* 63:327-339.
Pratt, J., H. Raiffa, and R. Schlaifer
    1995   *Introduction to Statistical Decision Theory*. Cambridge, Mass.: MIT Press.
Pratto, F., and O. John
    1991   Automatic vigilance: The attention-grabbing power of negative social information. *Journal of Personality and Social Psychology* 61(3):380-391.
Preston, S.H., and M.R. Haines
    1991   *Fatal Years: Child Mortality in Late Nineteenth Century America*. Princeton, N.J.: Princeton University Press.
Robbins, T.
    1996   Refining the taxonomy of memory. *Science* 273:1353-1354.
Sah, R.
    1991   The effects of child mortality changes on fertility choice and parental welfare. *Journal of Political Economy* 99(3):582-606.
Savage, I.
    1993   An empirical investigation into the effect of psychological perceptions on the willingness-to-pay to reduce risk. *Journal of Risk and Uncertainty* 6:75-90.
Schultz, T.P.
    1981   *Economics of Population*. Reading, Mass.: Addison-Wesley.
Simons, J.
    1989   Cultural dimensions of the mother's contribution to child survival. Pp. 132-145 in J. Caldwell and G. Santow, eds., *Selected Readings in the Cultural, Social and Behavioural Determinants of Health*. Health Transition Series No. 1. Canberra: Health Transition Centre, Australian National University.
Skowronski, J., and D. Carlston
    1989   Negativity and extremity biases in impression formation: A review of explanations. *Psychological Bulletin* 105(1):131-142.
Slovic, P.
    1987   Perception of risk. *Science* 236:280-285.

Taylor, S.
    1991   Asymmetrical effects of positive and negative events: The mobilization-minimization
            hypothesis. *Psychological Bulletin* 110(1):67-85.
Tversky, A., and D. Kahneman
    1974   Judgment under uncertainty: Heuristics and biases. *Science* 185:1124-1131.
Wright, G., and L. Phillips
    1980   Cultural variation in probabilistic thinking: Alternative ways of dealing with uncertainty.
            International Journal of Psychology 15:239-257.
Wright, G., L. Phillips, P. Whalley, G. Choo, K. Ng, I. Tan, and A. Wisudha
    1978   Cultural differences in probabilistic thinking. *Journal of Cross-Cultural Psychology*
            9(3):285-299.
Zellner, A., and P. Rossi
    1984   Bayesian analysis of dichotomous quantal response models. *Journal of Econometrics*
            25:365-393.

5

The Impact of AIDS Mortality on Individual Fertility: Evidence from Tanzania

Martha Ainsworth, Deon Filmer, and Innocent Semali

During the European demographic transitions, fertility decline was often but not always preceded by an aggregate decline in mortality (Matthiessen and McCann, 1978). In sub-Saharan Africa, high levels of child mortality are thought to be an impediment to fertility decline. Caldwell et al. (1992), for example, suggest that a decline in infant mortality to levels below 70 per 1,000 may be a prerequisite for the onset of fertility decline, based on the experience of Botswana, Kenya, and Zimbabwe.

Child mortality has declined and life expectancy increased in sub-Saharan Africa in recent decades, but the spreading AIDS epidemic threatens this progress. Nearly two-thirds of the 23 million people currently infected with human immunodeficiency virus (HIV) worldwide live in sub-Saharan Africa (UNAIDS data, cited in Ainsworth and Over, 1997). AIDS is fatal and is striking two key groups—sexually active adults who become infected through sexual relations and very young children who are infected from their mothers at birth or while breastfeeding. The impact of AIDS on mortality is difficult to measure, as vital registration systems in sub-Saharan Africa are subject to extensive underreporting (Stover, 1993). However, the U.S. Bureau of the Census predicts that the decline in African infant and child mortality will be stalled and reversed as a result of the AIDS epidemic (Way and Stanecki, 1994). Nicoll et al. (1994) predict that mortality of children under the age of 5 in severely affected urban areas will increase by one-third in eastern and central Africa and by as much as three-quarters in southern Africa, sharply diminishing the existing differentials in child mortality between urban and rural areas. Furthermore, levels of adult mortality in the age group 15-50 can be expected to double, triple, or even quadruple in some locales.

What will be the impact of heightened mortality from AIDS on fertility in sub-Saharan Africa? There is remarkably little empirical evidence on this issue. In fact, demographic modelers of the impact of the AIDS epidemic commonly assume no fertility response to AIDS mortality. For example, *The AIDS Epidemic and its Demographic Consequences* (UN/WHO, 1991) presents seven mathematical models for the demographic consequences of the spread of HIV, none of which includes an individual fertility response. The World Bank's AIDS-adjusted population projections assume no interaction between HIV prevalence and fertility (Bos and Bulatao, 1992).

In this chapter we review the channels through which we might expect both positive and negative fertility responses to the heightened mortality of the AIDS epidemic, summarize the evidence to date, and present new evidence of the response of individual fertility behavior to heightened mortality based on three data sets from Tanzania. In the next section we provide an overview of levels of HIV infection in sub-Saharan Africa and the relation between HIV infection and mortality. This is followed by a discussion of the channels through which heightened mortality from AIDS might induce changes in fertility. In the fourth section we present results of multivariate analysis of individual fertility using three data sets from Tanzania—two national and one from the severely affected Kagera region. The results suggest that, although there is evidence of a positive effect of heightened child mortality on fertility, adult mortality at the household and community level tends to be associated with lower individual fertility. These results are supported by an analysis of the effect of mortality on other indicators of fertility intentions, such as the desire for additional children and patterns of sexual behavior.

EXCESS MORTALITY FROM THE AFRICAN AIDS EPIDEMIC

Although sub-Saharan Africa has the highest number of current HIV infections of any region in the world, the prevalence of HIV varies considerably across the continent and within countries. Figure 5-1 shows the adult seroprevalence rate (the percentage of people aged 15-50 who are HIV-positive) for HIV-1 among "low-risk" urban populations, based on *HIV/AIDS Surveillance Data Base* (Bureau of the Census, 1995).[1] These data are drawn from samples of pregnant women attending antenatal clinics.[2] In 12 countries, over 10 percent of pregnant women in urban areas are infected with HIV. "High-risk" urban populations,

---

[1] The discussion focuses on HIV-1 infection, which is the most prevalent variant of HIV in sub-Saharan Africa (National Research Council, 1996).

[2] Note, however, that these data are not necessarily indicative of seroprevalence levels in a random sample of the population; women attending antenatal clinics are often better educated and have higher incomes than the general population.

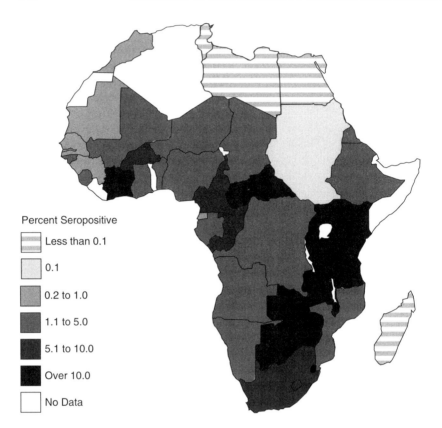

FIGURE 5-1 Percentage of the low-risk urban adult population infected with HIV-1, circa 1995. SOURCE: Bureau of the Census (1995:Map 2).

such as commercial sex workers and soldiers, have seroprevalence levels of 40 percent or higher in 12 countries (not shown in Figure 5-1). Prevalence is generally lower in rural areas. However, because in most countries the overwhelming share of the population is rural, even low rural rates of infection imply that the majority of AIDS deaths occur in rural areas. The number of these deaths is compounded by urban relatives who migrate to rural areas shortly before death, the magnitude of which is not known.

Heterosexual transmission accounts for approximately 80-90 percent of all adult HIV infections in sub-Saharan Africa (Mann et al., 1992; National Research Council, 1996). In many hard-hit countries, women are equally if not more likely to be infected than men. A second important transmission route is from mother to child. In Africa, roughly a quarter to a half of the children born to HIV-positive mothers themselves become infected, either through the birth process or through breastfeeding (Lallemant et al., 1994).

Thus, AIDS can be expected to increase mortality dramatically in Africa both among the very young and among adults in their prime childbearing and economically active years. Way and Stanecki (1994) show a profile of age-specific mortality rates in a population in which 20 percent of adults are infected with HIV (Figure 5-2). The baseline mortality in their comparison population without HIV is clearly not from sub-Saharan Africa, where infant mortality ranges from 70-150 per 1,000 and where prevailing mortality among prime-aged adults, which ranges between 5 and 8 per 1,000, is roughly eight times higher than in a developed country. Furthermore, their estimates of AIDS-related child mortality likely do not include the deaths of HIV-negative children who are put at greater risk because of the loss of their parents due to AIDS. Child mortality (ages 1-4) may be more sensitive to AIDS than is infant mortality since many infected children survive beyond 1 year of age (Valleroy et al., 1990; Way and Stanecki, 1994). Nevertheless, Figure 5-2 illustrates the substantial impact that AIDS can have on mortality early in life and in the prime age groups. Indeed, in many cities

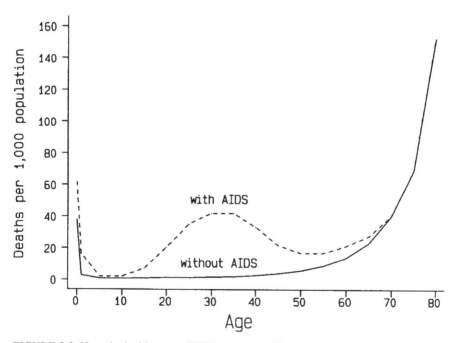

FIGURE 5-2 Hypothetical impact of HIV on age-specific mortality, assuming 20 percent of adults are infected. SOURCE: Way and Stanecki (1994:Fig. 11, p. 13).

in sub-Saharan Africa, seroprevalence rates among adults are even higher than the 20 percent assumed in Figure 5-2.

The United Nations (1995) estimates that AIDS will increase the cumulative mortality among children under the age of 5 by 7.8 percent in the 15 most seriously affected African countries from 1980-2005. The effect increases with age: Cumulative deaths among people aged 15-34 will be 25 percent higher and among 35-49 cumulative deaths will be 61 percent higher. Because of the way in which HIV is spread to children, households with AIDS-related child mortality will also likely experience AIDS-related adult mortality. The clustering of deaths of children and prime-aged adults in the same households distinguishes AIDS from other causes of child mortality that do not threaten adults. Thus, when we consider the effects of AIDS-related child mortality on fertility, we must at the same time consider the effects of AIDS-related mortality among adults in their prime years.

HOW AIDS-RELATED MORTALITY AFFECTS FERTILITY

Increased mortality due to the AIDS epidemic can induce changes in individual fertility through many different channels, some biological and some behavioral. The posited effect of higher levels of child mortality is to raise fertility and of higher adult mortality to lower fertility.

Child Mortality and Fertility

A couple's own child mortality can result in higher fertility through two channels: (1) abrupt cessation of breastfeeding following the child's death, which eliminates the protection afforded by breastfeeding's contraceptive effect and raises the risk of another pregnancy (the "interval effect"); and (2) by an increase in the number of births a couple must have to achieve a target number of surviving children (Preston, 1978). This latter behavioral response to child mortality may take two forms—"replacement" of young children who die through additional births or simply bearing more children than needed to "insure" against anticipated child mortality in the future.

The "interval" and "replacement" effects of child deaths that are due to AIDS are unlikely to be strong because the parents of these children themselves are infected. In fact, it is often due to the illness and death of a child that the parents learn of their own infection. The parents may attempt to prevent future births through abstinence, contraception, or abortion; abstinence to prevent re-infection with HIV would also make a subsequent birth unlikely. The mother may also succumb to AIDS before another pregnancy can come to term, making it unlikely that one would observe her or her children's deaths in a sample of women. Thus, elevated child mortality due to AIDS will probably exert a stronger positive effect on fertility through the "insurance" channel—by raising uninfected couples' perceptions of their probable child mortality experience, increasing their estimate of the number of excess births necessary to guarantee a target number of surviving children.

Multivariate studies of the relation between a couple's own child mortality and their fertility in African countries have generally confirmed a positive relationship (Ahn and Shariff, 1993; Anker, 1985; Benefo and Schultz, 1996; Farooq, 1985; Okojie, 1989; Snyder, 1974). However, most of these studies have treated the couple's child mortality as exogenously determined. If one accepts the proposition that child health and child mortality are the outcomes of household decisions on health "inputs," such as consumption of food and health care, then the exogeneity of child deaths is difficult to accept. Failure to take the endogeneity of child deaths into account leads to biased estimates of the relationship with fertility. Studies that examine the impact of a woman's own child mortality on fertility are also problematic because they are confined to samples of women who have had at least one live birth, which is in effect conditioning on an endogenous variable (fertility). At least two studies have taken the endogeneity of child mortality into account using African data. Okojie (1989) found in Bendel State, Nigeria, a negative relation between a woman's predicted child survival and fertility in rural areas and among women nearing the end of their reproductive lives. Benefo and Schultz (1996) tested for and were unable to reject the exogeneity of child mortality in Côte d'Ivoire and Ghana. When child mortality was treated as exogenous, they found a very weak replacement effect—an increase in fertility of one child in response to every 4-15 child deaths, depending on the country and region. Preston (1978) points out that such weak relationships should be expected in areas with a high demand for children; if couples want as many children as possible, then a reduction in child mortality will not reduce fertility. Although Ahn and Shariff (1993) did not account for the endogeneity of child mortality, they also examined the impact of community infant and child mortality rates, which can be considered exogenous to the household. They found high infant mortality to be associated with a higher hazard of subsequent birth in Togo, but high child mortality to be negatively associated with the hazard of subsequent births in Uganda. These studies collectively suggest a positive, if sometimes weak, relation between child deaths and fertility in sub-Saharan Africa.

Adult Mortality and Fertility

Heightened adult mortality due to AIDS may reduce desired family size and the observed demand for children of individual women through the following channels:

• AIDS mortality often occurs in young adulthood before the long-run benefits of earlier child investments can be realized by the parents of those infected. Heightened adult mortality rates due to AIDS will thus reduce the expected long-run benefits of children, in turn lowering desired family size. High adult mortality may also prevent parents from investing in their children's schooling and health care.

• Mortality of prime-aged adults in the household may reduce household income (at least temporarily) and raise the demand for labor of the surviving adults. This would raise the shadow cost of children and shrink the budget constraint, both of which would tend to reduce the demand for children.

• High adult mortality will also leave many orphaned children to be absorbed by the households of relatives. These orphaned children make additional claims on existing income and the time of adults and may reduce the demand for additional children of their own.

Other Channels Through Which AIDS Morbidity and Mortality May Affect Fertility

Any change in the demand for children or in biological factors affecting the supply of children because of the AIDS epidemic will be reflected in corresponding changes in the proximate determinants of fertility, such as contraceptive use, breastfeeding, marriage, abortion, infecundity, and sterility (Bongaarts, 1978). Changes in the proximate determinants reflect, in most cases, individual choices or their outcomes that are joint decisions with fertility. Gregson (1994) points out many of the following effects of AIDS on the proximate determinants and, jointly, with fertility:

• Fertility among infected women may decline because of illness, infertility induced by other sexually transmitted diseases (STDs), increased use of contraception, widowhood, and increased resort to abortion (Nicoll et al., 1994).

• The use of condoms to prevent the spread of STDs, including AIDS, may reduce unwanted births. At the same time, to the extent that condoms replace more effective methods of birth control, fertility may rise.

• One of the major strategies to slow the spread of AIDS is to offer treatment for other "conventional" STDs, such as syphilis and gonorrhea, thought to facilitate transmission of HIV. This intervention would have the beneficial side effect of reducing levels of pathological sterility in many countries, which could result in higher fertility.

• Other behavioral changes to prevent the spread of AIDS may include delayed age at marriage, monogamy, and increased celibacy (Caldwell et al., 1993). These changes would be associated with lower fertility. However, HIV is also spread through breast milk, and breastfeeding is a major determinant of the period of postpartum infecundability. Any reduction in breastfeeding could reduce the period of postpartum infecundability and raise fertility unless compensated for by higher contraceptive use or abstinence.

• In a review of the fertility effects of HIV counseling and testing programs,

Setel (1995) concludes that there is no evidence that women informed of their HIV-positive status accelerate childbearing, while a few studies show that they have somewhat lower subsequent fertility than women told they were HIV negative.

Finally, in the aggregate, AIDS mortality affects fertility through its impact on the age structure of women of reproductive age. But there are other aspects of the selective mortality of women of reproductive age that could affect aggregate fertility. For example, if the women who are becoming infected are also those who would have had fewer children in any event (for example, urban women), then the women with lower fertility are selectively dying and overall fertility may rise. Or, if these low-fertility women have already had the children they would have had, aggregate fertility may remain unchanged. Many demographic modelers have assumed that women who die of AIDS will have already borne most of the children they could expect in a lifetime and therefore would have very little effect on aggregate fertility (Bos and Bulatao, 1992; Way and Stanecki, 1994). However, infection rates in Africa are on the increase among young females, raising the possibility that many will die before having completed their lifetime fertility.

A few medical researchers have found lower fertility among HIV-positive women, although they have not been able to attribute the results to biological as opposed to behavioral causes. Ryder et al. (1991) found somewhat lower fertility and higher contraceptive use among HIV-positive women than among HIV-negative women in a sample of women followed over 3 years following delivery of a live-born child in Mama Yemo Hospital in Kinshasa, Zaire. Sewankambo et al. (1995), in a recent study of 1,860 households in the rural Rakai district in Uganda, found that the birth rate among HIV-positive women aged 15-49 was 169 per 1,000, whereas that for HIV-negative women was 213 per 1,000. Using data from the same region of Uganda, Gray et al. (1995) found the prevalence of pregnancy to be lower among HIV-infected women. In addition, there is some evidence that HIV-positive mothers have a higher likelihood of spontaneous abortion (Langston et al., 1995).

To the best of our knowledge, there has been no empirical study of the behavioral response of individual fertility to increased mortality due to AIDS. Among the reasons for the lack of empirical work is the difficulty of identifying AIDS mortality, the difficulty of observing a sufficient number of adult deaths to measure their impact, the lack of longitudinal data, and the absence of observations on community-level measures of mortality. An added complication is that the line of causation between child mortality and fertility runs in both directions—high levels of fertility and closely spaced births are thought to raise the risk of death to children and mothers. Indeed, as Nicoll et al. (1994) point out, the impact of the epidemic on child mortality depends heavily on fertility. If all infected women were to cease having children, then child mortality may increase very little. Thus, there is also the need for data with sufficient instruments to separately identify the two relationships.

INDIVIDUAL FERTILITY RESPONSE IN TANZANIA

Tanzania, on the eastern coast of Africa, stretches to Lake Victoria in the northwest, Lake Tanganyika in the west, and Lake Nyassa in the southwest. Per capita gross national product (GNP) in the early 1990s was on the order of $100, and about three-quarters of Tanzania's 24 million people live in rural areas (World Bank, 1995). The 1991/92 Demographic and Health Survey (DHS) estimated Tanzania's total fertility rate at 6.3, infant mortality at 92 per 1,000 and under-5 mortality at 141 per 1,000 for the 5 years preceding the survey (Ngallaba et al., 1993). Results from the 1988 census indicate relatively higher levels of both infant and under-5 mortality—15 and 191 per 1,000, respectively (Bureau of Statistics, undated).

Tanzania is among the countries most severely affected by the AIDS epidemic in Africa and in the world. The first case of AIDS was diagnosed in 1983 in the Kagera region, on the western shore of Lake Victoria and adjacent to Uganda and Rwanda. HIV was probably in the region for a decade or more before the first diagnosis. By 1992 there was a cumulative total of 38,416 reported AIDS cases from all regions of the country since the beginning of the epidemic (Ministry of Health, cited in Mukyanuzi, 1994). This was surely a gross undercount, but by how much we cannot be sure. As of 1990 it was estimated that between 400,000 and 800,000 people were infected, and it was anticipated that AIDS would shortly become the major cause of death among young children and prime-aged adults (World Bank, 1992).

No one has undertaken a nationally representative seroprevalence survey in Tanzania, so the true prevalence of HIV is unknown. Chin and Sonnenberg (1991) compiled a map of the estimated HIV prevalence among sexually active adults, by region, using the results of seroprevalence surveys of smaller, select samples and the reported number of cases (Figure 5-3). At that time, the highest levels of infection were thought to be in Dar es Salaam and Kagera, followed by Mwanza and Mbeya regions. Kagera, Mwanza, and Mbeya are all along major transportation routes to adjacent countries, over which much cross-border trade passes. A population-based seroprevalence survey of Kagera region in 1987 found an infection rate of 24.2 percent among adults aged 15-54 in the main town of Bukoba (on the lake and about 100 km south of the Uganda border) (Killewo et al., 1990a). Rural rates of infection were also high: 10 percent of adults in the rural areas surrounding Bukoba and next to the lake, 4.5 percent in the northwestern part of the region bordering Rwanda and Uganda, but less than half a percent in the southern part of the region. The infection rate among children 0-14 years of age was 3.9 percent in Bukoba, with the highest levels among the youngest children.

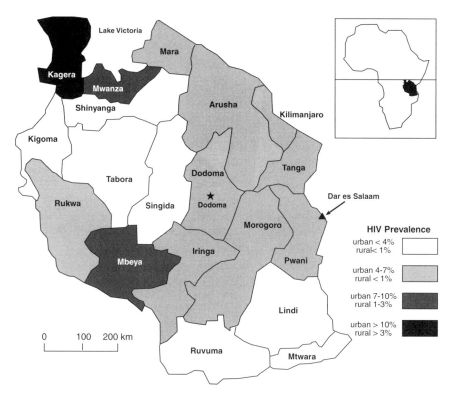

FIGURE 5-3 Estimated HIV prevalence among sexually active adults, Tanzania, 1989.
SOURCE: Chin and Sonnenberg (1991), cited in World Bank (1992).

    In Western countries, the median time between infection with HIV and de-
velopment of AIDS and death is roughly 10 years (Moss and Bachetti, 1989;
Rutherford et al., 1990). The incubation period is thought to be shorter in sub-
Saharan Africa because of higher underlying morbidity and lower nutritional
status (Killewo et al., 1990b; National Research Council, 1996). The extent to
which AIDS is contributing to overall mortality is not known. Results of the
1988 Tanzanian census reveal that the unadjusted death rates for adults aged 15-
49 ranged from 3.4 to 9.4 per 1,000 across the 20 regions of mainland Tanzania
(Ainsworth and Rwegarulira, 1992). These adult death rates are based on raw
census data, without any adjustments for internal consistency or underreporting.
Although the levels may be underestimates, the differentials in mortality across
regions point to the areas with relatively higher mortality. The highest adult
mortality was recorded in Kagera region; Mbeya and Dar es Salaam, where HIV
infection is also widespread, had relatively high adult death rates as well (6.3 and
6.5 per 1,000, respectively). The results reveal that under-5 mortality in 1985

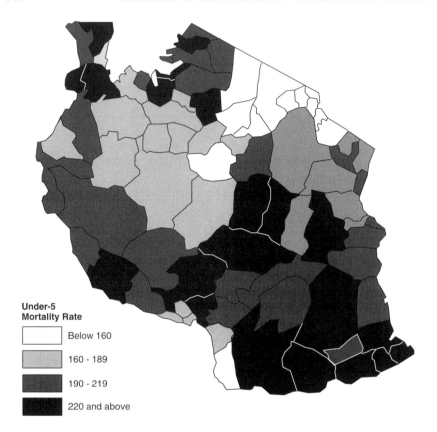

Under-5 Mortality Rate

- Below 160
- 160 - 189
- 190 - 219
- 220 and above

FIGURE 5-4 Under-5 mortality by district, Tanzania mainland, 1985. SOURCE: Data from Bureau of Statistics (no date).

was higher around Lake Victoria and in the southern parts of Tanzania (Figure 5-4). These regional differentials in mortality reflect not only the effect of the AIDS epidemic but the distribution of other underlying determinants of mortality and nutritional status, such as household incomes, food prices, disease vectors (such as mosquitos), and the availability of medical care.

The Model

Economic models of fertility in developing countries begin with a model of a household that both produces and consumes (Becker, 1993; Schultz, 1981). Household members derive utility from their children and from other consumption goods. However, children also have a potentially important contribution to household production activities and their future earnings may be an important long-term benefit to their parents and relatives. The demand for children is thus a function both of the benefits and the costs of raising or "producing" them. Among the costs are the value of the time of the mother or other female relatives, the costs of schooling, health care, food, clothing, and other essentials. In the more formal economic model, the "demand" for children varies with a number of factors exogenous to the household—wages, prices, nonlabor income, and unobserved preferences of the parents or household for children.

The supply of children is determined by biological factors such as fecundity, which varies with the woman's age. An important consideration in African settings (and in particular in light of the AIDS epidemic) is that the supply of children to the household is not necessarily dependent on fertility. Foster children and orphans can also be accepted into the household to raise the household's utility (Ainsworth, 1996).

Even though high levels of child mortality are likely to raise fertility among parents who wish to be assured of a target number of surviving births, community levels of adult mortality are likely to reduce the demand for children by lowering their long-run expected benefits. Deaths of adults in a given household may lower fertility through decreased income and household production. Deaths of adults outside the household—particularly among close relatives—might also generate an unanticipated supply shock as others' children must be absorbed into the household. We thus expect both male and female adult deaths in the household to lower fertility. To the extent that prime-aged males are engaged in market work, their deaths may be more likely to affect fertility through an income effect (regardless of their relation to female members of the household).[3] In addition, if the death is that of a husband or partner, we expect a negative relation because of widowhood and a socially determined delay in remarriage. Prime-aged females are likely to be substitutes for one another in household production (such as in child care, domestic tasks, and farming). Therefore, the death of a prime-aged female in the household will likely result in lower fertility for remaining members as the value of female time (which is scarcer within the household) increases and the cost of raising children increases indirectly.

We estimate a model of the determinants of births in the past 12 months among women of reproductive age. The dependent variable equals one if the woman has given birth in the 12 months before the interview and zero otherwise. The explanatory variables of key interest to this study include different measures of mortality at the household, community, and extended family level, all of which are assumed to be exogenous:

---

[3]The relation between income and fertility is theoretically indeterminate—it could be positive or negative.

- death of prime-aged adults in the same household according to the time since death,
  - death of adult relatives,
  - community child mortality,[4] and
  - community mortality of prime-aged adults.

A fairly standard set of fertility determinants that include factors affecting both the supply of and demand for children comprises the remaining explanatory variables. The variable definitions are somewhat specific to each data set, but include

- age and age squared, to control for exposure to the risk of pregnancy;
- variables that reflect the opportunity cost of a woman's time, such as her schooling and schooling squared;
  - variables that measure or represent the household's budget constraint; and
- variables that reflect prices, such as regional or national price indices, adult and child wages, the availability of health care, schooling, and family planning infrastructure.

With respect to measures of the budget constraint, two of the three data sets described below contain annual household consumption expenditure. We anticipate that a male death affects fertility by lowering income, for which household expenditures are a proxy. Thus, results are shown for two specifications of the determinants of a recent birth. The first specification is a reduced form, in which all of the explanatory variables are assumed to be exogenous and household consumption expenditure is excluded. These results can be compared across all three data sets. The second specification, estimated for only two of the data sets, includes an endogenous regressor, the log of annual household expenditures per adult. The latter has been replaced by its predicted value using as instruments the household head's characteristics (gender, age, and schooling), the value of household productive assets and dwellings, and the hectares of banana crop harvested. We estimate the relation between the probability of a live birth in the past 12 months and different indicators of adult and child mortality using probit (for the cross-sectional surveys) and random-effects probit (for the longitudinal survey)

---

[4]We do not examine the impact of women's own child mortality on their subsequent fertility because: (1) there are inadequate instruments to identify the woman's own child mortality, which is jointly endogenous with fertility; (2) the analysis would have to be limited to women who have had at least one child recently, which sharply reduces the sample and conditions the analysis on endogenous fertility; and (3) the likelihood of observing a fertility response of women whose children die of AIDS is low, since the mothers are infected, have higher mortality, and are less likely to be observed in the sample.

regression (Maddala, 1987). The probit coefficients have been transformed to facilitate interpretation. For continuous variables, the reported figures represent the percentage point increase in the probability of a birth in the past 12 months associated with a one-unit change in the explanatory variable. For binary explanatory variables, the coefficients have been transformed into the increase in the probability of birth when the variable equals one, compared with when it equals zero. Mortality variables are highlighted below; descriptive statistics for other variables are shown in Appendix 5-A and regression results for all variables are available from the authors.

The Data Sets

We use three household-level data sets collected in Tanzania in the early 1990s. Two are national and one is from the Kagera region, in the northwest. Although the three data sets are all for a single country, we are unaware of other countries with the requisite mortality data. The impacts in Tanzania are likely to be similar to those in other East African countries hard hit by the AIDS epidemic at equivalent points in the demographic transition and with similar levels of economic development. The dependent variables, measures of mortality, and other regressors in the three data sets are compared in Table 5-1.

The Kagera Health and Development Survey (KHDS), conducted as part of the research project "The Economic Impact of Fatal Adult Illness due to AIDS and Other Causes in sub-Saharan Africa," and funded by the World Bank Research Committee, the United States Agency for International Development, and the Danish International Development Agency (Over and Ainsworth, 1989), is a longitudinal living standards survey of more than 800 households in the Kagera region. The survey was conducted from 1991 to 1993, roughly 8-10 years after the first cases of AIDS were diagnosed in the region. The sample was heavily stratified so as to capture households at high risk of adult deaths. Each household was interviewed a maximum of four times at 6- to 7-month intervals. A total of 757 households completed all four waves of the survey. The questionnaire and sampling are described in Ainsworth et al. (1992).

The KHDS questionnaire included a list of children ever born for all females aged 15-50, which was updated every wave with information on new births and on women who joined the sample. The questionnaire also collected information on the death of all household members in the 24 months before the first interview and between interviews and the death of all relatives who were not living with the household at the time of death. In addition, the data set includes several indicators of community-level mortality rates based on three sources: ward-level rates from the 1988 census, an enumeration of all households in the 51 survey clusters in 1991, and the results of questionnaires administered to community informants. This information allows us to examine the probability of recent births as a function of adult mortality in the household and the extended household, as well as of

TABLE 5-1 Overview of Tanzania Data Sets and Mortality Variables

	Data Set		
Variables	Kagera Health and Development Survey (KHDS) 1991-1993 ($n = 2,896$)	Tanzania Human Resources Development Survey (THRDS) 1993 ($n = 6,234$)	Tanzania Knowledge, Attitudes and Practices Survey (TKAP)[a] ($n = 3,950$)
Dependent variables			
Birth in the past 12 months	✓	✓	✓
Desire for additional births			✓
Ever had sex, among subsample 15-19 years old			✓
Frequency of sexual intercourse, last 4 weeks			✓
Explanatory variables—mortality			
Adult death 15-50 in the household (reference period)	✓ (0-30 months ago)	✓ (0-12 months ago)	

Household member has AIDS or has died of AIDS			✓
Death of adult relative (15-50), past 30 months	✓	✓	
Adult mortality[b]	✓	✓	✓
(age)	(15+)	(15-49)	(15-49)
[level of aggregation]	[cluster]	[region]	[region]
Child death[b]	✓	✓	✓
(age)	(<15)	(<5)	(<5)
[level of aggregation]	[cluster]	[district]	[district]
Percentage of respondents in cluster who know anyone who died of AIDS			✓
Other explanatory variables[c]			
Consumption expenditure	✓	✓	
Assets/durable goods	✓	✓	✓
Community characteristics/services	✓	✓	✓

[a] This is the sample size for women. The TKAP also interviewed 1,948 men aged 15-59 with nonmissing data.

[b] The denominator for the KHDS adult and child death rates is 1,000 population (irrespective of age); the denominator for the rates for the other two surveys is 1,000 population *of the same age.*

[c] A complete list of all regressors for each data set is provided in Appendix 5-A.

community-level mortality of children and adults. The analysis is based on a pooled sample of 2,896 women aged 15-50 who were interviewed in waves 2-4 of the longitudinal survey. The first wave of data was dropped to permit study of the effect of a death as long ago as 30 months. On average, 13 percent of the women had given birth in the 12 months prior to each interview.

The Tanzania Human Resources Development Survey (THRDS), jointly undertaken by the Department of Economics of the University of Dar es Salaam, the Government of Tanzania, and the World Bank and funded by the World Bank, the Government of Japan, and the British Overseas Development Agency, collected information from a national cross-section of nearly 5,000 households in mainland Tanzania in 1993. It included questions on fertility as well as on household and individual economic variables, although less extensively than the KHDS. A module on the mortality of household members of all ages in the past 12 months makes it possible to examine the effect of recent adult death on fertility. Each observation can also be linked with its district-level child (under-5) mortality and its regional adult (15-49) mortality rate from the 1988 census.[5] The survey design and questionnaires of the THRDS are described in Ferreira and Griffin (1995). We use as our sample 6,234 women aged 15-50. An average of 10.4 percent of these women gave birth in the 12 months before the survey.

The Tanzania Knowledge, Attitudes and Practices Survey (TKAP) collected data from a national cross section of about 4,000 households in mainland Tanzania in 1994. The survey design and questionnaires are described in Weinstein et al. (1995). The TKAP has only a limited set of economic variables but a broader set of variables that reflect fertility intentions (for example, desire for an additional child and measures of sexual activity). Each respondent in the household was asked whether a household member has AIDS or has died of AIDS. If the answer was negative, respondents were asked whether they knew anyone who had AIDS or had died of AIDS. From these we construct the cluster proportion of women who report knowing anyone (including household members) who has AIDS or has died of AIDS. This variable, although not measuring actual mortality, reflects levels of perceived AIDS mortality in the survey communities. No other (adult) mortality questions were asked of the respondents so we cannot include deaths from other causes at the household or cluster levels. We do, however, link the data to the district child (under-5) mortality rate and the regional adult (15-49) mortality rate from the 1988 census. Approximately 7 percent of the women in the sample live in households in which a member has AIDS or has died of AIDS. This ranges from about 1 percent in the Dodoma

---

[5]The under-5 child mortality rate is from Bureau of Statistics (no date) and the adult mortality rate is from Ainsworth and Rwegarulira (1992). The THRDS covers 49 of 103 districts in all 20 regions of mainland Tanzania and the TKAP covers 83 districts.

region to almost 20 percent in the Kagera region. The sample mean of the cluster proportion of women respondents who knew anyone who had AIDS or had died of AIDS is equal to about 47 percent, with a range from about 29 percent in the Rukwa region to almost 88 percent in the Kagera region.

It should be noted that the TKAP did not include an income or expenditure module and therefore we are unable to condition on these variables in the analysis. The regressions do include some measures of household wealth (such as type of flooring in the dwelling, ownership of a bicycle or a car), which indicate to some extent potential income effects. Nor were community and facility data collected in the 1994 TKAP. However, in 1991 and 1992 all the clusters included in the TKAP were administered a community and health facility questionnaire as a part of the Tanzania Demographic and Health Survey (TDHS) whose sampling frame and questionnaire are described in Ngallaba et al. (1993). Therefore, the community and facility data included in the regressions are from approximately 2 years prior to the individual-level data. The community and facility variables used here are described in Beegle (1995). The sample used is that of 3,950 women aged 15-49. Of these women, 19.4 percent gave birth in the past 12 months.[6]

The Impact of Child Death Rates on Recent Fertility

The marginal effect of a one-unit change in the community-level child mortality on the probability of a birth in the past 12 months is presented in Table 5-2. Note that the child mortality variable for the THRDS and the TKAP is defined in the same way and comes from the same source, the 1988 census. An increase in the under-5 child mortality of 10 per 1,000 (from 177 to 187 per 1,000 in the THRDS, for example) is associated with an increase in fertility of 0.3 to 0.5 percent—not a very strong effect.

The KHDS child mortality variable is based on the ratio of the number of children who died who were under age 15 per 1,000 population in the community. The source of this information is the KHDS community questionnaire. In every wave, the community respondents were asked how many people of different ages had died in the community since the last wave (or in the case of wave 1, in the past 12 months). This information was divided by the total population of

---

[6]The means of the dependent variables are quite different across the three data sets, part of which can be accounted for by the stratification of the samples. When weighted, the mean percentage of women who gave birth in the past 12 months is 15.0 percent for the KHDS (wave 1), 11.4 percent for the THRDS, and 19.5 percent for the TKAP. An additional factor is the phrasing of the questions. Although the KHDS and TKAP variables were obtained from a full fertility history of each woman, the THRDS fertility variable is based on asking each woman whether she gave birth in the past 12 months.

TABLE 5-2 Marginal Effect[a] of Child Mortality on Recent Fertility, Women
Aged 15-50[b] (dependent variable: births in the past 12 months)

Data Set	Child Mortality Variable	Mean (Standard Deviation)	Marginal Effect of Child Mortality Rate	
			Excluding Expenditure	Including Expenditure[c]
KHDS, 1991- 1993	Death of children <15 per 1,000 population, community level	5.97 (5.42)	0.1133	0.0948
THRDS, 1993	Deaths of children <5 per 1,000, 1988 census, district level	177.15 (40.54)	0.0275[d]	0.0292[d]
TKAP, 1994	Deaths of children <5 per 1,000, 1988 census, district level	186.26 (40.52)	0.047[d]	—

NOTE: —, data not available.

[a]The derivative of the probability of birth in the past 12 months with respect to the explanatory variable, evaluated at the means of all of the independent variables and multiplied by 100 (see Appendix 5-B).

[b]For the TKAP survey, women aged 15-49.

[c]Predicted log expenditures per adult are included as an explanatory variable.

[d]Indicates probit parameter estimate is significantly different from zero at the 5 percent level.

the community from the door-to-door enumeration in early 1991, updated for in- and out-migration and births and deaths, and annualized. The average death rate in the sample of women was about 6 children under age 15 per 1,000 population. An increase in the child mortality rate of 10 children per 1,000 population would raise the probability of birth in the last 12 months by one percentage point, although this result is not statistically significant. The positive correlation for child deaths in all three samples is expected and consistent with the literature. The inclusion of controls for household expenditure per adult do not much alter the results.

The Impact of Adult Death Rates on Recent Fertility

Higher levels of adult mortality at the community level are associated with lower recent fertility in all three data sets (Table 5-3). However, the results are statistically significant only in the THRDS when the predicted log of expenditure per adult is included. An increase in the adult mortality of 5 per 1,000 would

TABLE 5-3 Marginal Effect[a] of Adult Death Rates on Recent Fertility, Women Aged 15-50[b] (dependent variable: births in the past 12 months)

Data Set	Adult Mortality Variable	Mean (Standard Deviation)	Marginal Effect of Adult Death Rate	
			Excluding Expenditure	Including Expenditure[c]
KHDS, 1991-1993	Deaths of adults 15 and older per 1,000 population, community level	9.73 (6.55)	–0.0343	–0.0540
THRDS, 1993	Deaths of adults 15-49 per 1,000, 1988 census, regional level	5.63 (1.34)	–0.551	–0.854[d]
TKAP, 1994	Deaths of adults 15-49 per 1,000 1988 census, regional level	5.46 (1.55)	–0.781	—

NOTE: —, data not available.

[a]The derivative of the probability with respect to the explanatory variable evaluated at the means of all the independent variables and multiplied by 100 (see Appendix 5-B).

[b]For the TKAP survey, women aged 15-49.

[c]Predicted log expenditures per adult are included as an explanatory variable.

[d]Indicates that the probit parameter estimate is significantly different from zero at the 5 percent level.

reduce the percentage of women giving birth from 10.4 to 6.2 percent. Such an increase would represent a doubling of adult mortality, which is not unexpected in areas hard hit by the AIDS epidemic. The community-level mortality for adults and children (Tables 5-2 and 5-3) are jointly significant at the 5 percent level for the THRDS and at 11 percent for the TKAP. For the KHDS, they are not jointly significant.

The Impact of Deaths of Household Members and Relatives

Higher levels of community adult mortality are associated with lower recent fertility in the Tanzanian data sets, possibly because of the reduced expected long-run benefits of children as adults. We would expect adult deaths in a particular household to lower the fertility of surviving women for additional reasons—lower income, greater demand on the time of surviving women in home production, and the need to care for orphaned children who may substitute for the woman's own children.

Only the KHDS and the THRDS collected information on deaths in the household. During all four waves of the KHDS, from 6 months before the first wave of household interviews until the end of the last interview, 268 household members died among households interviewed (Ainsworth et al., 1995). Of these, 47 percent (126 persons) were adults aged 15-50, and roughly half of them were reported by their relatives to have died of AIDS. One-third of adult deaths were attributed to other illness or unknown causes. The mean proportion of women in the KHDS with male and female adult deaths in their household in various time frames is reported in Table 5-4. Deaths of adult relatives include relatives who were household members as well as nonresident relatives.

The one-round THRDS recorded a total of 324 deaths of household members in the 12 months before the survey, of which only 118 (36 percent) were adults aged 15-50. The main causes of death among adults were illness (88 percent), traffic accidents (6 percent), and childbirth (3 percent). About 1.3 percent of the women lived in a household where there had been a male adult death and an equal number where there had been a female adult death (age 15-50) in the past 12 months.[7]

Because the birth and death variables used in this analysis are measured over discrete time intervals, it is not always obvious which of these two events occurred first. Adult deaths in the past 12 months (measured in both the KHDS and the THRDS) could have occurred before conception, during pregnancy, or after a recent birth. However, deaths more than 12 months in the past (measured in the KHDS only) occurred before any recent birth and in most cases before conception.

Turning first to the results for the KHDS, both the deaths of adult household members and the deaths of adult relatives are associated with lower recent fertility (see Table 5-5).[8] Only the death of women in the household and of both male and female relatives are significantly related to recent fertility, however. Women in households where another female adult died 0-12 months ago have a three

---

[7]The relative rarity of the deaths of prime-aged adults in the THRDS (with 5,000 households) underscores the difficulty of studying the impact of adult deaths from AIDS, even in a country with an AIDS epidemic. In contrast, the KHDS obtained information on 126 adult deaths (age 15-50) from a much smaller sample of about 800 households over a 2-year period by selecting areas with known high adult mortality and by stratifying the sample according to the anticipated risk of adult deaths. This required an extensive enumeration of 29,000 households, from which the survey sample was selected.

[8]The KHDS results are based on separate regressions using death of adult household members in one specification and death of relatives in another. The two sets of mortality variables were not entered in the same regression.

TABLE 5-4 Descriptive Statistics for Household-Level Mortality Variables, KHDS, Women 15-50 ($n = 2,896$)

Mortality Variable	Male Deaths		Female Deaths	
	Mean	Standard Deviation	Mean	Standard Deviation
Death of household member aged 15-50				
0-12 months ago	0.033	(0.178)	0.038	(0.191)
12-18 months ago	0.023	(0.150)	0.029	(0.168)
18-24 months ago	0.037	(0.220)	0.051	(0.220)
24-30 months ago	0.040	(0.197)	0.060	(0.238)
Death of a relative aged 15-50 last 30 months				
Sibling	0.078	(0.268)	0.090	(0.286)
Parent	0.016	(0.125)	0.024	(0.154)
Spouse	0.026	(0.159)	—	—

NOTE: —, data not available.

percentage point lower probability of having had a birth in the past year and for those in households where a female adult died 18-24 months ago the probability is two percentage points lower. These results are statistically significant and large compared with the average probability of a birth in the past year of 13 percent. The signs on the results for female deaths in other time periods are also negative, but not statistically significant. The results for male deaths are not statistically significant, although the effect of death in each period is negative. As a group, the female deaths are jointly significant at the 5 percent level; the male death variables are not jointly statistically significant.

The death of close relatives of both genders (siblings, husband, parents) in the past 30 months is associated with lower fertility. The death of an adult brother, sister, or husband leads to a drop in the probability of a birth in the past year of two to three percentage points. The results for deaths of parents and other relatives of the head or spouse (not shown) are not statistically significant. The death of a spouse is significantly associated with lower fertility, but loses the significance when household consumption per adult is included. The deaths of all relatives are jointly statistically significant, both with and without including the log of consumption per adult.

In summary, the deaths of female household members and close relatives are associated with lower recent fertility, whereas deaths of adult males in the household have no apparent relation with fertility, irrespective of whether controls for household resources are included. These results suggest that female deaths and

TABLE 5-5 Marginal Effect[a] of Household-Level Adult Mortality on Recent Fertility, Women Aged 15-50 (dependent variable: birth in the past 12 months)

Data Set and Mortality Variable	Male Deaths		Female Deaths	
	Excluding Expenditure	Including Expenditure[b]	Excluding Expenditure	Including Expenditure[b]
KHDS, 1991-1993				
Death of household member aged 15-50				
0-12 months ago	-0.608	0.538	-3.088**	-2.790*
12-18 months ago	-2.455	-2.249	-2.616	-2.703*
18-24 months ago	-1.835	-1.459	-2.269*	-2.510**
24-30 months ago	-0.588	-0.532	-1.217	-1.535
(Joint test *p* value)	(0.5415)	(0.6709)	(0.0404)	(0.0422)
Death of a relative aged 15-50 in last 30 months[c]				
Sibling	-3.422***	-3.324***	-2.471***	-2.461**
Parent	-1.507	-1.730	1.768***	-2.621
Spouse	-2.743*	-2.530	—	—
THRDS, 1993				
Death of household member age 15-50 in last 12 months	3.014	2.303	-0.279	0.215

NOTE: —, data not available.

[a]The change in the probability of having a birth in the past 12 months due to a change in the dummy variable from zero to one, evaluated at the means of all of the independent variables and multiplied by 100. ***, **, * indicate that the probit parameter estimate is significantly different from zero at the 1 percent, 5 percent, and 10 percent level, respectively.

[b]Predicted log expenditures per adult as included as an explanatory variable.

[c]The deaths of male and female relatives in the KHDS regressions are jointly significant (including other relatives, not shown) at $p = 0.0177$ without and $p = 0.0230$ with log expenditures per adult.

the deaths of adult siblings, in particular, raise the opportunity costs of time of surviving women, lowering their fertility. The negative (generally insignificant) effect of husband's death on fertility may be operating purely through lower exposure to the risk of pregnancy, but evidently not through its indirect effect on household resources.

In the lower half of Table 5-5, the coefficients on deaths of adults in the past 12 months for the THRDS are not individually statistically significant, nor are they jointly so. The signs and magnitudes of the (insignificant) marginal effects are greatly different from the KHDS results. What can account for this? It must be kept in mind that the marginal effects are evaluated at the mean values of the explanatory variables, so that samples with identical probit coefficients but different means on the independent variables may have very different marginal effects. Other factors explaining the difference in results are that deaths were far more prevalent in the KHDS survey, and the survey questions on adult deaths differed. The KHDS asked about the date of every death, on which basis the time since death could be determined. The THRDS simply asked for a list of all deaths in the past 12 months.

Mortality and Other Measures of Fertility Intentions

Results discussed in the previous section suggest a negative relation between adult mortality at the community and household level and fertility, but a positive relation between community levels of child mortality and fertility. However, the results are not always statistically significant. Conception and birth occur 9-months apart; retrospective data on deaths often do not extend back far enough in time to study this issue easily.

In this section we consider the impact of deaths on several "proximate" indicators of fertility intentions or outcomes that are likely to respond to mortality with a shorter lag:

- the desire for an additional child; and
- measures of recent sexual activity.

If mortality affects fertility outcomes through behavioral channels, then to be consistent with the results on fertility in the previous section, heightened adult mortality from AIDS or other causes would be associated with a reduction in desire for additional children and a reduction in sexual activity. Heightened child mortality would be associated with increased desire for additional children and greater sexual activity. Irrespective of whether a reduction in sexual activity is due to a change in fertility intentions or an attempt to prevent HIV infection, it can be expected to reduce fertility.

Among the three data sets, only the TKAP obtained information on these variables, but the questions were asked of both women and men. Table 5-6

TABLE 5-6 Marginal Effect of Mortality on Measures of Fertility Intentions and Sexual Activity[a]

Measure of Mortality	Mean	Standard Deviation	Dependent Variables		
			Would Like Another Child (0/1)	Ever Had Sexual Intercourse (0/1) (ages 15-19)	Frequency of Sexual Intercourse in Past 4 Weeks
Sample of women aged 15-49 (n = 3,950) or 15-19 (n = 810)					
Proportion in cluster who know someone who has AIDS or who has died of AIDS	0.468	(0.230)	−20.67***	0.245	0.710
Under-5 mortality[b]	186.3	(40.52)	0.013	−0.022	−0.003
Adult mortality, age 15-49[c]	5.46	(1.55)	0.819	4.166**	−0.231***
Joint test, mortality variables (*p* value)			0.4353	0.0431	0.0036
Mean of dependent variable			0.616	0.528	4.314

Sample of men aged 15-59 (n = 1,948) or (n = 394)

Proportion in cluster who know someone who has AIDS or who has died of AIDS	0.495 (0.223)	−5.72**	−14.08	−1.662**
Under-5 mortality[b]	187.6 (40.22)	0.022	0.081	0.005
Adult mortality, age 15-49[c]	5.57 (1.42)	0.116	0.040	−0.066
Joint test, mortality variables (p value)		0.3047	0.7269	0.6019
Mean of dependent variable		0.876	0.635	4.833

[a]Fertility intentions and sexual activity are shown as the derivative of the probability with respect to the explanatory variable evaluated at the means of all the independent variables and multiplied by 100. Among men and women aged 20-49, 98 percent have had sexual intercourse. The results are not substantially affected if the age cutoff is raised to 24 years. Estimates reported for frequency of sexual intercourse in the past 4 weeks are the marginal effects implied by Tobit parameter estimates, with a lower limit of zero, of changes of the independent variable on the expected value of the dependent variable, evaluated at the means of the regressors (see Appendix 5-B). ***, ** indicate that the parameter estimate is significantly different from zero at the 1 percent or 5 percent level, respectively.

[b]The under-5 mortality rate is defined as the number of deaths of babies and children under 5 years of age per 1,000 live births in the same calendar year. This variable is measured at the district level and is from the 1988 census.

[c]The adult mortality rate is the number of adults (age 15-49) who died in the previous 12 months per 1,000 population in the same age group. This variable is measured at the regional level and is from the 1988 census.

presents the relation between measures of mortality and three dependent variables:

- *Fertility intentions*: A dichotomous variable (0/1) equal to one if the respondent would ever like another child. For women, this variable is the answer to a direct question; for men, it is equal to one if the current family size is smaller than the respondent's ideal family size and zero otherwise.
- *Onset of sexual activities*: Among the sample of men and women aged 15-19, a dichotomous variable equal to one if the respondent has ever had sexual intercourse.
- *Recent sexual activity*: The frequency of sexual intercourse in the past 4 weeks.

Models for the first two of these dependent variables are estimated using a probit regression, whereas the models for the third dependent variable are estimated using a Tobit regression with a lower limit of zero. Among women aged 15-49 and men aged 15-59, 62 percent and 88 percent, respectively, would like another child. The mean number of acts of sexual intercourse in the past 4 weeks was 4.3 for women and 4.8 for men, including about 40 percent of female and 30 percent of the male respondents who reported no sexual intercourse in the past 4 weeks. Among those aged 15-19, 53 percent of women and 64 percent of men had ever had sexual intercourse.

These dependent variables are regressed on the same set of explanatory variables as in the fertility regressions and include three measures of adult mortality: the proportion of households in the sample cluster who know someone who has AIDS or who has died of AIDS, the district-level under-5 mortality rate, and the region-level adult (aged 15-49) mortality rate from the 1988 census.[9] Unfortunately, the regressions do not control for household resource availability because the TKAP survey did not collect consumption information. The results for women and men are reported in Table 5-6.

Among both men and women, perceptions of high mortality due to AIDS are associated with a significant reduction in the desire for additional children. Specifically, an increase of 0.10 in the proportion of respondents who know someone who has AIDS or has died of AIDS is associated with a reduction of 2.1 percentage points in the probability of wanting another child among women, and a 0.6 point fall for men. Child mortality, surprisingly, has no significant relation to the

---

[9]In a separate specification, the first of these variables was replaced by a dummy variable for whether a household member had AIDS or had died of AIDS. The coefficient was never significant in regressions for any of the three dependent variables, for men or women. The coefficients on the under-5 and adult mortality are qualitatively unaffected when the AIDS variables at the household and cluster level are excluded from the regressions.

desire for additional children among men or women, confirming the weak relationship found earlier and in other studies. The results for adult and child death rates are unaffected by exclusion of the AIDS awareness variable from the regression.

Among women aged 15-19, higher community adult death rates are associated with a significantly lower probability of ever having sexual intercourse. Anecdotes suggest that as the result of the AIDS epidemic, increasingly younger girls are being sought for sex because they are presumed to be uninfected. However, to the contrary, the results in Table 5-6 provide evidence that fewer teenage girls are sexually active in high-mortality communities. An increase in the adult mortality of 1 per 1,000 (about a 20 percent increase over the mean level) is associated with a four percentage point reduction in the probability of ever having sexual intercourse, from 53 to 49 percent. A doubling of the adult mortality rate, which is typical in hard-hit areas, would reduce the onset of sexual activity among women by about 20 percentage points. Adult mortality is not significantly correlated with the onset of sexual activity among men aged 15-59, however.

Finally, higher levels of adult mortality in the community are associated with a reduction in the frequency of sexual intercourse among women, whereas among men the perception of higher mortality due to AIDS is associated with less intercourse. An increase of 5 per 1,000 in the community adult mortality rate corresponds to a decrease in sexual activity from 4.3 to 3.3 in the past month among women. Among men, an increase of 0.10 in the proportion of those knowing of someone who has AIDS or has died of AIDS (from 0.5 to 0.6) is associated with a reduction in sexual activity from 4.8 to 4.5 in the past month. Thus, women's sexual activity responds to the adult mortality rate, whereas men's sexual activity responds to the perception of AIDS deaths in the community. The results in Table 5-6 suggest that greater personal experience with AIDS and AIDS mortality in the community leads to a lower reported desire for children among both men and women and a decrease in sexual activity among men. Higher adult mortality rates in the community, which are the result of high levels of HIV infection, are associated with delayed onset of sexual activity and a reduction in the frequency of sex among women. All of these outcomes would be associated with lower fertility.

CONCLUSIONS

This chapter has examined the impact of increased mortality that is due to the AIDS epidemic on individual fertility behavior. Models of the demographic impact of the epidemic have generally ignored the possibility of a behavioral fertility response to higher mortality from AIDS. The AIDS epidemic will raise mortality in two main groups—children under 5 and sexually active adults, generally in the age group 15-50. However, child mortality is already very high in most sub-Saharan countries, whereas adult mortality in the prime ages is among the lowest of any age group. The AIDS epidemic will marginally raise child mortality, but could as much as quadruple underlying mortality among prime-aged adults.

We use three recent data sets from Tanzania to explore the relation between various measures of mortality and the probability of a birth in the past 12 months. Individuals' perceptions of mortality trends are likely to be influenced by mortality in their communities as well as deaths in their households and extended family. The results confirm the positive but weak relation between community levels of child mortality and recent fertility found elsewhere in the literature. Thus, an increase in child mortality due to AIDS can be expected to contribute to higher fertility.

Community levels of adult mortality are negatively correlated with recent fertility (as expected), but are often not statistically significant at conventional levels. Deaths of female adults within the past 24 months are significantly associated with lower recent fertility of surviving women in the same household. However, a male death as long as 30 months ago is not correlated with the recent fertility of surviving women in the same household. It was not anticipated that very recent adult deaths would influence fertility, but this appears to be true for the deaths of women in the past 12 months. Because AIDS deaths are the outcome of extended illness, it is likely that mortality among household members and relatives can be anticipated. This could account for the unexpected finding that recent fertility responds to recent deaths. The relation of the deceased adult to the surviving woman does matter. Women who lost a brother or sister within the last 30 months had significantly lower recent fertility. The effect of the loss of a husband in the past 30 months was also negative, but only marginally significant.

Analysis of the impact of mortality on other indicators of fertility intentions tends to reinforce the hypothesis that higher adult mortality will lead to a decrease in fertility. Higher personal awareness of AIDS and AIDS mortality are associated with a reduced desire for additional children among both men and women and a decrease in sexual activity among men. Higher levels of adult mortality in the community are associated with a lower probability that women aged 15-19 have ever had sexual intercourse and with a reduction of sexual activity among women.

Taken together, these results suggest that there will indeed be a behavioral response to heightened mortality because of AIDS and that it will, on net, be negative. An important caveat is that the three data sets used in this study allowed us to consider the fertility response only within 30 months of an adult death in one sample, 12 months in another, and quite vaguely in the third. Conceivably, with a longer time lag, one might observe a compensating increase in fertility for the preceding period of low fertility. However, the negative relationship between recent fertility and community-level adult death rates is not subject to this problem and implies that even in the long run the fertility response to adult mortality will be negative. Although we have identified evidence of behavioral response, the total effect of heightened mortality due to AIDS on fertility will include both behavioral and biological components, the latter reflecting the impact of HIV infection on fecundity.

APPENDIX

Appendix tables begin on the following page.

APPENDIX 5-A:
SUMMARY STATISTICS FOR THE THREE SAMPLES

(a) Kagera Sample of Women Aged 15-50 in Waves 2, 3, and 4 ($n = 2,896$)

Variable	Mean	Standard Deviation
Woman-level variables		
Birth in the past 12 months (0/1)[a]	0.128	0.334
Age	27.064	10.18
Age squared	836.07	620.22
Years of education	4.907	2.965
Years of education squared	32.87	26.51
Household-level variables		
Water from closed source[b] (0/1)	0.126	0.332
Dwelling has a toilet or latrine (0/1)	0.967	0.18
No household member owns any land (0/1)	0.0317	0.175
Acres of land owned by all household members	5.413	5.763
Value of land owned by		
all household members (/1,000,000)	0.678	2.29
Community-level variables		
Dispensary in community (0/1)	0.307	0.461
Health center in community (0/1)	0.0849	0.279
Hospital in community (0/1)	0.0521	0.222
Urban community (0/1)	0.198	0.398
Motorable road in community (0/1)	0.963	0.19
Road is sometimes impassable (0/1)	0.46	0.5
Number of primary schools in community	1.315	0.542
Family planning within		
5 kilometers of community (0/1)	0.693	0.461
Price index	1.262	0.245
No child wage reported in community (0/1)	0.427	0.495
Child wage for clearing land		
in community (/1,000)	0.0869	0.0954
Adult male wage for clearing		
land in community (/1,000)	0.266	0.297
Karagwe district (0/1)	0.139	0.346
Muleba district (0/1)	0.157	0.364
Biharamulo district (0/1)	0.0808	0.273
Ngara district (0/1)	0.111	0.314
Household expenditure variables		
Log of annual household expenditure	−2.106	0.718
per adult		
Identifying variables for annual household (hh)		
expenditure per adult (not in fertility equations)		
Head of hh male (0/1)	0.762	0.426
Head's age	48.18	15.64
Head's age squared	2565.9	1593.9
Head's years of schooling	4.55	3.09
Head's schooling squared	30.28	34.46
HH member owns dwelling (0/1)	0.933	0.251

(a) Kagera Sample of Women Aged 15-50 in Waves 2, 3, and 4 (*n* = 2,896) (*continued*)

Variable	Mean	Standard Deviation
Value of owned and occupied dwelling		
(/1,000,000)	0.459	2.07
Value of farm equipment (/1,000,000)	0.0194	0.134
Value of farm buildings (/1,000,000)	0.00159	0.0145
Value of livestock (/1,000,000)	0.0732	0.328
Value of business assets (/1,000,000)	0.0382	0.472
Hectares of banana crop harvested		
(averaged over all waves observed)	0.888	0.776

[a](0/1), dummy variable.

[b]Closed source includes indoor plumbing, inside standpipe, water vendor, water truck or tanker service, neighboring household, private outside standpipe or tap, public standpipe.

(b) Tanzania National Sample, THRDS (*n* = 6,037)

Variable	Mean	Standard Deviation
Woman-level variables		
Birth last 12 months (0/1)	0.105	0.306
Age	27.75	9.098
Age squared	852.7	561.8
Years of schooling	5.625	3.331
Years of schooling squared	44.73	36.92
Household-level variables		
Toilet or latrine (0/1)	0.963	0.188
Water from closed source (0/1)	0.593	0.491
Any farmland owned by hh member (0/1)	0.350	0.477
Hectares of farmland owned by hh member	0.973	2.398
Male adult (15-50) death in household		
in past 12 months (0/1)	0.0129	0.113
Female adult (15-50) death in household		
in past 12 months (0/1)	0.0133	0.114
Community-level variables		
Distance to nearest public road		
(cluster median)	0.390	0.963
Land area (sq km)/population[a]	2.480	3.755
Number of primary schools/population[a]	4.272	1.622
Number of hospitals/population[a]	0.140	0.107
Number of health centers/population[a]	0.132	0.073
Number of doctors/population[a]	0.500	0.559
Number of nurses/population[a]	29.43	31.00
Rural cluster (0/1)	0.426	0.495
North highland zone[b] (0/1)	0.122	0.327

(b) Tanzania National Sample, THRDS ($n = 6,037$) (*continued*)

Variable	Mean	Standard Deviation
Central zone[b] (0/1)	0.061	0.239
South highland zone[b] (0/1)	0.135	0.342
Southern zone[b] (0/1)	0.100	0.300
Lake zone[b] (0/1)	0.251	0.434
Under-5 mortality rate	177.15	40.54
Adult mortality rate	5.632	1.341
Household expenditure variables		
Log of annual household expenditure per adult (/1000000)	−1.662	0.728
Identifying variables for annual household expenditure per adult (not in fertility equations)		
Head of hh male (0/1)	0.851	0.356
Head's age	43.91	12.76
Head's age squared	2090.8	1218.6
Head's years of schooling	5.519	3.783
Head's years of schooling squared	44.77	46.79
HH member owns dwelling (0/1)	0.699	0.459
Value of owned and occupied dwelling(/1,000,000)	0.004	0.010
Owned dwelling walls of mud or wood (0/1)	0.318	0.465
Owned dwelling floors of earth or wood (0/1)	0.463	0.4987
Owned dwelling roof of grass or mud (0/1)	0.335	0.472
Owned dwelling windows with glass or screens (0/1)	0.124	0.330
Total number of cows, bulls or oxen currently owned	2.622	12.78

[a]Variables calculated at the district level. Land per capita is scaled upward by a factor of 100; the other variables are scaled upward by a factor of 10,000.

[b]Coastal zone (Tanga, Morogoro, Coast, Dar es Salaam regions), north highland zone (Arusha and Kilimanjaro regions), central zone (Dodoma and Singida regions), south highland zone (Iringa, Mbeye, and Rukwa regions), southern zone (Lindi, Mtwara, and Ruvumba regions), lake zone (Tabora, Kigoma, Shinyanga, Kagera, Mwanza, and Mara regions).

(c) TKAP Sample of Women Aged 15-49 and Sample of Men Aged 15-59

Variable	Women Aged 15-49 (n = 3,950)		Men Aged 15-59 (n = 1,948)	
	Mean	Standard Deviation	Mean	Standard Deviation
Individual-level variables				
Birth in past year (0/1)	0.194	0.396		
Want another child (0/1)	0.616	0.486	0.876	0.329
Ever had sexual intercourse, ages 15-19 (0/1)	0.528	0.500	0.635	0.482
Frequency of sexual intercourse in past 4 weeks	4.314	5.943	4.833	7.159
Age	28.001	8.980	31.014	11.641
Age squared	864.68	546.19	1097.31	806.03
Years of schooling	4.485	3.926	5.710	4.368
Years of schooling squared	35.526	208.791	51.677	305.408
Household-level variables				
Water from closed source (0/1)	0.361	0.480	0.423	0.494
Flush or pit toilet facility	0.906	0.292	0.921	0.269
Floor of parquet, finished wood, or cement (0/1)	0.228	0.419	0.268	0.443
Household member owns a bicycle (0/1)	0.339	0.473	0.355	0.479
Household member owns a car (0/1)	0.019	0.136	0.017	0.128
Community-level variables				
Rural HH (0/1)	0.732	0.443	0.692	0.462
North highland zone (0/1)[a]	0.109	0.312	0.095	0.293
Central zone (0/1)[a]	0.087	0.281	0.093	0.290
South highland zone (0/1)[a]	0.148	0.355	0.184	0.388
Southern zone (0/1)[a]	0.079	0.271	0.082	0.275
Lake zone (0/1)[a]	0.368	0.482	0.278	0.448
Road is seasonal or is a path (0/1)[a]	0.238	0.426	0.216	0.411
Distance to primary school (km)[b]	0.660	1.907	0.724	2.007
Village has one or more health workers (0/1)[b]	0.375	0.484	0.365	0.481
Distance to nearest health facility[b]	4.372	7.071	4.543	7.490
Nearest health facility is a pharmacy (0/1)[b]	0.063	0.244	0.080	0.271

(c) TKAP Sample of Women Aged 15-49 and Sample of Men Aged 15-59
(*continued*)

Variable	Women Aged 15-49 (n = 3,950)		Men Aged 15-59 (n = 1,948)	
	Mean	Standard Deviation	Mean	Standard Deviation
Nearest health facility is a hospital (0/1)[b]	0.128	0.335	0.115	0.320
Nearest health facility is a health center (0/1)[b]	0.170	0.375	0.192	0.394
Number of family planning methods available at nearest facility[b]	2.209	1.486	2.204	1.534
Pill available at nearest facility (0/1)[b]	0.751	0.443	0.710	0.454
Injections available at nearest facility (0/1)[b]	0.298	0.457	0.327	0.469
Condoms available at nearest facility (0/1)[b]	0.799	0.401	0.809	0.393
IUD available at nearest facility (0/1)[b]	0.218	0.413	0.245	0.430

[a]Coastal zone (Tanga, Morogoro, Coast, and Dar es Salaam regions), north highland zone (Arusha and Kilimanjaro regions), central zone (Dodoma and Singida regions), south highland zone (Iringa, Mbeye, and Rukwa regions), southern zone (Lindi, Mtwara, and Ruvumba regions), lake zone (Tabora, Kigoma, Shinyanga, Kagera, Mwanza, and Mara regions).

[b]Community and facility data from 1991/92 Tanzania Demographic Health Survey (see Beegle, 1995, for details).

APPENDIX 5-B:
ESTIMATION OF THE DETERMINANTS OF FERTILITY

Specification and Estimation

The probit model assumes an underlying linear index function (B_i^*) for woman i of the following form:

$$B_i^* = \beta X_i + v_i, \tag{1}$$

where X_i is a set of explanatory variables and v_i is an error term that is distributed normally with mean 0 and with variance σ_v^2 (which is normalized to 1 in the estimation). Actual (observed) birth in the last 12 months (B_i) is given by

$$B_i = 1 \text{ if } B_i^* \geq 0, B_i = 0 \text{ otherwise.} \tag{2}$$

The probit model is a convenient (and commonly used) method to estimate a model with a dichotomous outcome. However, it is sensitive to misspecification. A non-normal distribution of v_i or omitted variables can cause the parameter estimates to be biased. In this chapter we check the robustness of our results to certain types of violations of the underlying assumptions (see below). However, we leave more formal tests for future work.

Two main issues arise in the estimation of this model. First, when including income in the analysis of fertility, it must be treated as (potentially) endogenous. Second, in the Kagera sample, the fact that there are as many as three observations per woman in the sample may affect our results. We address below how these problems were dealt with.

The Potential Endogeneity of Household Consumption

In the estimation of the determinants of having had a birth in the past 12 months for two of the data sets (KHDS and THRDS), we estimate models that include the effect of household permanent income. Consistent with what is done in this literature we use the log of total household consumption expenditures per adult as a proxy for income. Household expenditures cannot necessarily be assumed as exogenous to fertility decisions. For example, if children themselves contribute to household income then the causal relationship runs in both directions.[10]

Including an endogenous right-hand side regressor will lead to inconsistent probit parameter estimates. Smith and Blundell (1986) and Rivers and Vuong

---

[10]For recent discussions of these and other explanations of the endogeneity of income in African contexts see Benefo and Schultz (1996), as well as Montogomery et al. (1995).

(1988) propose an exogeneity test for a model with a dichotomous dependent variable and a potentially endogenous continuous explanatory variable. In the present case, we rewrite equation (1) to include the log of household expenditures per adult:

$$B_i^* = \beta X_i + \gamma E_i + v_i,$$ (3)

where $B_i = 1$ if $B_i^* \geq 0$, $B_i = 0$ otherwise.

$$E_i = \partial_1 X_i + \partial_2 Z_i + u_i,$$ (4)

where B_i is the event of having a birth, X_i is a set of exogenous variables, E_i is the log of household expenditure per adult, and β, γ, ∂_1, and ∂_2 are parameters to be estimated. The set of variables Z_i are the identifying instruments, that is they affect fertility only through their effect on E_i.

Smith and Blundell show that an exogeneity test for E is a t-test of the significance of the parameter α in the following probit regression:

$$B_i^* = \beta X_i + \gamma E_i + \alpha \hat{u}_i + v_i',$$ (5)

where $\hat{u}_i$ are the residuals estimated from equation (4). If the estimate of α is significantly different from zero then we must treat E_i as endogenous.

The set of instrumental variables we use differs somewhat for the two samples. They are in general, however, characteristics of the head of the household and the value and/or characteristics of household assets. In both analyses the set includes the sex, age squared, education, and education squared of the head of the household. For the KHDS it includes in addition to the head's characteristics the value of farm equipment, the value of farm buildings, the value of livestock, the value of business assets, a dummy for whether or not a household member owns the dwelling, and if so the value of the dwelling, and the area of banana crops harvested. For the THRDS it includes in addition to the head's characteristics the total number of cows, bulls, and oxen currently owned, a dummy for whether or not a household member owns the dwelling, and if so the value of the dwelling and a series of dummies equal to one if the dwelling has walls made of mud or wood, has a floor made of earth or wood, has a roof made of grass or mud, and has windows or screens.

The validity of these variables as instruments for income is dependent on the assumption that they affect the probability of a birth in the past year only through their impact on income (or its proxy, expenditures). The head of the household may or may not be the husband of the woman in question, and therefore his or her characteristics (conditional on the women's characteristics) are unlikely to affect the probability of a birth in the past 12 months directly. Characteristics and the value of the dwelling and productive assets are potentially good measures of "exogenous" wealth if there is a low turnover in the ownership of these assets, that is that they capture that part of income that is not endogenously related to the probability of birth in the past year. But, if only the characteristics of the head are used as instruments, none of the results of this chapter are substantially changed.

The first-stage regressions perform well in the sense that they explain a good part of the variance of the dependent variable. The adjusted R-squared in the KHDS sample is 0.32 and in the THRDS is 0.39. The instruments perform well in the sense that they explain a reasonable part of this variance. The incremental R square of adding the set of instruments in the first-stage regression is about 0.05 in the KHDS sample and about 0.08 in the THRDS sample. In addition, both sets of instruments are jointly significantly different from zero at the 99 percent level.

When the residual from the first-stage estimation is included in the second-stage probit regression for birth in the past year (equation 5), the t-tests reject exogeneity in both samples (and in both model specifications in the KHDS analysis).[11]

Therefore, to control for the endogeneity of expenditure, we estimate equation (2) in a first step and then use the predicted value of E_i (that is $\hat{E}_i$) to estimate

$$B_i^* = \beta X_i + \gamma \hat{E}_i + v_i'. \tag{6}$$

In the THRDS results, the asymptotic covariance matrix derived from this probit is then adjusted for the fact that $\hat{E}_i$ is a variable predicted from an auxiliary regression. This is done using the formula given in Maddala (1983:245).

Multiple Observations on a Single Woman in the KHDS

Random-Effects Probit

The KHDS data were collected over four interviews, separated by approximately 6 months each. In our current analysis we have pooled the data across waves 2, 3, and 4, and therefore a woman can appear up to three times in the sample. To be able to include deaths up to 30 months of age, we exclude wave 1 observations from this analysis. Estimating this model as a probit regression on pooled data produces consistent but inefficient estimates (Maddala, 1987). To improve the efficiency of the estimates, we estimate a random-effects probit model (reviewed in Maddala, 1987).

The random-effects probit model derives from a decomposition of the error

---

[11]In the KHDS model with deaths of household members, the t statistic has a value of 2.711 (t statistics derived from a pooled probit estimation with huber standard errors). In the THRDS it has a value of 2.903. We note that the derivation of this test was done under the assumption of cross-sectional data.

term given in equation (1). Including subscripts for time periods, equation (1) for woman i in time period t becomes

$$B_{it}^* = \beta X_{it} + w_i + v''_{it} ,\tag{7}$$

where $B_{it} = 1$ if $B_{it}^* \geq 0$, $B_{it} = 0$ otherwise, where w_i is a woman-specific time-invariant unobserved variable that is distributed normally with mean zero and variance σ_w^2. This model is estimated using a method proposed by Butler and Moffitt (1982).

In general these results are very similar to the pooled sample with simple probit estimation. The estimate of the share of the variance that is woman specific (ρ) is equal to approximately 0.34 and is significantly different from zero. However, the point estimates, as well as the statistical significance of these, are not very different.

One Observation per Woman

A woman can appear either one, two, or three times in the sample. If the number of times a woman is present in the sample is related to the issues under study, this could potentially bias our results. To investigate the sensitivity of our estimates to this, we estimate the models using only one observation, selected at random over the three waves, per woman.

The biggest difference between these estimates and those in the random-effects model is that the community mortality variables are no longer significant, although the signs remain. In general the household-level mortality variables exhibit the same patterns, although the effect of a female death in the past 18-24 months is no longer significant, and the effect of the death of a husband in the past 30 months is larger.

Transforming the Results from A Probit or Tobit Regression

In Tables 5-1 through 5-6, the probit parameter estimates have all been transformed to correspond to the marginal effect of a change in one of the independent variables on the expected value of the dependent variable (i.e., the probability that it equals one). If the underlying model for the observed variable B is

$$B_i^* = \beta X_i + v_i ,\tag{8}$$

where $B_i = 1$ if $B_i^* \geq 0$, $B_i = 0$ otherwise, then the change in the probability that B equals 1 due to a change in one of the X's, $\delta E(B)/\delta X^1$, is equal to $\beta^1 f(z)$, where β^1 is the probit parameter estimate on X^1, $f()$ is the standard normal probability density function, and z is equal to βX. In the reported results, βX is evaluated at the means of the X's.

The Tobit parameter estimates have been transformed to correspond to the marginal effect of a change in the independent variables on the expected value of the dependent variable. If the underlying model for the observed variable T is

$$T_i^* = \beta X_i + \varepsilon_i, \tag{9}$$

where $T_i = T_i^*$ if $T_i^* > 0$, $T_i = 0$ otherwise, then the change in the expected value of T due to a change in one of the X's, $\delta E(T)/\delta X^1$, is equal to $\beta^1 F(z)$, where β^1 is the Tobit parameter estimate on X^1, $F()$ is the standard normal cumulative distribution function, and z is equal to $X\beta/\sigma$, where σ is the standard deviation of ε. McDonald and Moffitt (1980) recommend evaluating this at the mean of the X's.

ACKNOWLEDGMENTS

We thank Ed Bos, Barney Cohen, Will Dow, Tom Merrick, Mark Montgomery, and participants in World Bank and Committee on Population seminars for comments on earlier drafts. The opinions expressed in this chapter are those of the authors and do not necessarily reflect the policy of The World Bank or its member governments. This research was financed by The World Bank Research Committee, RPO#680-46.

REFERENCES

Ahn, N., and A. Shariff
   1993   A Comparative Study of Fertility Determinants in Togo and Uganda: A Hazards Model Analysis. Paper prepared for the XIInd General Population Conference of the IUSSP, Montreal, Canada, August 24-September 1.

Ainsworth, M.
   1996   Economic Aspects of Child Fostering in Côte d'Ivoire. Pp. 25-62 in T. Paul Schultz, ed., *Research in Population Economics* volume 8. Greenwich, Conn.: JAI Press.

Ainsworth, M., and A.A. Rwegarulira
   1992   Coping with the Impact of the AIDS Epidemic in Tanzania: Survivor Assistance. AFTPN Working Paper no. 6. The World Bank, Washington, D.C.

Ainsworth, M., G. Koda, G. Lwihula, P. Mujinja, M. Over, and I. Semali
   1992   Measuring the Impact of Fatal Adult Illness in Sub-Saharan Africa: An Annotated Household Questionnaire. Living Standards Measurement Study Working Paper no. 90. The World Bank, Washington, D.C.

Ainsworth, M., S. Ghosh, and I. Semali
   1995   The Impact of Adult Deaths on Household Composition in Kagera Region, Tanzania. Paper presented at the Annual Meetings of the Population Association of America, San Francisco, Calif., April 6.

Ainsworth, M., and M. Over
   1997   *Confronting AIDS: Public Priorities in a Global Epidemic.* New York: Oxford University Press.

Anker, R.
  1985   Problems of interpretation and specification in analyzing fertility differentials: Illustrated
          with Kenyan survey data. Pp. 277-311 in G.M. Farooq and G.B. Simmons, eds., *Fertility
          in Developing Countries.* London: MacMillan Press.
Becker, G.S.
  1993   *A Treatise on the Family.* Cambridge, Mass.: Harvard University Press.
Beegle, K.
  1995   The Quality and Availability of Family Planning Services and Contraceptive Use in Tan-
          zania. Living Standards Measurement Study Working Paper no. 114. The World Bank,
          Washington, D.C.
Benefo, K.D., and T.P. Schultz
  1996   Fertility and child mortality in Côte d'Ivoire and Ghana. *World Bank Economic Review*
          10(1):123-158.
Bongaarts, J.
  1978   A framework for analyzing the proximate determinants of fertility. *Population and De-
          velopment Review* 4(1):105-132.
Bos, E., and R.A. Bulatao
  1992   The demographic impact of AIDS in sub-Saharan Africa: Short- and long-term projec-
          tions. *International Journal of Forecasting* 8(3):367-384.
Bureau of the Census, Health Studies Branch, International Programs Center, Population Division
  1995   HIV/AIDS in Africa. *Research Note* no. 20, December.
Bureau of Statistics, Government of Tanzania
  no date *Infant and Child Mortality in Tanzania, 1988 Population Census.* Dar es Salaam: Bu-
          reau of Statistics.
Butler, J.S., and R. Moffitt
  1982   A computationally efficient quadrature procedure for the one-factor multinomial probit
          model. *Econometrica* 50(3):761-764.
Caldwell, J.C., I.O. Orubuloye, and P. Caldwell
  1992   Fertility decline in Africa: A new type of transition? *Population and Development Re-
          view* 18(2):211-242.
Caldwell, J.C., P. Caldwell, E.M. Ankrah, J.K. Anarfi, D.K. Agyeman, K. Awusabo-Asare, and I.O.
Orubuloye
  1993   African families and AIDS: Context reactions and potential interventions. *Health Tran-
          sition Review* 3(Suppl.):1-16.
Chin, J., and F. Sonnenberg
  1991   The Epidemiology and Projected Mortality of AIDS in the United Republic of Tanzania.
          Background paper prepared for the Tanzania AIDS Assessment and Planning Study. The
          World Bank, Washington, D.C.
Farooq, G.M.
  1985   Household fertility decision-making in Nigeria. Pp. 312-350 in G.M. Farooq and G.B.
          Simmons, eds., *Fertility in Developing Countries.* London: MacMillan Press.
Ferreira, L., and C. Griffin
  1995   *Tanzania Human Resource Development Survey: Final Report.* Population and Human
          Resources Division, Eastern Africa Department. Washington, D.C.: The World Bank.
Gray, T.H., M.J. Wawer, N.K. Sewankambo, D. Serwadda, J.K. Konde-Lule, F. Nalugoda, C-J. Li,
L. Paxton, and D. McNaim
  1995   The Association between HIV Infection, Selected STDs, and Fertility in Rural Uganda.
          Abstract TuB121, IXth International Conference on AIDS and STDs in Africa, Kampala,
          Uganda, December 10-14.

Gregson, S.
    1994   Will HIV become a major determinant of fertility in sub-Saharan Africa? *Journal of Development Studies* 30(3):650-679.
Killewo, J., K. Nyamurayekunge, A. Sandstrom, U. Bredberg-Raden, S. Wall, F. Mhalu and G. Biberfeld
    1990a   Prevalence of HIV-1 infection in the Kagera region of Tanzania: A population-based study. *AIDS* 4(11):1081-1085.
Killewo, J., A. Sandstrom, U. Bredberg-Raden, K. Palsson, S. Wall, F. Mhalu, and G. Biberfeld
    1990b   Incidence of HIV infection in Kagera Region, Tanzania: A population-based study. Abstract T.O.B.2, presented at Vth International Conference on AIDS and STDs in Africa, Kinshasa, Zaire, October 10-12.
Lallemant, M.J., S. Lallemant-LeCoeur, and S. Nzingoula
    1994   Perinatal transmission of HIV in Africa. Pp. 211-236 in M. Essex, S. Mboup, P.J. Kanki, and M.R. Kalengayi, eds., *AIDS in Africa*. New York: Raven Press.
Langston, C., D.E. Lewis, H.A. Hammill, E.J. Popek, C.A. Kozinetz, M.W. Kline, C. Hanson, and W.T. Shearer
    1995   Excess intrauterine fetal demise associated with maternal human immunodeficiency virus infection. *The Journal of Infectious Diseases* 172:1451-1460.
Maddala, G.S.
    1983   *Limited-dependent and Qualitative Variables in Econometrics*. Cambridge, England: Cambridge University Press.
    1987   Limited dependent variable models using panel data. *Journal of Human Resources* 22(3):307-338.
Mann, J.M., D.J.M. Tarantola, and T.W. Netter, eds.
    1992   *AIDS in the World*. Cambridge, Mass.: Harvard University Press.
Matthiessen, P.C., and J.C. McCann
    1978   The role of mortality in the European fertility transition: Aggregate-level relations. Pp. 47-68 in S.H. Preston, ed., *The Effects of Infant and Child Mortality on Fertility*. New York: Academic Press.
McDonald, J.F., and R.A. Moffitt
    1980   The uses of Tobit analysis. *Review of Economics and Statistics* 62:318-321.
Montgomery, M., A. Kouamé, and R. Oliver
    1995   The Tradeoff Between Number of Children and Child Schooling: Evidence from Côte d'Ivoire and Ghana. Living Standards and Measurement Study working paper no. 112. Washington, D.C.: The World Bank.
Moss, A.R., and P. Bachetti
    1989   Natural history of HIV infection. *AIDS* 3:55-61.
Mukyanuzi, F.
    1994   Health Sector Overview Paper. Second draft, March. Tanzania Social Sector Review, The World Bank, Washington, D.C.
National Research Council
    1996   *Preventing and Mitigating AIDS in Sub-Saharan Africa*. Committee on Population, National Research Council. Washington, D.C.: National Academy Press.
Ngallaba, S., S.H. Kapiga, I. Ruyobya, and J.T. Boerma
    1993   *Tanzania Demographic and Health Survey, 1991/1992*. Dar es Salaam: Bureau of Statistics, Planning Commission. Calverton, Md.: Macro International.
Nicoll, A., I. Timaeus, R. Kigadye, G. Walraven, and J. Killewo
    1994   The impact of HIV-1 infection on mortality in children under 5 years of age in sub-Saharan Africa: A demographic and epidemiologic analysis. *AIDS* 8:995-1005.

Okojie, C.E.E.
   1989   Fertility response to child survival in Nigeria: An analysis of microdata from Bendel
           State. Pp. 93-112 in T.P. Schultz, ed., *Research in Population Economics*, Vol. 7.
           Greenwich, Conn.: JAI Press.

Over, M., and M. Ainsworth
   1989   The Economic Impact of Fatal Adult Illness due to AIDS and other Causes in Sub-
           Saharan Africa: A Research Proposal. The World Bank, Washington, D.C., October.

Preston, S.H., ed.
   1978   *The Effects of Infant and Child Mortality on Fertility.* New York: Academic Press.

Rivers, D., and Q.H. Vuong
   1988   Limited information estimators and exogeneity tests for simultaneous probit models. *Jour-
           nal of Econometrics* 39:347-366.

Rutherford, G.W., A.R. Lifson, N.A. Hessol, W.W. Darrow, P.M. O'Malley, S.P. Buchbinder, J.L.
Barnhart, T.W. Bodecker, L. Cannon, and L.S. Doll
   1990   Course of HIV-1 infection in a cohort of homosexual and bisexual men: An 11-year
           follow-up study. *British Medical Journal* 301(6762):1183-1188.

Ryder, R.W., V.L. Batter, M. Nsuami, N. Badi, L. Mundele, B. Matela, M. Utshudi, and W.L.
Heyward
   1991   Fertility rates in 238 HIV-1-seropositive women in Zaire followed for 3 years post-partum.
           AIDS 5:1521-1527.

Schultz, T.P.
   1981   *Economics of Population.* Reading, Mass.: Addison-Wesley.

Setel, P.
   1995   The effects of HIV and AIDS on fertility in East and Central Africa. *Health Transition
           Review* 5(Suppl.):179-189.

Sewankambo, N.K., M.J. Wawer, R.H. Gray, D. Serwadda, J.K. Konde-Lule, F. Nalugoda, and C-J.
Li
   1995   Demographic Effects of the HIV-1 Epidemic in Three Community Strata of Rural Rakai
           District, Uganda. Poster MoB440, IXth International Conference on AIDS and STDs in
           Africa. Kampala, Uganda, December 10-14.

Smith, R.J., and R.W. Blundell
   1986   An exogeneity test for a simultaneous equation Tobit model with an application for labor
           supply. *Econometrica* 54(3):679-685.

Snyder, D.W.
   1974   Economic determinants of family size in West Africa. *Demography* 11(4):613-627.

Stover, J.
   1993   The Impact of HIV/AIDS on Adult and Child Mortality in the Developing World. IUSSP
           Working Group on AIDS and Foundation Marcel Merieux, Seminar on AIDS Impact and
           Prevention in the Developing World: The Contribution of Demography and Social Sci-
           ence. Veyrier-du-Lac, France, December 5-9.

UN/WHO (United Nations, Department of International Economic and Social Affairs, and World
Health Organization, Global Programme on AIDS)
   1991   *The AIDS Epidemic and Its Demographic Consequences.* Proceedings of the UN/WHO
           Organization Workshop on Modeling the Demographic Impact of the AIDS Epidemic in
           Pattern II Countries. New York and Geneva: United Nations/WHO.

United Nations, Department for Economic and Social Information and Policy Analysis, Population
Division
   1995   *World Population Prospects: The 1994 Revision.* New York: United Nations.

Valleroy, L.A., J.R. Harris, and P.O. Way
   1990   The impact of HIV-1 infection on child survival in the developing world. *AIDS* 4(7):667-
           672.

Way, P.O., and K.A. Stanecki
  1994   *The Impact of HIV/AIDS on World Population.* Economic and Statistics Administration, Bureau of the Census, U.S. Department of Commerce. Washington, D.C.: U.S. Government Printing Office.
Weinstein, K.I., S. Ngallaba, A.R. Cross, and F.M. Mburu
  1995   *Tanzania Knowledge, Attitudes and Practices Survey, 1994.* Dar es Salaam: Bureau of Statistics and Planning Commission. Calverton, Md.: Macro International.
World Bank
  1992   *Tanzania: AIDS Assessment and Planning Study.* Washington, D.C.: The World Bank.
  1995   *World Development Report 1995: Workers in an Integrating World.* New York: Oxford University Press.

6
Infant Mortality and the Fertility Transition: Macro Evidence from Europe and New Findings from Prussia

Patrick R. Galloway, Ronald D. Lee, and Eugene A. Hammel

INTRODUCTION

Most attempts to understand secular fertility decline include some allusion to the European experience. It is generally thought that little or no relationship existed between fertility decline and infant mortality decline in Europe, or that the findings from relevant studies are inconsistent. We believe that these common perceptions are mistaken. When more attention is given to the varying methods of analyses, a more consistent picture emerges. We argue that it is particularly important to keep in mind whether studies are bivariate or multivariate; whether studies estimate cross-sectional relations between levels of fertility and of infant mortality, or instead focus on the relation of changes in these variables; and whether studies take into account the possibility that causality flows in both directions—from fertility to mortality as well as from mortality to fertility.

We estimate both the impact of infant mortality on fertility and the impact of fertility on infant mortality, using aggregate data from Prussia from 1875 to 1910 and fixed effects models with instrumental variables. This is followed by an extensive review of previous research on fertility and infant mortality within the historical European context.[1] By comparing our findings for Prussia with earlier research looking at both level and change effects, we find considerable evidence

---

[1]Our review of earlier research is restricted to those studies using aggregate data. There is a body of literature on fertility and infant mortality that uses micro-level data, see for example Knodel (1988). However, it is beyond the scope of this chapter to survey such studies.

for a positive association between the fertility level and the infant mortality level, as well as a positive association between fertility change and infant mortality change.

The Long Term

It is clear that in the very long run, in closed populations, fertility and mortality are linked because of the finiteness of the resource base, which implies that the average rate of natural increase n must not exceed zero more than slightly. This is an abstract argument. The historical reality has been that rapid natural increase sustained over long periods (say an average rate of natural increase greater than 0.02 over a period of more than two centuries) has not been observed except in frontier regions[2] such as North America. Much more typically, large populations appear to have had rates of natural increase of less than 1 percent per year until the Industrial Revolution, and usually with a strong positive statistical association between fertility and mortality in the cross section. Such a long-term positive association of fertility and mortality, and a limit to average rates of natural increase, can be explained in at least two ways. First, positive growth rates mean increasing population size and density, which under preindustrial conditions typically meant declining living standards. These in turn caused mortality to rise, or fertility to fall, and therefore growth rates to return toward zero. This is the Malthusian theory of population equilibration through negative feedback (Lee, 1987). Of course, emigration was another possible outcome, and technological progress or international trade might intervene between population growth and declining living standards. Second, it is sometimes argued that the sociocultural institutions governing fertility evolved in the context of some average mortality regime so as roughly to balance fertility and mortality on average, leaving rates of natural increase close to zero. In this version there is no feedback from population size to the vital rates; rather, growth rates themselves tend to have average levels not far above zero. Again, migration, technological progress, and international trade might play a role (Smith, 1977; Yule, 1906).

The constraint on average growth rates, and hence on fertility and mortality, implied by these theories and the positive association of fertility and mortality observed in the historical record, may also help to explain the long-run shape of the demographic transition (Lee and Bulatao, 1983, for example). Demeny (1968:502) gave a classic description of the transition: "In traditional societies, fertility and mortality are high. In modern societies, fertility and mortality are low. In between, there is demographic transition." In fact, in those national

---

[2]By frontier regions we mean from the point of view of agricultural populations, that is, not from the point of view of hunter and gatherer populations who may have occupied the area at relatively low density before the arrival of agriculturists.

populations that have "completed" the transition, fertility has dropped so low that growth rates may turn very substantially negative. Nonetheless, it is difficult to escape the conclusion that, in some vague and unspecified way, and despite all the accompanying structural changes in the economies and societies, the very long-term decline in fertility is ultimately due to a very long-term decline in mortality, or the two are interlinked. In fact, some theories link both declines to the same set of parental decisions concerning investment in children.

These very long-run relations, both theoretical and empirical, are based on some sort of slow-acting feedback operating through the macro-economic or macro-societal level. The posited mechanisms might be expected to operate over the course of a century or more, but not over the course of decades. For this reason, they are of little relevance for questions about the policy-relevant time frame of adjustment over the medium range of, say, 5-30 years.

The Short Term

Although the long-run historical relation of fertility and mortality is doubtless positive, it is equally true that the empirical relationship over short-run fluctuations has been consistently negative in historical populations. This has been established by a large number of studies of time series of births and deaths, once the long-term trends in the data have been statistically removed. It is easy to think of reasons to expect either a positive or a negative association of the two vital rates. For a positive relationship, note that high mortality will break many marriages, particularly those of older couples, and that the subsequent remarriages of widows and widowers might result in higher fertility than if the marriages had been unbroken. Furthermore, higher mortality would free land holdings and create other economic opportunities permitting new marriages that would have high fertility. In existing unions, high infant and child mortality would interrupt breastfeeding, eliminating its contraceptive effects, and therefore lead to earlier conceptions and a temporary increase in fertility. Reconstitution studies have often demonstrated this lactation interruption effect. On the behavioral side, if we are not dealing with a natural fertility regime, we might expect couples who have experienced the loss of a child to attempt to replace it with another birth sooner than they normally would have, or by having one more birth than originally intended. However, many historical demographers dispute that this actually occurs to any appreciable degree, except in special subpopulations (Knodel, 1978).

For a negative relationship, note that many factors that tended to raise mortality would also tend to reduce fertility. For example, low real incomes apparently had this effect, as did unusually hot summer months or unusually cold winter months (see Lee, 1981; Galloway, 1986, 1988, 1994). The variation of such factors in the short term would have led to a negative bivariate association of fertility and mortality, but if observable, they can be netted out in multivariate studies. Perhaps more important were unobservable influences, of which ill health dominated. Fluctuations in morbidity both raised mortality and reduced fertility, leading to a strong negative association of short-term fluctuations in fertility and mortality, even after controlling for observed fluctuations in real incomes or grain prices and temperature. The estimated, strongly negative association of short-run variations in fertility and mortality is not very informative about structural or causal influences of mortality on fertility or the reverse. The many short-run studies of the relation of fertility to mortality in historical populations will therefore not answer the question before us.

The Medium Term

For policy makers, the most relevant time frame for fertility and infant mortality interactions is probably the medium term, say 5-30 years. Assuming a couple has some notion of a desired number of surviving offspring, infant and child mortality should be positively associated with the number of births. A couple can assume that some unknown number of offspring will die, and then stop when they think they have enough children (often called hoarding behavior). Or the couple can wait to see if the last child born survives past a certain age. If the child dies, the couple can then engage in replacement reproductive behavior. Both strategies are types of "inventory control" (Preston, 1978:10) leading to some desired number of surviving offspring. Within either strategy, the number of births should decline as infant mortality declines.

There are also ways in which declining mortality might alter the desired number of surviving children. It reduces the costs of achieving a given target number, and therefore might raise the target by increasing discretionary income. Alternatively, declining mortality might raise the rate of return on investments in children, which could lead to a substitution of quality for quantity, and a reduced target. Here, however, we concentrate on the fixed target scenario.

Once infant mortality begins to decline, it might take some time for couples to perceive the effect of infant mortality on child survivorship, which would ultimately lead to changes in fertility. It is also possible, however, that the effect could be almost immediate, as couples hear about and read about mortality decline.[3]

---

[3]It would be difficult to test for very short lags because censuses (from which we derive most of our independent variables) are nearly always at least 5 years apart, and because it is very likely that the level of infant mortality rates at year t will be highly correlated with the level of infant mortality rates at years $t-2$, $t-3$, or $t-4$. Using Prussian data and the model shown in Appendix Table 6A-2, we added the variable infant mortality lagged 5 years and found that, in the fixed effects model, which estimates changes, the regression estimate on infant mortality with no lag was 0.267 whereas the regression estimate on infant mortality lagged 5 years was –0.062, suggesting that the lagged variable was relatively unimportant.

Elevated infant mortality tends to shorten the birth interval because the death of an infant curtails lactation amenorrhea along with its contraceptive effects. An increase in infant mortality will cause an increase in fertility, *ceteris paribus*, although few children may ultimately survive, of course. This short-term phenomenon can persist over time, becoming an important factor over both the medium and the long term.

Fertility variations, whether deliberate or accidental, can also affect infant and child mortality as demonstrated by a host of contemporary studies. There is good reason then to expect that exogenous increases in infant and child mortality caused increases in marital fertility and that exogenous increases in fertility caused increases in infant and child mortality. (However, this micro-level reasoning about motives and relations does not translate exactly to the macro level because of expected nonlinearities in the relationships.)

Infant and Child Mortality

Matthiessen and McCann (1978) provide a useful overview of the findings of historical studies of macro-level data, with an emphasis on the early results of the European Fertility Project. They are particularly critical of the use of infant mortality as the explanatory mortality index, because they find that in practice other more appropriate measures, such as mortality of children age 0-15, began to decline earlier than did infant mortality, so that the European Fertility Project's studies of timing, for example, are of little value. When they reexamine the timing of the fertility transition in relation to $_{15}q_0$, they find that mortality decline almost always preceded fertility decline. We believe that it is very difficult to estimate the onset of secular $_{15}q_0$ decline. In general, we suggest that there is often no clear point at which one can categorically state that mortality or fertility has begun to decline, a suggestion with which Matthiessen and McCann (1978:52) clearly agree. Concerning the onset of infant mortality decline, van de Walle is appropriately cautious, noting that "in most instances we are left ignorant of past trends: the data do not allow us to go back in time and the existence of an earlier decline cannot be ascertained" (1986:213).

It might be useful to address the issue of infant (under age 1) versus child (age 1-9) mortality in multivariate analyses of secular fertility decline. When a husband or wife thinks about procreation in terms of offspring survivorship, he or she considers both infant and child mortality (Matthiesson and McCaan, 1978:52). Although infant mortality rates can generally be found in most historical registration material, the more detailed measures of child mortality are often unavailable. However, in a high infant mortality regime, the bulk of infant and child deaths will be infant deaths, and infant mortality should be very highly correlated with infant and child mortality combined. Using 1890-1891 male mortality data for the 36 provinces (Regierungsbezirke) of Prussia, we find that the correlation r between $_1q_0$ and $_5q_0$ is 0.96, between $_1q_0$ and $_{10}q_0$ is 0.96, and between $_1q_0$ and

$_{15}q_0$ is 0.95 (Königliches Statistisches Bureau, 1904:135-147). The range of $_1q_0$ in the provinces is 109-273. A similar analysis of the 15 largest cities in Prussia from the same source reveals respective r's of 0.98, 0.97, and 0.91 with a range of $_1q_0$ of 170 to 326. Plots of each of the six graphs reveal essentially a straight line with no outliers. It seems likely that the infant mortality rate is an adequate proxy for infant and child mortality when using aggregate data in high infant mortality populations.

Although it is difficult to say much about the timing or onset of secular infant and child mortality decline, we can examine their relative speed. It is clear from Figure 6-1 that $_1q_0$ and $_{15}q_0$ generally declined at about the same rate over the decades from the 1870s to around 1925. The quality of German infant and child mortality data before 1875 is questionable. Such consistency lends further support to the notion that infant mortality is an adequate proxy for infant and child mortality, at least in Germany.

ANALYSIS OF PRUSSIAN DATA

From a theoretical perspective it seems likely that higher infant mortality should ultimately be associated with higher fertility, and vice versa. We attempt to evaluate both the effect of infant mortality on fertility and the effect of fertility on infant mortality using fixed-effects models and instrumental variables estimation applied to data from 407 Prussian Kreise (administrative districts) and 54 cities in Prussia from 1875 to 1910.[4]

The following equation system describes the structural relationships between fertility and mortality:

$$F_{i,t} = \alpha_1 Y_1^F + \alpha_2 X_{i,t} + \alpha_3 Z_{i,t}^F + \alpha_4 M_{i,t} + \tilde{\alpha}_{5,i} + \tilde{\delta}_t + \tilde{\varepsilon}_{i,t},$$

$$M_{i,t} = \beta_1 Y_1^M + \beta_2 X_{i,t} + \beta_3 Z_{i,t}^M + \beta_4 F_{i,t} + \tilde{\beta}_{5,i} + \tilde{\theta}_t + \tilde{\upsilon}_{i,t}.$$

Here F and M refer to appropriate measures of fertility and infant (and/or child) mortality in the subpopulation of region i at time t. Y is a matrix of unchanging characteristics of the regions that influence fertility or mortality (indicated by superscripts). X is a matrix of changing influences on both fertility and mortality in the regions. Z refers to changing variables in the regions that influence just fertility or just mortality, respectively. $\tilde{\alpha}_{5,i}$ and $\tilde{\beta}_{5,i}$ are disturbances or fixed effects in the two equations that do not change over time, but are specific to the regions. $\tilde{\delta}_t$ and $\tilde{\theta}_t$ are disturbances to the two equations that are the same across all regions, but that vary over time. Finally, $\tilde{\varepsilon}_{i,t}$ and $\tilde{\upsilon}_{i,t}$ are disturbances to the

---

[4]See Galloway et al. (1994, 1995) for details regarding these two data sets.

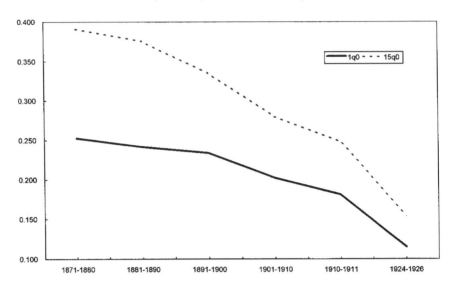

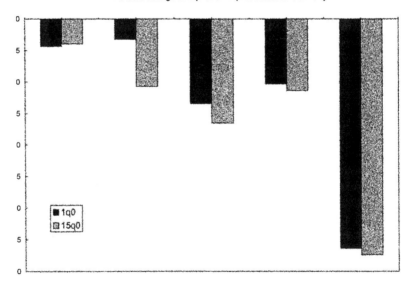

FIGURE 6-1 Level and change of male infant and child mortality rates in Germany, 1871-1926. SOURCE: Statistischen Reichsamt (1930:168).

equations that are specific to time period and to region. Because our data represent non-overlapping 5-year averages, the short-term relations will be largely masked, so long-term and medium-term relations will dominate the estimates.

We use this pair of equations to attempt to approximate a far more complicated dynamic pair of equations that would explicitly include the long-run adjustment processes that bring fertility and mortality to similar levels. In the given equations, the fixed-effect terms are used to represent the outcome of these long-term adjustment processes. The coefficients α_4 and β_4, which represent the influence of mortality on fertility and fertility on mortality, therefore abstract from these long-run adjustment processes and represent only the medium-term influences of one on the other. For example, they would not reflect the possible development of social institutions to motivate high fertility in the face of high mortality. When we estimate this model, which includes fixed effects, therefore, the estimated coefficients should reflect only the medium-term adjustment processes that we believe to be particularly informative for policy considerations. We often refer to such fixed-effect estimates as change estimates, because they are shaped entirely by the relation of changes over time within each Kreis, and not at all by differences in fertility and mortality between Kreise.

By contrast, estimates of these equations based on a single cross section, as are common in the literature, mainly reflect the outcome of the long-term adjustment processes and of correlations of right-hand variables with persistent features of the different geographic units, such as agrarian system, local culture, political orientation, or breastfeeding practices, yielding coefficient estimates that are inconsistent or irrelevant for policy. When suitable instruments are available, two-stage least squares can be used to avoid the biases arising from correlations of right-hand variables with persistent influences; however, suitable instruments can rarely be found in this context. Furthermore, instruments will not solve the problem that long-term adjustment processes probably dominate cross-sectional estimates.

We expect that over the long run, the levels of fertility and mortality will be positively correlated. These long-run correlations would show up in correlations of the fixed effect disturbances $\tilde{\alpha}_{5,i}$ and $\tilde{\beta}_{5,i}$. These correlations would bias any estimate of the structural coefficients relating fertility and mortality directly. Furthermore, the system described by these equations is simultaneous, with both fertility and mortality endogenous. Attempts to estimate the equations by ordinary least squares would yield biased estimates.

Now suppose we difference all the variables, representing the differenced values by lower case letters. We will actually be using fixed-effects estimators, but looking at the effects of differenced variables is a simple way to examine the consequences of using the fixed-effect model. Differenced disturbance terms are represented by the same Greek characters, but without the tildes. In this case, the region-specific disturbances that do not change over time disappear, as do all other variables that do not change over time. We then have

$$f_{i,t} = \alpha_2 x_{i,t} + \alpha_3 z_{i,t}^F + \alpha_4 m_{i,t} + \delta_t + \varepsilon_{i,t},$$

$$m_{i,t} = \beta_2 x_{i,t} + \beta_3 z_{i,t}^M + \beta_4 f_{i,t} + \theta_t + \upsilon_{i,t}.$$

The problem of correlated fixed effects has been removed, but the simultaneity remains. However, we can use the variables z to identify instrumental or two-stage least-squares estimates of the coefficients. These should, in principle, be unbiased—except that there is an additional problem: We do not observe all the relevant x variables. For example, breastfeeding behavior, which affects both fertility and infant mortality, is unobserved.[5] But extended breastfeeding reduces both fertility and infant mortality, and failure to control for its influence will lead to a noncausal positive association of fertility and mortality. Put differently, unobserved and therefore omitted variables in the x matrix will induce a correlation of the error terms in the two equations ε and υ. To be concrete, the omission of breastfeeding variables from the estimated model will lead to a positive correlation in the disturbances, resulting in an upward bias in the estimated structural coefficients on fertility and mortality; the omission of health and illness variables may have the opposite effect. This could be a serious problem for which we have no remedy. Therefore, this potential source of bias must be kept in mind when interpreting the results.

Two-Stage Least-Squares Estimation

Our estimation model reflects the general theoretical perspective outlined above in the use of fixed effects and controls for the endogeneity of infant mortality. However, we have taken a rather eclectic approach to inclusion of socioeconomic influences on fertility and have not imposed any mathematical structure on the relations to be estimated beyond the usual assumption that our linear model approximates some true but unknown nonlinear specification.

One of the findings from our review of earlier research on fertility decline in Europe is that many studies that purport to say something about fertility decline (change) only examine fertility level. Preston (1978:1) states "a central problem in modern population studies . . . is . . . the degree to which changes in mortality can be expected to induce changes in fertility." This clearly poses the question in terms of changes and not of levels. We believe that this is indeed the appropriate question, and that it is not an issue that can be resolved by studying the relationship between levels of fertility and mortality.

---

[5]In Prussia, longitudinal data on breastfeeding are available only for Berlin. Breastfeeding in Berlin decreased significantly from 1885 to 1910 (Kintner, 1985:169-170) while both marital fertility and infant mortality were declining substantially. It is not known whether other areas in Prussia experienced similar trends.

In our analyses of pooled cross-sectional time series we first examine the "between" estimators, regressions on the means over time of each Kreise or city, that give us level effects. We also generate "within" or "fixed-effects" estimators, regressions that allow each Kreis or city to have its own intercept. This effectively measures how changes in our independent variables affect changes in our dependent variable and is the more appropriate approach for explaining fertility change.[6]

We have dealt at length with the theoretical expectations and empirical findings of fertility decline in 407 Prussian Kreise (Galloway et al., 1994) and 54 cities (Galloway et al., 1995) using quinquennial data from 1875 to 1910[7] and pooled cross-sectional time series ordinary least-squares methods.[8] A detailed analysis of infant mortality decline in the Kreise and cities of Prussia is in progress (Galloway et al., 1996).[9] We expect fertility to influence infant mortality and simultaneously we expect infant mortality to influence fertility. Instrumental variables estimation, two-stage least squares in this case, appears to be an appropriate method for estimating these effects. All the variables in all the models are defined in Appendix Table 6-A1. Our fertility model is shown in Appendix Table 6-A2 followed by a summary of regression results in Appendix Tables 6-

---

[6]Brass and Barrett (1978:212) also favor pooled cross-sectional time series studies done of areas within a country.

[7]Prussia became a state within Germany in 1871, but continued to maintain its own statistical bureau that published detailed demographic and economic data until the early 1930s. In 1910 the population of Prussia was just over 40 million, about 70 percent of Germany. If Prussia had been a country, it would have been the largest country in Europe excluding Russia. It covered most of modern-day Germany north of the Main River and most of the western half and northern quarter of modern-day Poland. Registration data are available annually and census data quinquennially from 1875 to 1910 for Kreise and major cities. Kreise are administrative units similar to U.S. census tracts though much larger (average population 60,000) and, like census tracts, tended to split over time. There were about 400 Kreise in Prussia in 1875 and about 600 by 1910, with the total area of Prussia being virtually constant. To maintain spatial consistency over time, we combined many of the split Kreise. This resulted in 407 Kreise, each with a constant area, from 1875 to 1910. Only seven of the 407 Kreise were 100 percent urban. To examine fertility decline within a strictly urban setting, we created another data set consisting of 54 cities, whose area we allowed to change over time, realizing that any area incorporated into a city was itself likely to be highly urban.

[8]We use general marital fertility rate (GMFR) as our measure of marital fertility in this and in all our previous analyses of Prussian Kreise. GMFR is defined as the number of legitimate births per 1,000 married women aged 15-49. A 5-year average centered on the census year is used. More detailed marital age structure data are not available. Coale and Treadway (1986:153) note that there would have been little difference in their findings if GMFR had been used instead of Ig. In fact we find that in 54 Prussian cities from 1875 to 1910 where data are available to calculate both Ig and the GMFR that Ig and GMFR are highly correlated ($r = 0.97$) and that the two measures are virtually interchangeable.

[9]The average infant mortality rate in Prussia in 1900 was 179, somewhat above that found in most less developed countries today. In 1992 Mozambique had an estimated infant mortality rate of 162, the highest of any county in the world (World Bank, 1994:214).

A3 and 6-A4. The infant mortality model can be found in Appendix Table 6-A5 with regression results summarized in Appendix Tables 6-A6 and 6-A7. We focus on the relationship between fertility and infant mortality. The findings for the other right-hand side variables have been discussed elsewhere (Galloway et al., 1994, 1995, 1996).

Estimation of the Fertility Equation

High fertility and the shorter birth intervals it involves might well cause higher infant and child mortality. To avoid the possible bias associated with ordinary least-squares estimation, we need instruments for infant mortality that are correlated with infant mortality but not correlated with the component of its variance that might be influenced by fertility. We believe that male mortality at older ages provides a nearly ideal instrument in this case. Fertility should affect only the mortality of children. We do not know the upper limit of the range of ages that might be affected by high fertility, so we avoided using the mortality even of teenagers. The mortality of women depends in part on maternal mortality, which would depend on fertility, so we avoided using female mortality. For these reasons, we decided to use the mortality of adult males. Because of the cost of data entry, we limited ourselves to male mortality in the 30-34 age group. This choice was based in part on an examination of a correlation matrix for mortality at different ages for both Prussian Regierungsbezirke and historical Swedish data, which showed that death rates at age 30-34 were relatively highly correlated with infant mortality. Other age groups had correlations that were nearly as high, so the exact choice makes little difference, and ideally we would have used mortality over a broader range.

The idea is that male mortality at age 30-34 is a useful index of the general level of mortality in the population, reflecting all local factors that influence mortality, such as standard of living, nutrition, general sanitary conditions, ecological and epidemiological conditions, and the quality of health care. At the same time, it does not reflect the particular influence of either breastfeeding conditions or of fertility and therefore should not correlate with marital fertility.

Unfortunately, age-specific death rates are available only for Regierungsbezirke (very large areas, similar to provinces) of which there were 36 in Prussia. Given 407 Kreise in Prussia, there were on average about 11 Kreise per Regierungsbezirk. We applied Regierungsbezirk male mortality at age 30-34 for each of the eight quinquennial periods from 1875 to 1910 to the Kreise or city within the Regierungsbezirk. This instrument captures only broad regional variations in mortality, but not local differences, reducing its usefulness.

Appendix Table 6-A3 presents the ordinary least-squares and two-stage least-squares findings for Kreise, for both levels and changes. Looking at levels, we find that when we use ordinary least squares the estimated coefficient on infant mortality is negative and marginally significantly different from zero, but, using two-stage least squares the coefficient switches to positive (as we would expect from theory) but is still only marginally significant. Looking at changes, two-stage least-squares estimates of infant mortality are four times higher than in ordinary least squares and highly significantly different from zero.

In the analysis of 54 Prussian cities (Appendix Table 6-A4), we have an additional instrument for infant mortality. The variable sanitation represents cumulative municipal sanitation bond debt per capita[10] and represents a rough measure of the development of sanitation infrastructure. It is available only for cities. It is difficult to see any reason why this variable would have a direct effect on fertility (unless by raising the healthiness of women it increased their fecundity, which seems unlikely). Looking at levels, there is little difference between ordinary and two-stage least-squares estimates, with the estimated coefficient on infant mortality being negative and not significantly different from zero in both cases. In the more relevant estimates of change, the estimate on infant mortality is positive and highly significantly different from zero and quite a bit larger than the ordinary least-squares estimate.

To sum up, we find little evidence of any statistically important influence of infant mortality on fertility in our analysis of levels. On the other hand, infant mortality has a very strong and positive impact on fertility if we consider changes.

Estimation of the Infant Mortality Equation

The infant mortality models are shown in Appendix Table 6-A5. Instruments for the general marital fertility rate include proportion of workers employed in religious occupations, mining, and manufacturing; measures of the development of financial services; and the married sex ratio (a measure of spousal separation). All these are theoretically related to fertility, but probably have little effect on infant mortality. Using the two-stage least-squares regressions for Kreis levels, the effect of fertility on infant mortality is insignificant. However, in our regressions on changes, the estimate is positive and highly significant. Similar results are found in our analysis of cities (Appendix Table 6-A7).[11]

---

[10]The variable's definition is based on a listing of municipal debt outstanding by purpose of loan (e.g., sanitation), date of loan, and amount of loan. The source was published in 1906, included loans through 1905, and covered all large cities in Prussia, including our 54. There was virtually no sewage construction in Germany before 1875, most loans were long term (over 30 years), and we assumed that it took about 5 years at most to complete construction on the project. Thus, the sanitation variable is cumulative municipal debt outstanding for sanitation loans per capita, calculated for each census period, and then lagged 5 years to allow for construction. For details see Galloway et al. (1996).

[11]Our theoretical models include both areal fixed effects and period fixed effects; however, we prefer to estimate the coefficients using only areal fixed effects. When only areal fixed effects are

Simultaneous Equation Bias

The most intuitive interpretation of simultaneous equation bias would be the following. A regression of fertility on mortality (and other variables) yields a positive coefficient. But perhaps this is because high fertility is causing high mortality, rather than the other way around. This would lead the estimated coefficient to overstate (be more positive than) the true effect of mortality on fertility; that is, it would have a positive bias. In this case, dealing with the simultaneity by means of instrumental variables or in some other way should reduce the size of the positive coefficient on mortality. But in fact, in our instrumental variable estimates, the size of the estimated coefficient on mortality gets larger, not smaller (i.e., the bias is apparently negative, not positive).

This unexpected outcome does not mean that something is necessarily wrong with our analysis, such as an inappropriate choice of instruments or a misspecified

---

included, then the coefficients are estimated so as to explain optimally the pattern of changes over time within each Kreis, regardless of the overall levels of fertility and infant mortality in the Kreis. Therefore, the coefficients can be thought of as being based on the individual histories of each Kreis, with each taken as a case study. When both areal and period fixed effects are included in the estimation, the interpretation is somewhat changed. Now the coefficients are estimated so as to explain optimally the differences between changes over time in each Kreis and those changes that occurred nationally, or in the average of all the individual Kreise. Therefore, the overall national (or average across Kreise) trends in fertility and infant mortality have no effect on the estimates. Fertility could be rising in every Kreis at the same time that infant mortality was falling, to take an extreme example, but the estimated coefficients could still indicate a positive effect of one on the other. For this reason, our preferred estimates are those that include areal fixed effects, but not period fixed effects. Nonetheless, given that both fertility and mortality did decline in Prussia over this period (counter to the extreme example given above), some readers may believe that the model that includes period effects provides a more rigorous test and cleaner estimate than our preferred model.

We estimate the model with and without period effects. The effects of infant mortality on fertility differ as follows. The ordinary least-squares estimate using 407 Kreise with areal effects is 0.242 (Appendix Table 6-A3), with areal and period effects 0.140. The two-stage least-squares estimate using 407 Kreise with areal effects is 1.028 (Appendix Table 6-A3), with areal and period effects 0.709. The ordinary least-squares estimate using 54 cities with areal effects is 0.337 (Appendix Table 6-A4), with areal and period effects 0.165. The two-stage least-squares estimate using 54 cities with areal effects is 1.836 (Appendix Table 6-A4), with areal and period effects –0.036. All estimates are highly significant, except the last which is insignificant.

For the Kreise-based estimates, inclusion of period effects leaves the coefficients highly significantly greater than zero, but reduces their size by 30-40 percent, for both ordinary and two-stage least-squares estimates. For the smaller sample of cities, however, the changes are greater: The ordinary least-squares coefficient is reduced by a half, while remaining highly significantly greater than zero, but the two-stage least-squares coefficient now becomes very slightly negative (and its difference from zero is insignificant). All estimated coefficients for the effect of fertility on infant mortality (not shown) remain highly significantly greater than zero, but they also are decreased in size by 30 or 40 percent. Although our preferred estimates are those with only areal fixed effects, those with period effects also indicate a positive influence of infant mortality on fertility, on the whole.

model. The direction of bias is much more complicated than the intuitive interpretation would suggest.[12] If the true effect of mortality on fertility is α and of
fertility on mortality is β, and if the errors in the fertility and mortality equations
are ε and υ, respectively, then the sign of the bias is given by the sign of
$\beta\sigma_\varepsilon^2 / (1 - \alpha\beta) + \sigma_{\varepsilon\upsilon}^2 / (1 - \alpha\beta)$ We strongly expect α and β to be positive. If
there is no correlation of errors across the two equations, so that $\sigma_{\varepsilon\upsilon}^2 = 0$, then the
sign of the bias depends on whether $\alpha\beta$ is greater than 1, in which case it is
negative, or less than 1, in which case it is positive. (If $\alpha\beta$ is greater than unity,
then the system is dynamically unstable.) However, because potentially impor-
tant variables are omitted from the equations, it is quite possible that $\sigma_{\varepsilon\upsilon}^2$ does
not equal zero. Breastfeeding presumably reduces both fertility and mortality,
and therefore its omission leads to a positive covariance. Variations in health and
morbidity might reduce fertility and raise mortality, so their omission might lead
to a negative covariance. For these reasons it is not clear a priori whether the
correction for simultaneous equation bias should increase or reduce the estimated
effect of mortality on fertility.

OVERVIEW OF PREVIOUS RESEARCH

Nearly all earlier studies of European historical fertility decline regress levels of fertility on levels of independent variables. Although this strategy does tell
us something about fertility levels, it tells us little about fertility change.

We assess earlier studies on marital fertility[13] level and change in Europe
using regional units of analysis (e.g., districts, counties, provinces) of countries
or large portions of countries where some attempt has been made to employ
multivariate techniques.[14] We restrict our overview to published research. Those
studies that do not examine infant, child, or general mortality are of course

---

[12]The following discussion is based on a communication from Mark Montgomery, whom we
thank.

[13]We review research that examines only marital fertility, with one exception. The study of
Netherlands analyzes only crude birth rate, but we decided to include it because it is the only study of
fertility change in the Netherlands. By focusing on marital fertility we are abstracting from any
response of nuptiality to changed mortality. However, if nuptiality responded strongly positively to
mortality change, so that the period of exposure to risk of childbearing within marriage did likewise,
possibly even overcompensating, then focusing on marital fertility could be misleading. It might be
useful to study the two together.

[14]F. van de Walle (1986:225-227) examined fertility levels and changes in relation to infant
mortality levels and changes in historical European countries. She shows bivariate correlations of
$_1q_0$ with I_g and I_f and I_m across countries of Europe and also across provinces within Europe. She
also looks at bivariate correlations of changes in $_1q_0$ and I_g and claims these to be inconclusive, but
in fact every significant correlation is positive in both periods (first period is 1870-1900 or so; the
second is 1900-1930 or so). Cross-period correlations, for which there are no apparent justifications,
sometimes have perverse signs. In another study, Fialová et al. (1990:102) present only bivariate
correlations between levels of independent variables and marital fertility level in their analysis of

excluded. Urban and rural differences are shown where available. We differentiate between analyses of level effects and change effects.[15]   Generally, we examine only those periods before World War II.

Tables 6-1 and 6-2 list summaries of previous research according to level and change, respectively, in alphabetical order by country. In all cases but one, marital fertility is the dependent variable. The author, date of publication, fertil-

---

fertility in Czechoslovakia. Bivariate correlations are at best suggestive, and useful conclusions for the analysis of theoretically complex models cannot be drawn from them.

Some examine fertility decline using time series techniques applied to one region (i.e., only one unit of analysis). For example, Lutz (1987:84) examines annual estimates of the Coale-Trussell index of family limitation m for Finland from 1873 to 1917 along with age at marriage, education, gross domestic product, marriage rate, life expectancy at age 5, and infant mortality (which showed a positive, but insignificant association with m). Crafts (1984b:583) examined GMFR in England and Wales from 1877 to 1938 along with measures of wages, income, prices, illegitimate fertility, and child mortality (which was positively related to GMFR, but not significant). Haynes et al. (1985:560-565) examined annual crude birth rate and crude death rate data, but no other variables, in four countries. Because these studies use annual data, important factors such as sectoral employment, female labor force participation, urbanization, religion, language, and other census-derived variables are usually missing from the models. Furthermore, it is difficult to know what to say about long-term fertility decline when looking at the results from short-run time series analysis where the long-term trend has been necessarily removed. See Galloway (1994) for a review of the literature on short-run fluctuation analyses and the various interactions among annual variations in fertility, mortality, nuptiality, migration, wages, and weather.

There are many articles about fertility and infant mortality based on data from family reconstitution or genealogical studies, but few attempt to estimate the influence of infant or child mortality on fertility (Knodel, 1978). Furthermore, most of these are about one parish, most use little data beyond the demographic indices generated by family reconstitution, and very few cover the period of the fertility transition. Most are plagued by the usual problems of family reconstitution: no subsequent information on persons who leave the parish, no information on those who lived in the parish but who were not born or married or did not die there, a lack of total population counts and age structure for the entire parish population, possible selectivity based on the fact that the only registers analyzed are those that survived. See Flinn (1981) for an old but still useful overview of family reconstitution studies. For more recent analyses of both fertility and infant mortality using micro-level data see Knodel (1988).

[15]The few attempts to derive a measure of the "onset" of long-term fertility decline are particularly problematic. The Princeton European Fertility Project's definition based on a 10 percent decline in fertility seems arbitrary, and the plateau from which fertility is supposed to have declined is typically based on only a few observations. Teitelbaum (1984:178-179) looked at his estimate of onset of fertility decline in Great Britain using the period around 1851-1931, along with income, urbanization, females not in the labor force, sectoral employment, religion, ethnicity, and infant mortality rate (which was significantly negatively associated with onset of fertility decline). Knodel (1974:238-239) examined fertility decline using his estimate of secular fertility decline in 71 provinces of Germany for the period 1875-1910, along with levels of religion, bank account, sectoral employment, literacy, and the infant mortality rate (which was sometimes positively and sometimes negatively associated with I_g decline, depending on which measures of fertility decline from onset that Knodel used).

In some studies, we find analyses of fertility change in relation to levels of the independent variables (Knodel, 1974; Lesthaeghe, 1977; Benavente, 1989; Reher and Iriso-Napal, 1989; Haines, 1989). These results are difficult to interpret.

ity measure, number of units of analysis, periods analyzed, independent variables, and sign and significance of the mortality variable are discussed. In the following overview, the estimated mortality coefficient is considered statistically significant, that is, statistically different from zero, if the t statistic probability is 5 percent or less.[16] It should be understood that it may be difficult to compare findings directly because of differences in definitions of variables, number and type of control variables, and methods used.

Level of Fertility and Levels of Independent Variables

Belgium

Lesthaeghe (1977:213) examined I_g in the 22 arrondissements of Flanders in four periods between 1880 and 1910 along with language, industrialization, literacy, political affiliation, and infant mortality rate. He did the same for the 19 arrondissements of Wallonia. Infant mortality rate was significantly positively associated with I_g only in Flanders in 1880 and was insignificant otherwise, perhaps a result of the small sample sizes involved. We note that seven of the eight estimated infant mortality coefficients were positive.

England and Wales

Haines (1979:68) examined marital fertility in a random sample of 125 registration districts in England and Wales in 1851, 1861, and 1871 along with sectoral employment, female employment, urbanization, net migration, sex ratio, and infant mortality rate. He found that infant mortality was negatively associated with fertility in all three periods, but insignificant in 1851. Haines notes, "Although several adjustments were tried to correct for underreporting of infant deaths, it was felt safest simply to divide uncorrected infant deaths by uncorrected live-births to obtain the infant mortality rate" (1979:60-62). It seems likely that the degree of underreporting of infant deaths and live births varied independently, and perhaps substantially, from district to district. As a consequence, it is difficult to interpret these infant mortality regression estimates.

Crafts (1984a:94,98) studied the general marital fertility rate (GMFR) in 619 urban districts of England and Wales for four periods from 1871 to 1911, along with single woman labor force participation rate, income, migration, literacy, sectoral employment, and child mortality (which was significantly positively associated with the GMFR in 1911, but negative and insignificant in 1871, 1881,

---

[16]In much of the earlier research (Livi Bacci, 1971, on Portugal, Knodel, 1974, on Germany, and Coale et al., 1979, on Russia) partial correlation coefficients were published, but not t statistics. We have calculated the t statistics using the published partial correlation coefficients (Wonnacott and Wonnacott, 1979:180) so as to obtain some idea of the statistical significance of the estimates.

TABLE 6-1 Sign and Statistical Significance of Estimates, Elasticity, and $(dF/dq)/F$ from Regressions of Marital Fertility Level on Infant or Child Mortality Level in Multivariate Studies of European Fertility Decline

Country and Region	Number of Districts	Method	Year 1851	1860	1870
Belgium					
Flanders	22	TSLS			
Wallonia	19	TSLS			
England and Wales					
National	125	OLS	(neg) (−0.03)	(NEG) (−0.06)	(NEG) (−0.06)
Urban	619	OLS			(neg)
National	590	OLS			
Urban	222	OLS			
Rural	368	OLS			
Towns	101	OLS			
National	600	OLS			
France	81	OLS		POS	
Germany					
National	71	OLS			
National	71	OLS			
Prussian Kreise	407	OLS			
Prussian Kreise	407	TSLS			
Prussian cities	54	OLS			
Prussian cities	54	TSLS			
Italy					
North and central	53	OLS			
South	34	OLS			
Veneto	57	OLS			
Netherlands	375	OLS		POS	POS
Portugal	18	OLS			
Russia					
Rural	50	OLS			
Urban	50	OLS			

1880	1890	1900	1910	1920	1930	Source
POS	pos	pos	neg			1
0.17 *0.88*	0.10 *0.52*	0.07 *0.37*	0.03 *−0.18*			
pos	pos	pos	pos			1
0.21 *1.62*	0.13 *1.00*	0.57 *4.63*	0.30 *3.09*			
						2
(neg)	(neg)		POS			3
			0.07			
	(NEG)		(NEG)			4
	(NEG)		(POS)			4
	(NEG)		(NEG)			4
			POS			5
POS						6
						7
POS						8
	POS					9
	0.05 *0.25*					
	neg					10
	−0.04 *−0.22*					
	pos					11
	0.17 *0.95*					
	neg					12
	−0.04 *−0.20*					
	neg					13
	−0.16 *−0.82*					
neg			POS		POS	14
NEG			POS		POS	14
(neg)						15
POS	POS					16
			pos		pos	17
		pos			POS	18
		pos			POS	18

continued on next page

TABLE 6-1 (*continued*)

Country and Region	Number of Districts	Method	Year 1851	Year 1860	Year 1870
Spain					
Catalonia	84	OLS		(neg)	
Rural	50	OLS			
Capital cities	50	OLS			
Sweden					
National	25	OLS			
Rural	25	OLS			
Urban	25	OLS			

NOTES: OLS, ordinary least squares. TSLS, two-stage least squares. POS, estimated coefficient is positive and significant within 5 percent. pos, estimated coefficient is positive but not significant within 5 percent. NEG, estimated coefficient is negative and significant within 5 percent. neg, estimated coefficient is negative but not significant within 5 percent. Parentheses mean that the estimated coefficient is difficult to interpret. See text for explanation. The number below the sign is the elasticity, defined as the estimated coefficient multiplied by the mean of infant or child mortality divided by the mean of marital fertility. It is calculated wherever possible. The number in italics next to the elasticity is $(dF/dq)/F$ where F is a measure of marital fertility and q is infant mortality. It is calculated wherever possible. For clarity in the table, I used the opposite sign of the author's estimate where the infant or child mortality measure is life expectancy at birth or some measure of survivorship.

and 1891). However the 1871-1891 regressions suffer from important data limitations, using 1911 data for four variables (Crafts, 1984a:97-99). In a later study, Crafts (1989:332-333) restricted his analysis to 1911 data in 101 towns using similar variables along with age of wife at first marriage and found that births per woman was significantly and positively associated with infant mortality.

Woods (1987:302) studied I_g in 590 districts of England and Wales for 1891 and 1911 along with coal miners, farm servants, females employed in textiles and as servants, literacy rate, and the probability of a child surviving from age 1 to 10 in 1861, defined by Woods as l_{10}/l_1 (1987:301). He used this 1861 child survivorship measure (which excludes infant mortality) as his mortality variable in his 1891 and 1911 fertility regressions (Woods 1987:301). It seems risky to try to estimate fertility using a child mortality measure lagged 30 and 40 years. It seems likely that districts experienced varying rates of mortality decline during

1880	1890	1900	1910	1920	1930	Source
						19
	(POS)	(pos)		POS		20
	(0.28)	(0.18)		0.31		
	(neg)	(NEG)		POS		20
	(−0.19)	(−0.61)		0.53		
			POS	POS		21
			0.45 *6.80*	0.39 *7.62*		
		POS				21
		0.36 *4.47*				
		pos				21
		0.06 *0.52*				

SOURCES: 1: Lesthaege (1977:106, 172, 213); 2: Haines (1979:63, 68); 3: Crafts (1984a:94, 98); 4: Woods (1987:302-304); 5: Crafts (1989:332-333); 6: Friedlander et al. (1991:341); 7: van de Walle (1978:287); 8: Knodel (1974:238); 9: Richards (1977:543-546). Results are based on a regression of pooled data for 1880, 1885, 1890, 1900, and 1910; 10: Galloway et al. (1994:143-152). Results are based on regressions using the average of data over the periods 1875, 1880, 1885, 1890, 1895, 1900, 1905, 1910. Also Appendix Table 6-A3, Equation 1, level; 11: Appendix Table 6-A3; 12: Galloway et al. (1995:38-39). Results are based on regressions using the average of data over the periods 1875, 1880, 1885, 1890, 1895, 1900, 1905, 1910. Also Appendix Table 6A-4, Equation 2, level; 13: Appendix Table 6A-4, Equation 2, level; 14: Livi Bacci (1977:194, 198); 15: Castiglioni et al. (1991:114); 16: Boonstra and van der Woude (1984:23, 34); 17: Livi Bacci (1971:122); 18: Coale et al. (1979:65); 19: Benavente (1989:229); 20: Reher and Iriso-Napal (1989:408, 412, 419, 420); 21: Mosk (1983:186, 252, 254, 257) and Sweden Central Bureau of Statistics (1969:115).

this period of 30-40 years. In both 1891 and 1911, Woods' 1861 measure of child survivorship was positively and significantly associated with I_g, although it is difficult to know what to make of this finding.

Woods (1987:303) examined 222 urban districts using the above data and found that the estimated coefficient on 1861 child survivorship ages 1-10 was significantly positive in 1891 but shifted to significantly negative in 1911. Woods (1987:304) analyzed 368 rural districts using the above data and found a significantly positive association between I_g and 1861 child survivorship ages 1-10 for both periods.

Friedlander et al. (1991:341) examined I_g in 600 districts of England and Wales for the period around 1870-1890 along with density, sectoral employment, females not in the labor force, urban proximity, and life expectancy at birth (which was significantly and negatively associated with I_g). We expect varia-

TABLE 6-2 Sign and Statistical Significance of Estimates, Elasticity, and $(dF/dq)/F$ from Regressions of Marital Fertility Change on Infant Mortality Change in Multivariate Studies of European Fertility Decline

Place	Number of Districts	Method	Period	Estimate	Elasticity	$(dF/dq)/F$	Source
Germany							
Prussian Kreise	71	OLS	1880-1910	POS	0.39	1.96	Richards (1977:543, 545)
Prussian Kreise	407	OLS	1875-1910	POS	0.17	0.95	Galloway et al. (1994:143, 152) and Appendix Table 6-A3, Equation 1, change
Prussian Kreise	407	TSLS	1875-1910	POS	0.70	3.92	Appendix Table 6-A3, Equation 1, change
Prussian cities	54	OLS	1875-1910	POS	0.29	1.49	Galloway et al. (1995:38, 39) and Appendix Table 6-A4, Equation 2, change
Prussian cities	54	TSLS	1875-1910	POS	1.55	7.97	Appendix Table 6-A4, Equation 2, change
Italy							
North and central	53	OLS	1880-1910	pos			Livi Bacci (1977:194, 199)
North and central	53	OLS	1911-1931	POS			Livi Bacci (1977:194, 199)
South	34	OLS	1880-1910	pos			Livi Bacci (1977:194, 199)
South	34	OLS	1911-1931	pos			Livi Bacci (1977:194, 199)
Netherlands	375	OLS	1871-1890	POS			Boonstra and van der Wonde (1984:36)
Sweden							
Urban	25	OLS	1900-1920	POS	0.09	1.15	Mosk (1983:257)
Urban	25	OLS	1900-1930	POS	0.15	2.00	Mosk (1983:254, 257) and Sweden Central Bureau of Statistics (1969:115)

NOTES: OLS, ordinary least squares. TSLS, two-stage least squares. POS, estimated coefficient is positive and significant within 5 percent. pos, estimated coefficient is positive but not significant within 5 percent. Elasticity is the estimated coefficient multiplied by the mean of infant mortality divided by the mean of marital fertility. It is calculated wherever possible. In the expression $(dF/dq)/F$, F is a measure of marital fertility and q is infant mortality. It is calculated wherever possible. Richards' results for Germany are based on a regression of pooled data for 1880, 1885, 1890, 1900, and 1910 using fixed effects. Galloway et al.'s results for Prussian Kreise and Prussian cities are based on regressions of pooled data for 1875, 1880, 1885, 1890, 1895, 1900, 1905, and 1910 using fixed effects. The Netherlands' regressions use crude death rate and crude birth rate instead of infant mortality and marital fertility.

tions in life expectancy at birth to be dominated by variations in overall child mortality, although a measure of overall child mortality would have been preferred.

At first glance, the picture for England and Wales appears confusing. However, it seems appropriate to be highly skeptical about Haines' and Woods' interpretations of their mortality estimates. Half of the variables in Crafts' 1871-1891 regressions used 1911 data. Thus, we are left with Crafts' analysis of 1911 data and Friedlander et al.'s study. Both find the expected significant and positive relationship between overall child mortality and fertility.

France

Van de Walle (1978:287) examined I_g in 81 departments in France for five periods from 1841 to 1851 along with religion, rural land revenue per capita, urbanization, and life expectancy at birth which was probably significantly negatively[17] associated with I_g. Watkins (1991:161) and Lesthaeghe (1992:275-317) did some research along these lines but neither included any measure of mortality in their analyses.

Germany

Knodel (1974:238-239) studied I_g in 71 provinces for the one period 1875-1910 along with religion in 1880, bank accounts in 1900, sectoral employment in 1882, literacy in 1875, and infant mortality rate in 1875 (which was positively and significantly associated with I_g). Knodel used maximum I_g in the interval as his dependent variable so caution must be used in interpreting these results.

Richards (1977:546) examined I_g in 71 provinces for five periods from 1880 to 1910 along with net migration, religion, urbanization, sectoral employment, and infant mortality rate (which was significantly and positively associated with I_g).

Galloway et al. (1994:152) analyzed general marital fertility in 407 Kreise covering all of Prussia using the average of quinquennial data from 1875 to 1910 along with religion, ethnicity, education, health, female labor force participation, income, mining, urbanization, financial, insurance, communication, sex ratio, and legitimate infant mortality variables. Legitimate infant mortality was negatively, but insignificantly, associated with fertility. However, using two-stage least squares the sign shifted to positive (see Appendix Table 6-A3).

Using the same periods and variables, but excluding urbanization and includ-

---

[17]Van de Walle (1978:287) suggests, "On the face of it, we end up with an 'explanation' of the fertility decline along the line of population transition theory, with a major role played by the decline of mortality and with an independent influence of income."

ing manufacturing and population size variables, Galloway et al. (1995:39) found that legitimate infant mortality in the 54 largest cities of Prussia was negatively related to general marital fertility, but not statistically significant. The same results were found using two-stage least squares (see Appendix Table 6-A4).

Italy

Livi Bacci (1977:198) examined I_g in 92 provinces for the periods 1881, 1911, and 1931 along with urbanization, sectoral employment, literacy, proportion married, and infant mortality rate in north and central Italy and south Italy. In north and central Italy infant mortality rate was insignificant in 1881, but positively and significantly associated with I_g in 1911 and 1931. In south Italy infant mortality rate was significantly negatively associated with I_g in 1881, but positively and significantly associated with I_g in 1911 and 1931.

Castiglioni et al. (1991:114) examined I_g in 1881 in 57 districts in Veneto along with topography, occupation, females employed in agriculture, migration, and infant mortality rate. Infant mortality was negatively associated with I_g, but test statistics were not provided.

Netherlands

Boonstra and van der Woude (1984:34, 40, 44, 51) examined the crude birth rate in 375 districts for eight periods from 1851 to 1890 along with net migration, religion, density, literacy, soil type, and crude death rate. The crude death rate was significantly and positively associated with the crude birth rate in each of the eight periods. Unfortunately, more refined measures of fertility and infant or child mortality were not available (Boonstra and van der Woude, 1984:24), but because this appears to be the only study of Netherlands fertility decline using multivariate analysis, we decided to include it.

Portugal

Livi Bacci (1971:122) analyzed I_g in 18 provinces in 1911 and 1930 along with sectoral employment, literacy, and infant mortality rate, which was positively associated with I_g in both periods, but significant only in 1930.

Russia

Coale et al. (1979:65) examined I_g for 50 provinces in rural and urban sectors in 1897 and 1926 along with urbanization, sectoral employment, literacy, and infant mortality rate. In each case, infant mortality rate was positively associated with I_g, but the estimates were significant only in 1926.

Spain

Reher and Iriso-Napal (1989:412) examined I_g in the rural sector of 50 provinces for 1887, 1900, and 1920 along with sectoral employment, migration, urbanization, 1936 political election results, literacy, female nuptiality, and $_5q_0$, which was positively associated with I_g in all periods, but significant only in 1887 and 1920.

Reher and Iriso-Napal (1989:420) also examined I_g in the 50 provincial capital cities for the same three periods along with sectoral employment, females in labor force, migration, city size, 1936 political election results, literacy, female nuptiality, and $_5q_0$, which was insignificantly related to I_g in 1887, significantly negatively associated with I_g in 1900, and significantly positively associated with I_g in 1920.

In the 1887 and 1900 regressions, $_5q_0$ was the average of 1860 and 1900 data (Reher and Iriso-Napal, 1989:410). As a consequence it is difficult to know what to make of the regression estimates. In general it seems unwise to use only two data points, 1860 or 1900, to create a child mortality variable covering 40 years. Even if one had $_5q_0$ data for intervening years, a 40-year average centered around 1880 seems an inappropriate indicator of child mortality when trying to explain 1887 and 1900 fertility. Therefore, we have strong reservations about the $_5q_0$ estimates from the regressions for the first two periods.

Benavente (1989:229) studied I_g in 84 selected local areas, not necessarily representative, of Catalonia in 1857 along with nuptiality, sectoral employment, proximity to France, and child mortality, which was negatively associated with I_g, but insignificant. The child mortality measure is number of deaths per 1,000 for children under age 7 in 1837 (Benavente, 1989:227). It is not clear whether this measure included infant deaths, which are known to be severely under-registered during this period. Furthermore, the 84 local areas analyzed are those areas in which registration data have survived, suggesting additional caution in interpreting the regression finding.

Sweden

Mosk (1983:252) examined I_g in 25 counties in Sweden in 1910 and 1920 along with sectoral employment, wage, primary school attendance, and legitimate infant mortality rate, which was significantly positively associated with I_g.

Mosk (1983:256-257) also studied I_g in the rural sector of 25 Swedish counties in 1900 along with sectoral employment, agricultural wage, social structure, and legitimate infant mortality rate, which was significantly positively associated with I_g. He also examined I_g in the urban sector of 25 Swedish counties in 1900 along with nonagricultural wages and legitimate infant mortality rate. The estimate on infant mortality was positive, but not significantly associated with I_g.

Fertility Change and Changes in Independent Variables

Germany

Using a fixed-effects model, Richards (1977:545) examined I_g in 71 provinces for five periods from 1880 to 1910 along with province dummy variables, net migration, religion, urbanization, sectoral employment, and infant mortality rate, which was significantly and positively associated with I_g.

Galloway et al. (1994:152) analyzed GMFR in 407 Kreise covering all of Prussia using quinquennial data from 1875 to 1910. Independent variables included religion, ethnicity, education, health, female labor force participation, income, mining, urbanization, financial, insurance, communication, sex ratio, legitimate infant mortality, and 407 Kreis dummies. From this fixed-effects model, changes in legitimate infant mortality were found to be positively and significantly associated with changes in fertility. Among all the independent variables, legitimate infant mortality was the fourth most important in terms of contribution to predicted change in average GMFR from 1875 to 1910, just behind female labor force participation, insurance, and communication variables (Galloway et al., 1994:156). A two-stage least-squares model also yielded a positive and significant association between fertility change and infant mortality change (see Appendix Table 6-A3).

Using the same periods and variables, but excluding urbanization and the 407 Kreise dummies variables, and including manufacturing, population size, and 54 city dummy variables, Galloway et al. (1995:39) found that change in legitimate infant mortality in the 54 largest cities of Prussia was positively and significantly related to changes in the GMFR. In terms of components of predicted change in average GMFR from 1875 to 1910, legitimate infant mortality was second only to female labor force participation in importance among all the variables considered (Galloway et al., 1995:41). Our two-stage least-squares model also revealed a positive and significant association between changes in fertility and changes in infant mortality (see Appendix Table 6-A4).

Italy

Livi Bacci (1977:199) examined change in I_g in 92 provinces for the periods 1881-1911 and 1911-1931 along with changes in urbanization, sectoral employment, literacy, proportion married, and changes in infant mortality rate in north-central and southern Italy. Changes in infant mortality were not significantly associated with changes in I_g in either region from 1881 to 1911, insignificant in the south from 1911 to 1931, but significantly positively associated with I_g in north-central Italy from 1911 to 1931. Each of the four estimated infant mortality change coefficients was positive.

Netherlands

Boonstra and van der Woude (1984:36) examined change in the crude birth rate in 375 districts for the period from 1871 to 1890 along with change in density; change in crude death rate; and levels of net migration, religion, density, literacy, and soil type. Change in the crude death rate was significantly and positively associated with change in the crude birth rate.

Sweden

Mosk (1983:257) examined changes in I_g in the urban sector of 25 Swedish counties from 1900 to 1920 and 1900 to 1930 along with changes in nonagricultural wages and changes in legitimate infant mortality, which were positively and significantly associated with changes in I_g in both periods.

Interpretation Problems and Some Suggestions

Interpretation problems in the analyses of level effects generally revolve around questionable definitions of the infant and child mortality variables, the use of explanatory variables in inappropriate time frames, and reliance on strictly bivariate correlations. We suspect that most of these problems result from data limitations in the original source material. Nonetheless, we found it necessary to address these problems to obtain a reasonably convincing overall picture of previous findings.

It would be useful if future researchers would include a detailed discussion of the quality of the data, especially of infant mortality, and would provide the reader with an unambiguous explanation of each variable's construction. In many cases we simply were not told what period was covered by the mortality variable. For example, was an infant mortality variable for 1890 based on the average of annual rates from 1888 to 1892, the average from 1889 to 1891, or simply the one year 1890? If the latter, then there are serious questions about the variable's relevance because we know that infant mortality rates can vary substantially from year to year.

Rather than divide a data set into two groups, and then run regressions for each group separately as some authors have done, it might be more instructive simply to create a dummy variable for each group and interact each independent variable with the dummy. This would preserve sample size and enable the researcher to determine whether the estimates for a given group are significantly different from the estimates for another group. Of course the best approach is to operationalize the variable that theoretically distinguishes the groups from each other, rather than rely on a dummy.

We found that using appropriate instruments for the infant mortality variable actually shifted the estimated impact of infant mortality on fertility from negative in our ordinary least-squares regression to positive using two-stage least squares in our analysis of Kreis levels (Appendix Table 6-A3). There was no difference in sign or significance in the ordinary least-squares and two-stage least-squares estimates in terms of change (Appendix Tables 6-A3 and 6-A4). Theory suggests that it is necessary to use statistical methods, such as instrumental variables, which can deal with problem of simultaneity.

Finally, we believe that the appropriate model for analyzing fertility decline involves the regression of changes in fertility on changes in the explanatory variables. We use a fixed-effects model. Although this places greater demands on the data set, both in terms of quality and quantity, it yields the most relevant results.

FINDINGS

Signs and Significance of Estimates

Table 6-1 summarizes the results of the regressions of the infant mortality level on the fertility level. If we discount the estimates that are difficult to interpret, and use our two-stage least-squares estimates for Prussian Kreise and cities instead of our ordinary least-squares estimates, we see that for levels nearly all the estimates are positive (34 of 38), as theory would predict. Of the 24 statistically significant estimates, 23 have positive signs. Of the 14 estimates that are not statistically significant, 11 are positive. Of these 11, 8 had relatively small samples sizes (*n* less than 26).

Although the study of fertility level may be interesting, analysis of fertility change is most relevant to demographic transition theory. Table 6-2 summarizes the ten regressions that examine the effects of changes in infant and child mortality on changes in fertility. Again we use the two-stage least-squares estimates instead of the ordinary least-squares estimates for Prussian Kreise and cities, although in this case it makes no difference because they have the same signs and significance. For changes the estimates are positive in every case (ten of ten), and significant in seven of them.

Elasticities

To compare the magnitude of the impact of infant mortality on fertility across countries, we calculated, where possible, the elasticity of fertility with respect to mortality. Figure 6-2 presents the distribution of elasticities for level effects for all interpretable estimates.[18] The average elasticity for levels is 0.21 (0.13 if we include the seven estimates that are difficult to interpret). In other

---

[18]The two-stage least-squares estimates, rather than the ordinary least-squares estimates, are used for Prussia in this and all subsequent discussion.

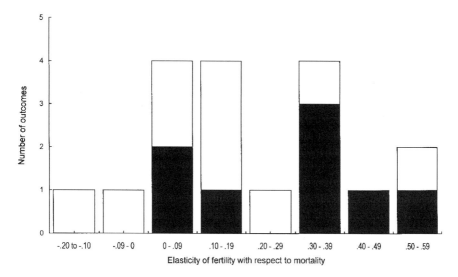

FIGURE 6-2 Distribution of elasticities of fertility with respect to mortality, level effects. NOTES: Only interpretable estimates are included. Mean is 0.21. The dark shading indicates statistically significant estimates. The light shading indicates statistically insignificant estimates. Only the two-stage least-squares estimates are used for Prussia.

words, on average a 10 percent decrease in infant mortality leads to about a 2.1 percent decline in fertility.

We are much more interested in the elasticities derived from studies that examine the effect of changes in infant mortality on fertility. We have such elasticity data for Germany, Prussian Kreise, Prussian cities, and urban Sweden (Table 6-2). The average elasticity is 0.58 and the distribution is shown in Figure 6-3. Elasticities of infant mortality and fertility change models appear to be much higher than in the level models. The elasticity in Germany was 0.39, 0.79 in Prussian Kreise, and 1.55 in Prussian cities. This suggests that the fertility of urban populations in Prussia was much more responsive to mortality changes than that of rural populations. A possible explanation for the high urban elasticity might be that urban couples may have become relatively more aware of infant mortality decline and its relation to infant and child survivorship, which may in turn have caused them to reduce fertility at a relatively faster rate (as measured by elasticity). This increased awareness may have been a result of a greater access to information about infant mortality decline from newspapers, pamphlets, books, organizations, peers, or health workers found in the cities.

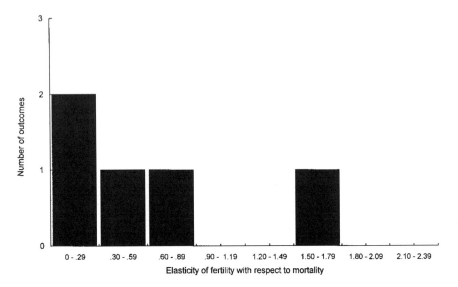

FIGURE 6-3 Distribution of elasticities of fertility with respect to mortality, change effects. NOTES: Only interpretable estimates are included. Mean is 0.58. All estimates are statistically significant. Only the two-stage least-squares estimates are used for Prussia.

Child Replacement and Lactation Interruption

There are two important points of reference for interpreting the size of the estimated effects. First, how large a response of fertility to infant mortality would be required to leave the population growth rate unaffected? And second, how large an effect can be expected from lactation interruption alone?

Let the number of children surviving to some age, say 15 years, be $SF = (1 - Q)F$, where F is the total number of births born over the reproductive years of a woman, and S is the survival probability from birth to age 15. Whereas in earlier equations M referred to general child mortality, here we use $Q = {}_{15}q_0$ and $q = {}_1q_0$ for specific measures, and $S = 1 - {}_{15}q_0$ and $s = 1 - {}_1q_0$ for their complements. The effect on the number of surviving children of a variation in mortality before this age, Q, is $d(SF)/dQ = dF/dQ\,(1 - Q) - F$. There is said to be complete replacement when this is zero, and this corresponds roughly to the situation in which a change in mortality does not affect the long-term population growth rate. In our data we observe marital fertility, not total fertility F, but let us for now ignore this fact. In our data we also observe the infant mortality rate q rather than mortality to age 15, Q. Fortunately, q and Q are fairly closely linked, so we may use q as a proxy for Q. The question then becomes: How sensitively must F respond to q for SF, the number of surviving children, to be constant when q varies? Or what is the benchmark value of $(dF/dq)/F$, call it $[(dF/dq)/F)]^*$, such that $d(SF)/dq$ is 0? Differentiating and solving, we find that $[(dF/dq)/F)]^* = (dQ/dq)/(1 - Q)$, which is the desired benchmark.

To attach an actual number to this benchmark we need to know dQ, dq, and Q. In principle, the relation of Q to q could be anything, and indeed over relatively short periods there can be a great deal of variation in the relation of changes in the two measures. For example, $(dQ/dq)/(1 - Q)$ in Germany is 2.30 in the 1870s, 8.22 in the 1880s, 2.65 in the 1890s, 2.12 in the 1900s, and 1.87 from 1910 to 1925 (Statistischen Reichsamt, 1930:168). However, over a series of longer periods, or for general tendencies as expressed in model life tables, the relation is much more regular. An examination of the Coale and Demeny (1983) Model West Female life tables shows that $\ln(1 - Q)$ is nearly linear in q, with a slope of about 2.5; that is, $\ln(1 - Q) = k - 2.5q$. Differentiating this expression, we find that $(dQ/dq)/(1 - Q) = 2.5$, which is the break-even point. The significance of this convenient empirical fact is that the break-even value is roughly constant over the course of the demographic transition and does not vary with the general level of fertility or mortality. This value of 2.5 agrees well with the value of 2.44 calculated over the entire period 1870-1925 for Germany (Statistischen Reichsamt, 1930:168). Table 6-1 provides $(dF/dq)/F$ for levels, where calculable, and these are plotted in Figure 6-4. The average is about 2.11. The

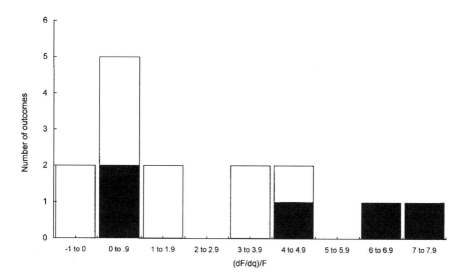

FIGURE 6.4 Distribution of sensitivities of fertility to mortality measured by $(dF/dq)/F$ level effects. NOTES: Only interpretable estimates are included. Mean is 2.11 The dark shading indicates statistically significant estimates. The light shading indicates statistically insignificant estimates. Only the two-stage least-squares estimates are used for Prussia.

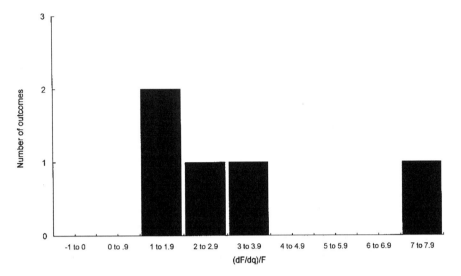

FIGURE 6-5 Distribution of sensitivities of fertility to mortality measured by $(dF/dq)/F$ change effects. NOTES: Only interpretable estimates are included. Mean is 3.40. All estimates are statistically significant. Only the two-stage least-squares estimates are used for Prussia.

distribution of $(dF/dq)/F$ for changes is shown in Figure 6-5 which is based on data in Table 6-2. For changes, the mean of $(dF/dq)/F$ is about 3.40.

It is worth considering the possible role of the lactation interruption effect in bringing about a positive causal effect of infant mortality on marital fertility. Preston (1978:8) gives a useful analysis of this question. He concludes that $(dF/dq)/F = (P2 - P1)/I$, where $P1$ is the average period of sterility following a live birth that results in an infant death, and $P2$ is the average period of sterility following a live birth that results in a surviving infant, while I is the overall average length of a birth interval. $P1$ and $P2$ will differ due to the lactation interruption effect and also because of the effect of practices and taboos such as prescription of intercourse while breastfeeding, or spending time following delivery with the mother's family. In the context of Europe, it is mainly the lactation interruption effect that is likely to have mattered.

Knodel (1978:25) provides a useful summary of evidence from European micro-level family reconstitution studies. The lactation interruption effect ($P2 - P1$) varies widely from 12 months to no months, apparently due to wide differences in breastfeeding practices. Average birth intervals (I) are about 30 months. The values of $(dF/dq)/F$ will thus range from 0 to 0.4. We use our calculation of $(dF/dq)/F$ from German data discussed above, and let $P2 - P1$ be on average about 6 months and I about 30 months, all reasonable averages for Prussia. Recall from above that the value of $(dF/dq)/F$ for complete offset is 2.44. The value of $(dF/dq)/F$ from lactation interruption alone is 0.2. Thus, lactation interruption accounts for only one-twelfth of the effect needed for full replacement. This is far too low to account for the size of response of fertility to infant mortality change that we observe in our data, and which has typically been found in studies of historical Europe.

Dynamic Stability

If the product of the estimated structural coefficients indicating the effect of fertility on infant mortality, and indicating the effect of infant mortality on fertility, is greater than unity, then the system they describe is dynamically unstable. In this case, an external shock that raised mortality, for example, would lead to an increase in fertility, which would lead to an increase in mortality larger than the first, and initiate an explosive spiral. One might take the view that because history has not been explosive, the product of the true coefficients must be less than unity. This would also imply that the first term in the bias expression given earlier is positive, and thereby remove one possible source of negative bias, making it more difficult to explain the direction of bias we have found in our estimates. However, one might equally take the view that in fact history has been explosive. Wolpin (in this volume) describes such a view, suggesting that an exogenous decrease in infant and child mortality may have set off a downward spiral of fertility and mortality. This would imply that the first term in the bias expression is negative, making it easier to explain the direction of bias we found. In our actual two-stage least-squares estimates, we find that this product in Prussian Kreise is 0.53 (Appendix tables 6-A3 and 6-A6) and in Prussian cities 0.95 (Appendix tables 6-A4 and 6-A7), suggesting dynamic stability in both areas, but with the cities bordering on instability.

Perhaps it is more interesting to examine the ultimate effect on fertility of an exogenous change in mortality, taking the coefficient estimates at face value. Let fertility F be a linear function of infant mortality q with coefficient b, and let q be a linear function of f with coefficient d. Let intercepts be a and c, respectively. Then c is the shifter to represent an exogenous change in q. We can solve for the equilibrium level of F, say F^*, after all changes have worked their way through the system. This is

$$F^* = (a + bc)/(1 - bd).$$

The estimated coefficient b gives the initial impact of q on F, while the factor $1/(1 - bd)$ accounts for the feedback cycle. With two-stage least-squares estimates, b is 1.03 in Kreise and 1.84 in cities, d is 0.51 in Kreise and 0.52 in cities, so that bd is 0.53 in the Kreise and 0.95 in the cities, as mentioned in the preceding paragraph. The multiplier $1/(1 - bd)$ in Kreise is about 2 and in the cities about 20. This suggests that the cities are very near to dynamic instability, whereas in the more rural areas the feedback is also important, but not so much as in the cities. With ordinary least-squares estimates the feedback multipliers are about 1.1 for both Kreis and cities, which seems more realistic.

We do not want to make too much of these results because our analysis lacks dynamic structure. The important point is that estimates of impacts do not tell the entire story. The full effects may be larger by a lot or by a little as the feedbacks play out.

CONCLUSIONS

According to theory, fertility and infant mortality should affect each other simultaneously, and these effects should be positive. A review and assessment of published research on European marital fertility and infant mortality suggest that there is a generally consistent, significant, and positive association between infant mortality level and marital fertility level. The evidence for this positive association of levels is stronger than has been realized. However, we argue that this association of levels is largely irrelevant for the policy issues of interest.

The evidence appears even stronger in studies that examine the association of changes in infant mortality with changes in marital fertility, which is more appropriate for examining secular fertility decline and most relevant for policy issues. In every case, changes in infant mortality are positively associated with changes in fertility and most are significant. However, there are important issues of causality that must be resolved before drawing conclusions. The few studies that attempted to disentangle the direction of causality using instrumental variables estimation found, as we did, that important causality was operating in both directions.

If we take these estimates of association at face value, then they are mostly far larger than could be explained by lactation interruption. They are also substantial relative to the size necessary to bring about a complete offset of fertility when mortality changes, leaving growth rates unchanged. Some are smaller than this offset level, some about equal to it, and some are larger than it. We are suspicious of estimates that indicate more than completely offsetting changes in fertility, which we find in our own two-stage least-squares estimates.

In general, parameter estimates using instrumental variables techniques are sensitive to the specific choice of instruments. Although we cannot be sure that the instruments we used in our estimation are the most appropriate, we believe they are the best given the data that are available. Furthermore, we cannot completely rule out the possibility that the estimated associations of fertility and mortality, even when using instrumental variables and fixed-effects methods, actually reflect a spurious association induced by unobserved variables that influence both fertility and mortality and that change over time. These variables might include breastfeeding, health conditions, nutrition, or unobserved aspects of economic development and modernization.

Nonetheless, we believe that the repeated estimation of positive associations, particularly with instrumental variables and fixed-effects models, likely does reflect a true and substantial effect of mortality change on fertility change. In the case of Prussia, we have been able to include an unusually extensive array of variables measuring differing aspects of socioeconomic change, and we still find strong positive effects of mortality change on change in fertility. Uncertainty arising from possible unobserved time-varying factors is a problem when making inferences from any time series analysis, not just this one, and there are corresponding problems with any cross-sectional analysis. On balance, then, we believe that there is substantial evidence that mortality decline was an important cause of fertility decline in Europe.

APPENDIX

Appendix tables begin on the following page.

TABLE 6-A1 Definitions of Variables Used in the Analysis

Variable	Definition
GMFR	General marital fertility rate (legitimate births per 1,000 married females 15-49).
Catholic	Catholics per 100 total population.
Slav	Slavic speakers per 100 total population.
Church	Employees in religious occupations per 100 population over age 20.
Education	Teaching employees per 100 population aged 6-13.
Health	Health employees per 100 total population.
FLFPR	Female labor force participation rate (employed females per 100 female population aged 20-69) (excludes agriculture and service).
Income	Average real income of male elementary school teachers in Deutsche marks as of 1900.
Mining	Mining employees per 100 employed persons.
Manufacturing	Manufacturing employees per 100 employed persons. Used only in the city model
Urban	Urban population per 100 total population. Used only in the Kreis model.
Bank	Banking employees per 100 population over age 20.
Insurance	Insurance employees per 100 population over age 20.
Communications	Post, telegraph, and railway employees per 100 population over age 20.
Population	Population, in thousands. Used only in the city model.
Infant mortality	Legitimate infant mortality rate (legitimate deaths under age one per 1,000 legitimate births).
Married sex ratio	Married males/married females.
Kreis born	Population born in Kreis per 100 total population. Used only in the Kreis model.
City born	Population born in city per 100 total population. Used only in the city model.
Sanitation	Cumulative municipal sanitation bond debt per capita in Deutsche marks. Available only for cities.
ASDR	Age-specific death rate for males aged 30-34. Data are available only for Regierungsbezirke.

NOTES: For details and sources see Galloway et al. (1994, 1995, 1996). Data are available quinquennially from 1875 to 1910. Vital registration variables are based on 5-year average centered around each quinquennial year. Stillbirths are excluded throughout. There are 36 Regierungsbezirke and 407 Kreise in Prussia. We also examined 54 cities. In general, the German occupational censuses do not lend themselves to calculation of economic sector variables because of a peculiar redefinition of female agricultural laborers that leads to an improbable 2 million increase in the category between 1895 and 1907 (Tipton, 1976:153-158). However, city populations were probably not affected by this problem because there were few agricultural workers in the cities. This is the reason the variable Manufacturing is available only in the cities. Mining is available for both Kreise and cities because virtually all miners were men.

TABLE 6-A2 Models Used in the Fertility Analysis

Variable	Kreis Fertility Model (equation (1))	City Fertility Model (equation (2))	Expected Sign
Dependent	GMFR	GMFR	
Independent	Catholic	Catholic	+
	Slav	Slav	+
	Church	Church	+
	Education	Education	−
	Health	Health	−
	FLFPR	FLFPR	−
	Income	Income	−
	Mining	Mining	+
		Manufacturing	+
	Urban		−
	Bank	Bank	−
	Insurance	Insurance	−
	Communications	Communications	−
		Population	−
	Infant mortality	Infant mortality	+
	Married sex ratio	Married sex ratio	+

NOTES: In equation (1) two-stage least-squares age specific death rate (ASDR) for males aged 30-34 is used as an instrument for Infant Mortality. In equation (2) two-stage least-squares Sanitation and ASDR are used as instruments for Infant Mortality.

TABLE 6-A3 Equation (1): Summary of Ordinary and Two-Stage Least-Squares Fertility Regression Results for Kreise in Prussia, 1875-1910 (dependent variable is GMFR)

Variable	Expected Sign	Level		Change	
		OLS	TSLS	OLS	TSLS
Constant		189.374**	258.026**		
Catholic	+	0.693**	0.716**	−2.138**	−1.654**
Slav	+	0.348**	0.137	−0.283	−1.161**
Church	+	1.013	10.586	23.231**	38.721**
Education	−	−5.488‡	−5.816	−9.075**	−7.164**
Health	−	−32.456*	−42.767*	−6.596	24.430‡
FLFPR	−	−0.529‡	−2.296*	−1.235**	−1.153**
Income	−	−0.014	0.032	−0.002	0.004
Mining	+	1.032**	1.251**	0.757**	0.430
Urban	−	0.034	−0.089	0.107	−0.385‡
Bank	−	−36.020	1.850	−55.325**	−26.903‡
Insurance	−	29.251	−48.872	−133.466**	−66.125*
Communications	−	−0.453	5.708	−7.333**	−1.799
Infant mortality	+	−0.052‡	0.478‡	0.242**	1.028**
Married sex ratio	+	91.828‡	−107.824	40.674*	−57.928

NOTES: OLS, ordinary least squares. TSLS, two-stage least squares. The unit of analysis is the Kreise. The level regressions use averages of each variable over eight quinquennial periods from 1875 to 1910. The change regressions are fixed-effects models using data for eight quinquennial periods from 1875 to 1910. Estimates for the 407 Kreis dummy variables are omitted. In the level regressions n = 407 and OLS R^2 = 0.681. In the change regressions n = 3,256 and OLS R^2 = 0.920. **, *, ‡ indicate that the coefficient is statistically significant at the 1 percent, 5 percent, and 10 percent levels, respectively, two-tailed test. Age-specific death rate for males aged 30-34 is used as an instrument for Infant Mortality in the two-stage least-squares regressions for both level and change. The two-stage least-squares t statistics are based on the structural residuals (Hall et al., 1992:133-134) and are asymptotically correct. The ordinary least-squares results are discussed at length in Galloway et al. (1994).

TABLE 6-A4 Equation (2): Summary of Ordinary and Two-Stage
Least-Squares Fertility Regression Results for Cities in Prussia, 1875-1910
(dependent variable is GMFR)

Variable	Expected Sign	Level		Change	
		OLS	TSLS	OLS	TSLS
Constant		422.365*	448.292*		
Catholic	+	0.581**	0.628**	−0.044	2.354‡
Slav	+	0.275	0.218	2.010*	−1.990
Church	+	25.989	18.053	−2.113	25.009
Education	−	−4.064	−4.589	−4.585**	−4.809‡
Health	−	−1.314	−1.618	7.693	96.812**
FLFPR	−	−1.264*	−0.976	−3.571**	−0.919
Income	−	0.004	−0.004	−0.022**	−0.030**
Mining	+	1.828**	1.616*	0.161	−1.221
Manufacturing	+	0.761*	0.468	0.357	−0.221
Bank	−	−44.682*	−53.788*	−11.139	54.861‡
Insurance	−	17.901	23.651	−43.001**	11.970
Communications	−	−5.276*	−6.122‡	−5.959*	−0.045
Population	−	−0.007	0.002	−0.041**	0.056
Infant mortality	+	−0.042	−0.187	0.337**	1.836**
Married sex ratio	+	−193.165	−163.150	354.038**	194.328

NOTES: OLS, ordinary least squares. TSLS, two-stage least squares. The unit of analysis is the
city. The level regressions use averages of each variable over eight quinquennial periods from 1875
to 1910. The change regressions are fixed-effects models using data for eight quinquennial periods
from 1875 to 1910. Estimates for the 54 city dummy variables are omitted. In level regressions $n =$
54 and OLS R^2 = 0.888. In the change regressions n = 432 and OLS R^2 = 0.896. **, *, ‡ indicate
that coefficient is statistically significant at the 1 percent, 5 percent, and 10 percent levels, respectively, two-tailed test. Sanitation and age-specific death rate for males aged 30-34 are used as
instruments for Infant Mortality in the two-stage least-squares regressions for both level and change.
The two-stage least-squares t statistics are based on the structural residuals (Hall et al., 1992:133-
134) and are asymptotically correct. The ordinary least-squares results are discussed at length in
Galloway et al. (1994).

TABLE 6-A5 Models Used in the Infant Mortality Analysis

| Variable | Infant Mortality Model | | Expected Sign |
	Kreis (equation (3))	City (equation (4))	
Dependent	Infant mortality	Infant mortality	
Independent	Catholic	Catholic	+
	Slav	Slav	+
	Education	Education	−
	Health	Health	−
	FLFPR	FLFPR	+
	Income	Income	−
	Urban		+
	Communications	Communications	−
		Population	+
	GMFR	GMFR	+
	Kreis born	City born	−
		Sanitation	−

NOTES: In equation (3) two-stage least squares, Church, Mining, Bank, Insurance, and Married sex ratio are used as instruments for GMFR. In equation (4) two-stage least squares, Church, Mining, Manufacturing, Bank, Insurance, and Married sex ratio are used as instruments for GMFR.

TABLE 6-A6 Equation (3): Summary of Ordinary and Two-Stage
Least-Squares Infant Mortality Regression Results for Kreise in Prussia,
1875-1910 (dependent variable is infant mortality rate)

Variable	Expected Sign	Level		Change	
		OLS	TSLS	OLS	TSLS
Constant		656.315**	723.051**		
Catholic	+	0.325**	0.475	0.109	0.639**
Slav	+	0.087	0.132	0.898**	0.925**
Education	–	−15.705**	−18.071**	−0.483	1.892
Health	–	−7.386	−14.945	−43.048**	−35.017**
FLFPR	+	2.567**	2.364**	0.050	0.362‡
Income	–	−0.110**	−0.111**	−0.009**	−0.007*
Urban	+	−0.256	−0.286	0.366**	0.392**
Communications	–	−12.640**	−12.368**	−5.862**	−3.967**
GMFR	+	−0.304**	−0.503	0.297**	0.512**
Kreis born	–	−3.418**	−3.559**	−0.333**	−4.10**

NOTES: OLS, ordinary least squares. TSLS, two-stage least squares. The unit of analysis is the Kreis. The level regressions use averages of each variable over eight quinquennial periods from 1875 to 1910. The change regressions are fixed-effects models using data for eight quinquennial periods from 1875 to 1910. Estimates for the 407 Kreis dummy variables are omitted. In the level regressions $n = 407$ and ordinary least-squares $R^2 = 0.432$. In the change regressions $n = 3,256$ and $R^2 = 0.922$. **, *, ‡ indicate that the coefficient is statistically significant at the 1 percent, 5 percent, and 10 percent levels, respectively, two-tailed test. Church, Mining, Bank, Insurance, and Married sex ratio are used as instruments for GMFR in the two-stage least-squares regressions for both level and change. The two-stage least-squares t statistics are based on the structural residuals (Hall et al., 1992:133-134) and are asympototically correct. These results are discussed at length in Galloway et al. (1996).

TABLE 6-A7 Equation (4): Summary of Ordinary and Two-Stage Least-Squares Fertility Regression Results for Cities in Prussia, 1875-1910 (dependent variable is infant mortality rate)

Variable	Expected Sign	Level		Change	
		OLS	TSLS	OLS	TSLS
Constant		459.350**	455.027**		
Catholic	+	0.621‡	0.609	−1.345**	−1.296*
Slav	+	−0.737	−0.743	1.983**	1.287
Education	−	−0.082	0.104	0.207	1.954
Health	−	−51.765	−51.793	−58.008**	−52.045**
FLFPR	+	0.977	1.002	−0.547	0.614
Income	−	−0.073**	−0.073**	0.009*	0.014**
Communications	−	−7.184	−7.084	−7.551**	−3.649
Population	+	0.053*	0.053*	−0.053**	−0.033‡
GMFR	+	−0.198	−0.183	0.247**	0.517**
City born	−	−2.215**	−2.220**	−0.852*	−0.289
Sanitation	−	−0.906	−0.910	−0.434**	−0.287*

NOTES: OLS, ordinary least squares. TSLS, two-stage least squares. The unit of analysis is the city. The level regressions use averages of each variable over eight quinquennial periods from 1875 to 1910. The change regressions are fixed-effects models using data for eight quinquennial periods from 1875 to 1910. Estimates for the 54 city dummy variables are omitted. In the level regressions $n = 54$ and ordinary least-squares $R^2 = 0.412$. In the change regressions $n = 432$ and $R^2 = 0.903$. **, *, ‡ indicate that the coefficient is statistically significant at the 1 percent, 5 percent, and 10 percent levels, respectively, two-tailed test. Church, Mining, Manufacturing, Bank, Insurance, and Married sex ratio are used as instruments for GMFR in the two-level least-squares regressions for both level and change. The two-stage least-squares t statistics are based on the structural residuals (Hall et al., 1992:133-134) and are asympototically correct. These results are discussed at length in Galloway et al. (1996).

ACKNOWLEDGMENTS

We are grateful for helpful comments from Barney Cohen, Mark Montgomery, Ken Wachter, and two anonymous reviewers on an earlier version of this chapter. The research on which this chapter was based was funded by grants HD25841 and HD07275 from the U.S. National Institute of Child Health and Human Development.

REFERENCES

Benavente, J.
   1989   Social change and early fertility decline in Catalonia. *European Journal of Population* 5:207-234.
Boonstra, O.W.A., and A.M. van der Woude
   1984   Demographic transition in the Netherlands, a statistical analysis of regional differences in the level and development of the birth rate and of fertility 1850-1890. *A.A.G. Bijdragen* 24:1-57.
Brass W., and J.C. Barrett
   1978   Measurement problems in the analysis of linkages between fertility and child mortality. Pp. 209-233 in S.H. Preston, ed., *The Effects of Infant and Child Mortality on Fertility.* New York: Academic Press.
Castiglioni, M., G. Dalla Zuanna, and S. La Mendola
   1991   Differenze di feconditá fra i distretti del Veneto attorno al 1881. Analisi descrittiva e ipotesi interpretative. Pp. 73-149 in F. Rossi, ed., *La Transizione Demografica nel Veneto, Alcuni Spunti di Ricerca.* Bassano: Infosfera.
Coale, A.J., and P. Demeny
   1983   *Regional Model Life Tables and Stable Populations.* New York: Academic Press.
Coale, A.J., and R. Treadway
   1986   A summary of the changing distribution of overall fertility, marital fertility, and the proportion married in the provinces of Europe. Pp. 31-181 in A.J. Coale and S.C. Watkins, eds., *The Decline of Fertility in Europe.* Princeton, N.J.: Princeton University Press.
Coale, A.J., B.A. Anderson, and E. Härm
   1979   *Human Fertility in Russia since the Nineteenth Century.* Princeton, N.J.: Princeton University Press.
Crafts, N.F.R.
   1984a   A cross-sectional study of legitimate fertility in England and Wales, 1911. *Research in Economic History* 9:89-107.
   1984b   A time series study of fertility in England and Wales, 1877-1938. *Journal of European Economic History* 13(3):571-590.
   1989   Duration of marriage, fertility and women's employment opportunities in England and Wales in 1911. *Population Studies* 43:325-355.
Demeny, P.
   1968   Early fertility decline in Austria-Hungary: A lesson in demographic transition. *Daedalus* 97(2):502-522.
Fialová, L., P. Pavlík, and P. Veres
   1990   Fertility decline in Czechoslovakia during the last two centuries. *Population Studies* 44:89-106.
Flinn, M.W.
   1981   *The European Demographic System, 1500-1820.* Baltimore, Md.: Johns Hopkins University Press.

Friedlander, D., J. Schellekens, and E. Ben-Moshe
  1991   The transition from high to low marital fertility: Cultural or socioeconomic determinants. *Economic Development and Cultural Change* 39(2):331-351.

Galloway, P.R.
  1986   Annual variations in deaths by age, deaths by cause, prices, and weather in London 1670 to 1830. *Population Studies* 39(3):487-505.
  1988   Basic patterns in annual variations in fertility, nuptiality, mortality, and prices in pre-industrial Europe. *Population Studies* 42(2):275-303.
  1994   Secular changes in the short-term preventive, positive, and temperature checks to population growth in Europe, 1460-1909. *Climatic Change* 26:3-63.

Galloway, P.R., E.A. Hammel, and R.D. Lee
  1994   Fertility decline in Prussia 1875 to 1910: A pooled cross-section time series analysis. *Population Studies* 48(1):135-158.

Galloway, P.R., R.D. Lee, and E.A. Hammel
  1995   Urban versus Rural: Fertility Decline in the Cities and Rural Districts of Prussia, 1875 to 1910. Unpublished manuscript, Demography Department, University of California, Berkeley.
  1996   Infant Mortality Decline in the Cities and Rural Districts of Prussia 1875 to 1910. Unpublished manuscript, Demography Department, University of California, Berkeley.

Haines, M.
  1979   *Fertility and Occupation, Population Patterns in Industrialization.* New York: Academic Press.
  1989   Social class differentials during fertility decline: England and Wales revisited. *Population Studies* 43:305-323.

Hall, B.H., C. Cummins, and R. Schnake
  1992   *Time Series Processor Version 4.2 Reference Manual.* Palo Alto, Calif.: TSP International.

Haynes, S.E., L. Phillips, and H.L. Votey
  1985   An econometric test of structural change in the demographic transition. *Scandinavian Journal of Economics* 87(3):554-567.

Kintner, H.J.
  1985   Trends and regional differences in breastfeeding in Germany from 1871 to 1937. *Journal of Family History* 10(2):163-182.

Knodel, J.
  1974   *The Decline of Fertility in Germany, 1871-1939.* Princeton, N.J.: Princeton University Press.
  1978   European populations in the past: Family-level relations. Pp. 21-45 in S.H. Preston, ed., *The Effects of Infant and Child Mortality on Fertility.* New York: Academic Press.
  1988   *Demographic Behavior in the Past: A Study of Fourteen German Village Populations in the Eighteenth and Nineteenth Centuries.* Cambridge, England: Cambridge University Press.

Königliches Statistisches Bureau
  1904   Rückblick auf die Entwickelung der preussischen Bevölkerung von 1875 bis 1900. *Preussische Statistik* 188:1-160.

Lee, R.D.
  1981   Short-term variation: Vital rates, prices and weather. Pp. 356-401 in E.A. Wrigley and R.S. Schofield, *The Population History of England 1541-1871, A Reconstruction.* London: Edward Arnold.
  1987   Population dynamics of humans and other animals. *Demography* 24(4):443-466.

Lee, R.D., and R.A. Bulatao
  1983   The demand for children: A critical essay. Pp. 233-287 in R.A. Bulatao and R.D. Lee,
          eds., *Determinants of Fertility in Developing Countries*. New York: Academic Press.
Lesthaeghe, R.
  1977   *The Decline of Belgian Fertility, 1800-1970*. Princeton, N.J.: Princeton University Press.
  1992   Motivation et légitimation: Conditions de vie et régimes de fécondité en Belgique et en
          France du XVIe au XVIIIe siècle. Pp. 275-317 in A. Blum, N. Bonneuil, and D. Blanchet,
          eds., *Modèles de la Demographie Historique*. Paris: Presses Universitaires de France.
Livi Bacci, M.
  1971   *A Century of Portuguese Fertility*. Princeton, N.J.: Princeton University Press.
  1977   *A History of Italian Fertility during the Last Two Centuries*. Princeton, N.J.: Princeton
          University Press.
Lutz, W.
  1987   *Finnish Fertility Since 1722*. Helsinki, Finland: The Population Research Institute.
Matthiessen, P.C., and J.C. McCann
  1978   The role of mortality in the European fertility transition: Aggregate-level relations. Pp.
          47-68 in S.H. Preston, ed. *The Effects of Infant and Child Mortality on Fertility*. New
          York: Academic Press.
Mosk, C.
  1983   *Patriarchy and Fertility: Japan and Sweden, 1880-1960*. New York: Academic Press.
Preston, S.H.
  1978   Introduction. Pp. 1-18 in S.H. Preston, ed., *The Effects of Infant and Child Mortality on
          Fertility*. New York: Academic Press.
Reher, D.S., and P.L. Iriso-Napal
  1989   Marital fertility and its determinants in rural and in urban Spain, 1887-1930. *Population
          Studies* 43:405-427.
Richards, T.
  1977   Fertility decline in Germany: An econometric appraisal. *Population Studies* 31(3):537-
          553.
Smith, D.S.
  1977   A homeostatic demographic regime: Patterns in west European family reconstitution
          studies.   Pp. 19-52 in R.D. Lee, ed., *Population Patterns in the Past*. New York:
          Academic Press.
Statistischen Reichsamt
  1930   *Statistik des Deutschen Reichs*, Vol. 360. Berlin: Hobbing.
Sweden Central Bureau of Statistics
  1969   *Historical Statistics of Sweden. Part 1. Population. 1720-1967*. Stockholm: Beckmans.
Teitelbaum, M.S.
  1984   *The British Fertility Decline: Demographic Transition in the Crucible of the Industrial
          Revolution*. Princeton, N.J.: Princeton University Press.
Tipton, F.B.
  1976   *Regional Variations in the Economic Development of Germany during the Nineteenth
          Century*. Middletown, Conn.: Wesleyan University Press.
van de Walle, E.
  1978   Alone in Europe: The French fertility decline until 1850. Pp. 257-288 in C. Tilly, ed.,
          Historical Studies of Changing Fertility. Princeton, N.J.: Princeton University Press.
van de Walle, F.
  1986   Infant mortality and the European demographic transition. Pp. 201-233 in A.J. Coale and
          S.C. Watkins, eds., *The Decline of Fertility in Europe*. Princeton, N.J.: Princeton Uni-
          versity Press.

Watkins, S.C.
  1991   *From Provinces into Nations: Demographic Integration in Western Europe, 1870-1960.*
          Princeton, N.J.: Princeton University Press.
Wonnacott, R.J., and T.H. Wonnacott
  1979   *Econometrics.* New York: John Wiley & Sons.
Woods, R.I.
  1987   Approaches to the fertility transition in Victorian England. *Population Studies* 41:283-
          311.
World Bank
  1994   *World Development Report 1994.* Oxford, England: Oxford University Press.
Yule, G.U.
  1906   On the changes in the marriage and birth rates in England and Wales during the past half
          century; with an inquiry as to their probable causes. *Journal of the Royal Statistical
          Society* 69:88-132.

7

The Relationshp Between Infant and Child Mortality and Fertility: Some Historical and Contemporary Evidence for the United States

Michael R. Haines

INTRODUCTION

The demographic transition from high to low levels of fertility and mortality is a defining characteristic of the development process. Historically, the precise timing of both the fertility and mortality transitions has varied considerably. Furthermore, there are important questions as to how fertility and mortality interact during this process. The writings of Thomas R. Malthus (1830) are an early example of this inquiry. One area of particular interest has been the relationship of birth rates to infant and early childhood mortality, which has occasioned a number of studies on developing nations since World War II (e.g., Hobcraft et al., 1985; Potter, 1988; Lloyd and Ivanov, 1988). There has also been some inquiry into the historical experience of European nations that have passed through the demographic transition (for a survey, see Galloway et al., in this volume), notably in the context of the European Fertility Project (e.g., van de Walle, 1986) and other projects using micro-data sources (e.g., Knodel, 1988:Chap. 14). Finally, there has been some work on more recent history of developing nations (Pampel and Pillai, 1986).

Much of the recent interest has centered on the following questions: Might exogenously caused declines in infant and child death rates induce partially or wholly offsetting declines in birth rates? Or will mortality-reducing programs, valuable in and of themselves, simply exacerbate already high rates of population growth? These questions form the focus in this volume.

There is, however, the complicating issue of reverse causality (or endogeneity). Lower (or higher) mortality might induce lower (or higher) fertility, but it is well established that higher birth rates lead to higher infant and child mortality. This higher mortality is related to the effect on infants and children of earlier weaning and reduced care from mothers. When the evidence is simply bivariate in nature (as the zero-order correlations used to an extent in this chapter), the causal paths cannot be disentangled. But treating them separately is possible, and this is investigated here as well.

REVIEW OF THE LITERATURE: EVIDENCE FOR THE UNITED STATES

The number of studies dealing with the interaction between fertility and infant (or child) mortality for the United States is surprisingly small. This contrasts with historical research for Europe and for contemporary developing nations. (See essays by Cohen and Montgomery and by Galloway et al., in this volume.)

Among the few historical studies is a recent work using the Utah Population Database of genealogies collected by the Mormon Church (Bean et al., 1992; Lynch et al., 1985). Bean et al. (1992) looked at the reasons why high fertility rates may have resulted in high infant mortality rates for the western United States in the nineteenth and early twentieth centuries. They propose three possibilities (not mutually exclusive): the contagion and competition hypothesis, the biological insufficiency hypothesis, and the maternal depletion hypothesis. The first (contagion and competition) argues that more siblings disadvantage a recent birth by way of increased risk of infectious disease and increased competition for family resources. The second (biological insufficiency) links higher fertility to higher-risk young mothers and hence higher infant mortality. This is both a physiological and socioeconomic argument, since young mothers may not have acquired as many childrearing skills. The third (maternal depletion) asserts that higher fertility is related to more births among older women (age 35 and over) who also have increased risk of infant death for both physiological and social reasons. The results of the study show that, over time, birth intervals lengthened and (by the late nineteenth century) ceased to have a major effect on infant mortality. There was also some evidence for the biological insufficiency and maternal depletion views as fewer births occurred to older women and as age at marriage rose. Bean et al. (1992:344, Figure 1) also found that the infant mortality rate had a curvilinear relation to mother's age (highest at the youngest and oldest ages), an inverse relationship to birth interval length (lowest at longest intervals), an increasing relationship to birth order after the first two children, and a strongly positive relation to parity. This covered the mid-nineteenth to the early twentieth centuries.

A substantial group of studies was conducted earlier in this century by the Children's Bureau using matched birth and infant death records over the period 1911-1915 for eight cities (Johnstown, Pennsylvania; Manchester, New Hampshire; Saginaw, Michigan; Brockton, Massachusetts; New Bedford, Massachusetts; Waterbury, Connecticut; Akron, Ohio; and Baltimore, Maryland). These were summarized in a monograph by Woodbury (1926) (see Table 7-1). These studies reported information on 22,967 births and 2,555 linked infant deaths for which data on the families were obtained by interviews. Several relationships were uncovered that echo the findings from the genealogical data. Infant mortality increased with birth order with the exception of a decline between the first and second births. Infant mortality was also strongly inversely related to birth interval. The characteristic curvilinear pattern of infant mortality and mother's age is also seen in these data—higher rates at the youngest and oldest ages. Father's income (both total and per family member) had a strong inverse association with infant mortality. These fascinating studies include some data on breastfeeding, one piece of evidence pertinent to the influence of infant mortality on fertility. Panel C of Table 7-1 presents information on breastfeeding by race and nativity. Higher levels of artificial feeding were associated with higher infant mortality. Greater incidence of breastfeeding partly offset the negative effects of lower income among several of the foreign-born groups (Italian, Jewish, Polish) and among blacks. Here we have some direct evidence that breastfeeding is associated with lower infant mortality risk, although the data are only suggestive. No tabulations were presented, however, on differences in birth intervals for breastfeeding versus artificial feeding, so it is not possible to see the joint association with fertility.

A more recent set of matched birth and death records (from the National Infant Mortality Survey of 1964-1966) have been analyzed by MacMahon and his colleagues (MacMahon, 1974; MacMahon et al., 1973). As of the 1960s, some of the effects that were seen earlier still persist. The infant mortality rate did increase with birth order, albeit not until parity six and above. Mother's age still had the same curvilinear relation to probability of infant death. Also, a previous infant or fetal death substantially increased the risk of subsequent infant death. This may have been because of shorter birth intervals, but more likely it reflected higher-risk mothers. This is a recurring finding in studies of developing nations (e.g., Hobcraft et al., 1985).

In general, however, work on this topic for the United States has been sparse. There have been numerous studies of fertility and of infant mortality separately, but few have attempted to link the two. Furthermore, previous studies have stressed the path from fertility to mortality rather than that from infant and child mortality to fertility.

THE DEMOGRAPHIC TRANSITION IN THE UNITED STATES

The study of the transition from high to low levels of fertility and mortality in the United States is bedeviled by lacunae in the data. The United States was early in the activity of taking national censuses (decennially from 1790), and the census did provide useful published age and sex distributions from 1800 onward.

TABLE 7-1 Mortality Analysis, Eight American Cities, 1911-1915

Panel A: Infant Mortality by Birth Order

| Birth Order | Infant Mortality Rate | Ratio to Average | Eliminating Influence of Mother's Age | | |
			Actual Deaths	Expected Deaths	Ratio Actual/ Expected
1	104.6	94.1	652	704.1	92.7
2	95.7	86.1	474	538.6	88.0
3	104.6	94.1	348	356.8	97.6
4	108.8	97.8	270	266.5	101.2
5	118.8	106.8	210	192.7	109.0
6	122.7	110.3	155	141.2	109.7
7	136.8	123.0	126	106.2	118.4
8	135.9	122.2	92	79.9	115.2
9	146.8	132.0	69	57.3	120.2
10 and over	181.5	163.2	159	112.0	142.0
Total	111.2	100.0	2555	2555.3	100.0

Panel B: Birth Interval since Preceding Birth (Baltimore only)

Birth Order/ Interval Length	Infant Mortality Rate	Ratio to Average
Birth order		
First birth	94.8	91.6
Second and later	106.6	103.0
Interval length		
1 year	146.7	141.7
2 years	98.6	95.3
3 years	86.5	83.6
4+ years	84.9	82.0
Total	103.5	100.0

TABLE 7-1 (*continued*)

Panel C: Infant Mortality Related to Breastfeeding and Ethnicity

| | | | Ratio Actual/Expected Death | | |
| | | | | | |
Ethnicity	Artificial Feeding (%)	Income <$650 (%)	Infant Mortality Rate	Partly Breastfed	Entirely Artificial
White	25.2	39.6	108.3	139.2	410.5
Native	28.3	27.4	93.8	170.7	534.5
Foreign born	21.2	55.3	127.0	125.1	327.4
Italian	13.1	70.5	103.8	85.9	219.0
Jewish	11.3	44.5	53.5	46.9	290.9
French					
Canadian	44.0	43.2	171.3	182.7	241.1
German	21.5	41.2	103.1	125.0	564.5
Polish	11.1	78.3	157.2	159.8	487.8
Portuguese	31.9	78.5	200.3	237.6	429.4
Other	23.2	45.0	129.6	102.3	325.4
Colored	19.7	81.9	154.4	82.2	315.8
Total	24.9	42.4	111.2	129.5	400.8

NOTE: Cities were Johnstown, Pennsylvania; Manchester, New Hampshire; Saginaw, Michigan; Brockton, Massachusetts; New Bedford, Massachusetts; Waterbury, Connecticut; Akron, Ohio; and Baltimore, Maryland. The study was based on samples totaling 22,967 live births and 2,555 infant deaths.

SOURCE: Woodbury (1926).

This allowed the study of fertility by way of the use of child/woman ratios (Yasuba, 1962; Forster and Tucker, 1972; Okun, 1958; Schapiro, 1986). As can be seen in Table 7-2, these results point to a consistent decline in fertility from at least 1800, as measured by child/woman ratios or by crude birth rates or total fertility rates derived from them.

Unfortunately, collection of vital statistics was left to individual states and municipalities, which resulted in tardy and uneven coverage. Massachusetts was the first to begin this activity at the state level in 1842 and achieved relatively good coverage by about 1855 (Abbott, 1897:714-715). But the official Death Registration Area was not formed until 1900 with ten states and the District of Columbia, comprising about a quarter of the nation's population. The official Birth Registration Area was not defined until 1915. Both were not comprehensive until 1933 with the admission of Texas. Hence, what we know about mortality before the 1930s, and infant mortality in particular, is limited to smaller

TABLE 7-2 Fertility and Mortality in the United States, 1800-1990

Date	Birth Rate[a]		Child/Woman Ratio[b]		Total Fertility Rate[c]		Expectation of Life[d]		Infant Mortality Rate[e]	
	White	Black[f]	White	Black[f]	White	Black[f]	White	Black[f]	White	Black[f]
1800	55.0		1000		7.04					
1810	54.3		1001		6.92					
1820	52.8		950	915	6.73					
1830	51.4		877	938	6.55					
1840	48.3		837	887	6.14					
1850	43.3	58.6[g]	692	837	5.42	7.90[g]	38.9		217.4	
1860	41.4	55.0[h]	709	818	5.21	7.58[h]	40.9[k]		196.9[k]	
1870	38.3	55.4[i]	641	782	4.55	7.69[i]	44.1		176.0	
1880	35.2	51.9[j]	615	848	4.24	7.26[j]	39.6		214.8	
1890	31.5	48.1	543	702	3.87	6.56	45.7		150.9	
1900	30.1	44.4	533	658	3.56	5.61	49.6	41.8[l]	120.1	170.3[l]
1910	29.2	38.5	508	586	3.42	4.61	51.9	47.0	113.0	131.7
1920	26.9	35.0	495	485	3.17	3.64	57.4	48.5	82.1	99.9
1930	20.6	27.5	405	444	2.45	2.98	60.8	53.9	60.1	73.8
1940	18.6	26.7	340	415	2.22	2.87	65.0	60.8	43.2	44.5
1950	23.0	33.3	490	581	2.98	3.93	69.1	63.6	26.8	43.2
1960	22.7	32.1	546	694	3.53	4.52	70.7	65.2	22.9	30.9
1970	17.4	25.1	392	490	2.39	3.07	71.7	68.1	17.8	21.4
1980	14.9	22.1	300	367	1.75	2.32	74.4	69.1	11.0	18.0
1990	15.5	23.8	298	385	1.96	2.58	76.1		7.6	

^{a}Births per 1,000 population per annum.

^{b}Children aged 0-4 per 1,000 women aged 15-44. Taken from Thompson and Whelpton (1933:Table 74). Adjusted upward 5 percent for relative underenumeration of white children aged 0-4 and 13 percent for black children for the censuses of 1800-1950. Based on corrections made in Grabill et al. (1958:Table 6).

^{c}Number of births per woman if she experienced the current period age-specific fertility rates throughout her life.

^{d}Expectation of life at birth.

^{e}Infant deaths per 1,000 live births per annum.

^{f}Black and other populations.

^{g}Average for 1850-1859.

^{h}Average for 1860-1869.

^{i}Average for 1870-1879.

^{j}Average for 1880-1884.

^{k}For the total population.

^{l}Approximately 1895.

SOURCES: Bureau of the Census (1975, 1985, 1994); Coale and Zelnick (1963); Coale and Rives (1973); Haines (1979:289-312); Preston and Haines (1991:Table 2.5).

geographic areas or to estimates. Some of these data are also presented in Table 7-2.

The United States was one of those cases of prior sustained fertility decline in which fertility and infant mortality exhibited little or no relationship. From Table 7-2 it is apparent that fertility had been falling since at least 1800. Mortality, in contrast, did not exhibit a sustained decline until about the 1870s. Table 7-2 does not show an unambiguous decline in expectation of life at birth of the infant mortality rate until 1880, although that date could have been an outlier with a decline occurring earlier. This does not appear to have been the case, however. Other mortality data, based on genealogies, and information on human stature, point to deteriorating mortality in the several decades before the American Civil War (Pope, 1992; Fogel, 1986), illustrated in Figure 7-1. The shorter life expectancy is consistent with anthropometric data showing declining heights of West Point cadets in the decades before the Civil War (Komlos, 1987). Thus, the United States constitutes a case in which, during the nineteenth century, fertility was being controlled, mostly by adjustments in marital fertility (Sanderson, 1979), whereas mortality came under control only very late. Under the circumstances, it is not surprising that there was little relation between fertility and infant mortality over time. It has been posited that only where there has been a prior decline in infant and childhood mortality would there likely be any replacement or insurance effect on fertility. If the relationship were from fertility to infant mortality and if infant mortality were mostly subject to exogenous environmental influences (e.g., summer gastrointestinal infections and winter respiratory infections), then the reduced birth ratios would have had only a damped effect on infant and child mortality.

The official data for the United States (from 1909) are presented in Figure 7-2. There it is apparent that the infant mortality rate was declining from 1915 onward, while fertility as measured by the general fertility ratio (births per 1,000 women aged 15-49) continued its decline until the baby boom.[1] The baby boom may have retarded the decline in the infant mortality rate, which essentially plateaued in the 1940s and 1950s, but it certainly did not raise it. In sum, there appears to be little relationship between the birth rate and the infant mortality rate in aggregate time series data for the United States from the early twentieth century.

To go back to the nineteenth century requires narrowing the geographic focus. Massachusetts is the best choice, because it had the longest continuum of data of reasonable quality. Some of these data are presented in Figure 7-3 for the

---

[1]It should be noted that the Birth Registration Area was changing in composition from 1915 to 1933 as it was being augmented. The pattern for the original Birth Registration Area of 1915 was virtually the same, however (Linder and Grove, 1947:Table 27).

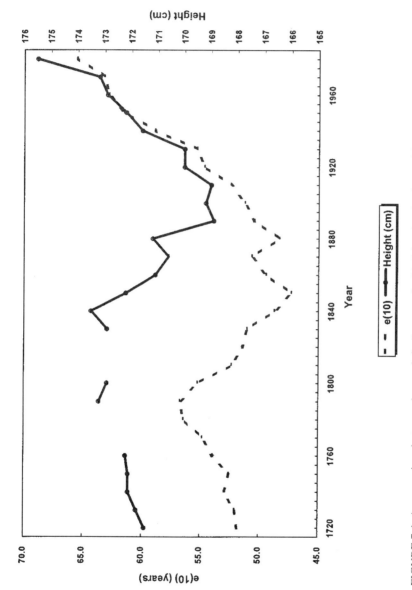

FIGURE 7-1 A comparison between the trends in the mean final height of native-born white males and the trend in life expectancy at age 10 (e^{10}) (height by birth cohort; e^{10} by period). SOURCE: Fogel (1986).

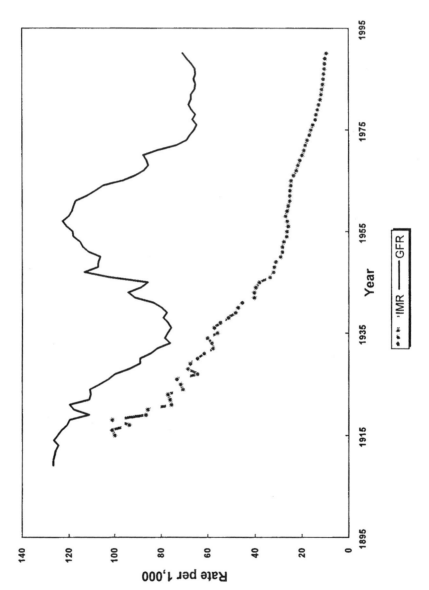

FIGURE 7-2 Fertility ratio and infant mortality rate, United States, 1909-1990.

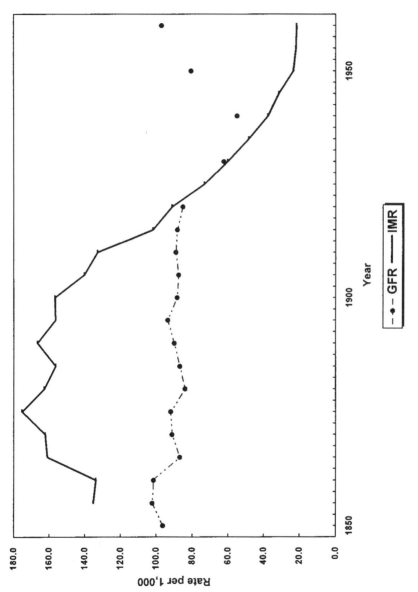

FIGURE 7-3 Fertility ratio and infant mortality rate, Massachusetts, 1850-1960.

state as a whole for the period 1842 to 1960. Massachusetts was certainly not typical of the United States during that period. It was more urban and industrial and had a higher percentage of foreign-born population. For example, in 1900 Massachusetts was 86 percent urban as compared with 40 percent for the United States as a whole. About 30 percent of the Massachusetts population was foreign born at that date in contrast to 13 percent for the nation. On the other hand, Massachusetts was a forerunner in its process of urbanization and structural change. In any event, Figure 7-3 indicates that fertility (as measured by the general fertility rate) had leveled off by the 1870s whereas the infant mortality rate did not commence its decline until the 1890s. One interpretation is that further fertility declines awaited declines in infant mortality, but the birth rate then remained quite steady from the 1890s until the early 1920s, at which point fertility recommenced its decline until World War II. In the meantime, the infant mortality rate continued to be reduced steadily from the 1890s through the baby boom until 1960. Although this could be interpreted as a lack of a relationship between birth rates and death rates, it can also be seen as a lagged response of parents to the changing mortality environment. Parents could well have been waiting to see if the mortality decline was permanent. Meanwhile they practiced hoarding (the insurance motive).

Cross-sectional relationships across space are also revealing. For example, the simple zero-order correlations between the infant mortality rate and the general fertility rate for the counties and towns (or cities for 1905 and 1915) of Massachusetts are given in Table 7-3, along with the state levels of the general fertility rate and the infant mortality rate for the counties and towns (or cities) of Massachusetts. The correlations by county exclude the small (and unusual) islands of Martha's Vineyard and Nantucket. The correlations are always positive (in the expected direction), but are weak and rather unstable until the late nineteenth century. They then become quite strongly positive (e.g., 0.878 for counties in 1915), and only weaken again in the 1920s and 1930s (0.137 for counties in 1940). The town-level correlations are presented both unweighted and weighted by population size. Unfortunately, town-level data on infant deaths cease to be available after 1890. Shortly thereafter, reporting by cities was done, so those are the units given for 1905 and 1915. Again, the picture is rather unclear until the early twentieth century. The correlations all have the expected positive sign, but the results are unstable. Sometimes the weighted and sometimes the unweighted results are significant. By the early twentieth century, both county and city data exhibit larger, positive, significant correlations.[2] These results are also consistent with the view that there is a connection between birth rates and mortality during periods of transition—especially mortality transition —although the response of birth rates may be delayed.

---

[2] It does not make a difference if only the larger cities are used in 1855 and 1885.

TABLE 7-3 Infant Mortality Rates, General Fertility Ratios, and Their
Correlation, Counties, Towns, and Cities of Massachusetts, 1855-1941

Zero-Order Correlations

| Years | Counties | Towns[a] | | General Fertility Rate | Infant Mortality Rate |
		Unweighted	Weighted		
1855-1856	0.3534	0.2177***	0.1773***	102.3	128.8
	(12)	(322)	(322)		
1859-1861	0.3747	0.2134***	0.0526	101.6	132.5
	(12)	(328)	(322)		
1864-1866	0.0670	0.2625***	0.0312	87.0	150.5
	(12)	(329)	(329)		
1874-1876	0.4994*	0.2625***	0.0312	92.3	166.2
	(12)	(335)	(335)		
1884-1886	0.5433*	0.0382	0.2767***	86.9	156.6
	(12)	(340)	(329)		
1894-1896	0.5819**			93.8	160.6
	(12)				
1904-1906	0.8260***	0.4061***	0.5256***	87.7	137.3
	(12)	(56)	(56)		
1914-1916	0.8785***	0.4439***	0.4958***	88.3	102.5
	(12)	(54)	(54)		
1929-1931	0.5955**			74.5	56.9
	(12)				
1939-1941	0.1368			55.0	36.7

NOTES: Numbers in parentheses below correlations are sample sizes. *, p < 0.10. **, p < 0.05.
***, p < 0.01.
  [a]Cities after 1904.

SOURCE: State and federal censuses; state and federal vital statistics publications.

Similarly, the simple correlations between the infant mortality rate and the
general fertility rate for the states of the Birth Registration Area of the United
States in the twentieth century are −0.3315 (1915), −0.1287 (1920), 0.6200 (1930),
and 0.6750 (1940), the latter two data points being significant at the 1 percent
level. Thus, once again, only later in the process did a significant positive
relationship appear. Thus, only as both fertility and infant mortality became quite
thoroughly under control did any perceptible positive association appear. This
was apparently not the case during the earlier period of the fertility transition in
the nineteenth century.

EVIDENCE FROM THE PUBLIC USE SAMPLES OF 1900 AND 1910

The availability of public use micro-data samples of the U.S. censuses of 1900 and 1910 (Graham, 1980; Strong et al., 1989) also affords an opportunity for further exploration of the fertility-childhood mortality relationship. The usefulness of these censuses lies in the inclusion of questions on children ever born, children surviving, and the duration of current marriage for adult women. These questions were not tabulated at the time, and only some results from 1910 were used in connection with the 1940 census. Analysis of childhood mortality using various indirect methods has now been conducted with both of these micro samples (e.g., Preston et al., 1981, 1994; Preston and Haines, 1991). As part of that work, an index of childhood mortality has been developed (Trussell and Preston, 1982; Preston and Haines, 1991:Chap. 3 and Appendix C; Preston et al., 1994:75-79). The index is based on the ratio of actual to expected child deaths for individual women or groups of women. Actual child deaths are calculated as the difference between stated children ever born and children surviving. Expected child deaths are calculated by multiplying children ever born for each eligible woman by the expected child mortality based on a national average or each marriage duration group (0-4, 5-9, 10-14, . . ., 30-34). It is a way of comparing actual child mortality to that expected by the national average. The use of marriage duration categories in calculating the index is a means of standardizing for the length of exposure to risk of mortality for the children. The overall totals (see Table 7-4) are close to the national average. That is, the ratio is close to unity (0.9894 for 1900 and 0.9800 for 1910). It is calculated only for once married, or currently married women for whom children ever born, children surviving, and marriage duration were known. The intuitive interpretation is that ratios above 1 showed greater than average mortality and vice versa.

Some tabulations of the child mortality index by marriage duration, woman's age, and parity are given in Table 7-4. The results are presented for the total and for white and black populations. It is important to note that mortality was declining rapidly over this period. Hence, some of the increases in the index by marriage duration, age, and parity reflect the time trend. That is, the children of women who were older, married longer, and at higher parity had been exposed, on average, to earlier, higher mortality regimes. That being said, the relationship of childhood mortality to parity was increasing and the curvilinear pattern with age observed elsewhere is repeated.

Table 7-5 attempts to look at this in a multivariate framework to examine the robustness of the results. These regressions examine only the issue of the influence of fertility on childhood mortality. The child mortality index for individual women is on the left-hand side and woman's age, age squared, parity, and years married are on the right-hand side. The regressions are weighted by children ever born to bring the analysis closer to the unit of the child (rather than the woman) and to correct partially for heteroskedasticity. The problem with doing this is that

TABLE 7-4 Fertility and the Child Mortality Index, United States, 1900 and 1910

Marriage Duration, Age, and Fertility	Child Mortality Index					
	Total		White		Black	
	1900	1910	1900	1910	1900	1910
Marriage Duration						
0-4	0.7413	0.9769	0.7132	0.8475	1.0769	1.8905
5-9	0.8277	0.9274	0.7610	0.8475	1.3134	1.3938
10-14	0.9923	0.9342	0.9263	0.8772	1.4028	1.4013
15-19	0.9572	0.9526	0.9363	0.9094	1.1192	1.3990
20-24	1.0157	1.0232	0.9713	0.9830	1.3611	1.3953
25-29	1.0635	1.0124	1.0247	0.9835	1.3817	1.2714
30-34	1.0438	1.0153	1.0070	0.9683	1.3742	1.4132
Woman's Age						
15-19	1.2000	0.9799	1.4167	0.8783	0.3333	1.2727
20-24	0.8899	0.9525	0.7831	0.8361	1.3667	1.5000
25-29	0.8620	0.8896	0.8028	0.8138	1.1269	1.3739
30-34	0.8874	0.9480	0.8321	0.8899	1.3624	1.4223
35-39	0.9590	0.9385	0.9287	0.8913	1.1896	1.3627
40-44	0.9770	0.9973	0.9320	0.9569	1.3383	1.3730
45-49	1.0445	1.0145	1.0000	0.9779	1.4309	1.3800
50-54	1.0580	1.0159	1.0434	0.9852	1.1939	1.4313
55-59	1.1601	1.1114	1.1118	1.0489	1.6591	1.6628
Parity						
1	0.5128	0.6117	0.4739	0.5560	1.0000	1.3258
2	0.6155	0.6747	0.5759	0.6342	1.2292	1.2000
3	0.7689	0.8029	0.7189	0.7676	1.3000	1.4036
4	0.8458	0.8922	0.8236	0.8560	1.1667	1.3144
5	0.9587	0.9224	0.9287	0.8808	1.1961	1.4128
6	1.0084	1.0057	0.9675	0.9688	1.3942	1.3805
7	0.9864	1.0381	0.9669	0.9960	1.1321	1.3913
8	1.0613	1.0566	1.0394	1.0229	1.2921	1.4064
9+	1.2663	1.2601	1.2237	1.2117	1.4389	1.4716
Total	0.9894	0.9800	0.9458	0.9300	1.3250	1.4093

SOURCE: Public use micro samples of the 1900 and 1910 U.S. censuses.

the time trend is still present. Also, it is clear that the coefficients will be biased since parity (on the right-hand side) is endogenous. Nonetheless, introducing these variables, as well as a dummy variable for race, did reveal that the curvilinear pattern of child mortality with age persisted and had the correct orientation (convex from below). Child mortality did increase with parity and black child

TABLE 7-5 Mortality Analysis, United States, 1900 and 1910

Explanatory Variable	Dependent Variable: Child Mortality Index	
	1900	1910
Constant	1.1627*	1.0610*
Woman's age	−0.0322*	−0.0239*
Woman's age squared	0.0006*	0.0005*
Parity	0.0863*	0.0874*
Marriage duration	−0.0280*	−0.0301*
Black	0.2379*	0.3359*
Sample size	11,562	43,299
Adjusted R^2	0.063	0.050
F ratio	156.20	455.44

NOTE: *denotes significance at the 1 percent level.

SOURCE: Public use micro samples of the 1900 and 1910 U.S. censuses.

mortality significantly exceeded that of the white population (by about 24 percent in 1900 and 34 percent in 1910 when controlling for age, parity, and marriage duration). The relationship of marriage duration now becomes negative, however, which is puzzling.

Finally, at each census date there was a positive zero-order correlation between the child mortality index and fertility (as measured by average parity): 0.1784 in 1900 and 0.1292 in 1910 for the same group of women in Table 7-4. Looking at aggregation data by state, the correlation between the child mortality index and average parity was weak in 1900 (-0.0132 unweighted and 0.1010 when weighted by population size). In 1910 the same exercise revealed a stronger positive correlation between the child mortality index and average parity (0.1669 unweighted and 0.3136 weighted) and between the index and estimated gross reproduction rates taken from the 1940 U.S. census (0.2627 unweighted and 0.3126 weighted) (Bureau of the Census, 1944). Again, there is evidence for the positive association, which appears to be strengthening over time.

EVIDENCE FOR THE EFFECT OF INFANT AND CHILD MORTALITY ON FERTILITY

The public use micro samples of 1900 and 1910 also afford the possibility of examining the interesting and pertinent opposite causal path: the replacement and hoarding effects. How extensively do couples replace an actual infant or child death with a new birth? Do families, even those who have not experienced a child death, have births in excess of the number that would be desired in the absence of child loss (hoarding)? It has already been mentioned that it is of interest whether reductions in infant and child mortality in developing nations, undertaken in conjunction with general public health programs or with specialized maternal and child health initiatives, might help reduce fertility and the population growth consequences of the mortality reduction (Lloyd and Ivanov, 1988:157-158). Typically the observed replacement effects have been small, in the range 0.1 to 0.4 for proportions adjusted for demographic and other covariates (Lloyd and Ivanov, 1988:Table 6).[3]

A method of estimating the pure replacement effect from basic data on children ever born and children surviving (or children dead) for individual women has been constructed by Olsen (Olsen, 1980; Trussell and Olsen, 1983; see also Mauskopf and Wallace, 1984).[4] The idea is that simply regressing the number of births on the number of child deaths (i.e., $CEB_i = \alpha_0 + \alpha_1 * D_i$ where CEB_i is births to woman i and D_i is child deaths to woman i, will yield a biased and inconsistent estimate of replacement (α_1)). As an alternative, an instrumental variable (IV) technique can be used. In stage one, children dead is regressed on the proportion dead (i.e., $D_i = \beta_0 + \beta_1 * P_i$, where P_i is the proportion dead to woman i). At stage two, the predicted value of child deaths from stage one is used in a regression with births (i.e., $CEB_i = \gamma_0 + \gamma_1 * \hat{D}_i$, where $\hat{D}_i$ is predicted child deaths). The coefficient γ_1 is a good predictor of the replacement effect (net of hoarding) if the number of births (CEB) and the proportion of children dead (P) are uncorrelated. If this condition is not met, further corrections are necessary.

The basic correction uses the observed child mortality rate and the mean and variance of the birth distribution (which can be calculated from the data) to estimate a "true" replacement coefficient (γ_1'). The final correction (IV[adj]) was done taking Olsen's assumption that births and the proportion dead have a joint bivariate lognormal distribution (Olsen, 1980; Trussell and Olsen, 1983). The corrected IV coefficient has been arbitrarily chosen in preference to the corrected ordinary least-squares estimate.[5]

---

[3]In a survey of the literature to the mid-1970s, Preston (1975) found that the proportion of child deaths replaced by a subsequent live birth was about 0.25 in high-fertility populations (Bangladesh, Senegal, Morocco) where many women were not using contraception and were also breastfeeding. It was even lower in populations in the early states of the fertility transition (Mexico, Peru, Colombia). This rose again for countries with more advanced demographic transitions (e.g., Costa Rica, Taiwan) and was still higher for developed countries (e.g., 0.33 in France in 1962).

[4]For a discussion and critique of these models and methods, see the chapter by Wolpin in this volume.

[5]Where there is observable heterogeneity in the underlying mortality risk (e.g., by geographic area, rural or urban residence, racial or ethnic group), the estimates can be made separately for those groups, areas, etc. Where the underlying mortality risk varies across individuals and groups but is unobserved (e.g., by income), the Olsen correction may not be entirely sufficient. (See Wolpin in this volume for a discussion of this.) Trussell and Olsen (1983) conducted some simulations of this and found the effects to be small.

Estimates of the replacement effect are presented in Table 7-6 for the simple ordinary least-squares (OLS) regression of births on child deaths, the two-stage instrumental variable approach (IV), and for the instrumental variable method corrected for the correlation between births and the proportion death (IV[adj]).[6] The bias in the instrumental variable estimate of replacement (that is, (IV-IV[adj]) in Table 7-6) is a measure of the correlation between fertility and child mortality and hence the extent to which high infant and child death rates could induce higher birth rates, that is, hoarding. The assumption is that couples are aware of the ambient child mortality rates. The results are given for women of all ages. Analysis (not shown) was also done for women of age groups 25-29 through 45-49. In addition, the population has been divided by race, nativity (native versus foreign-born white), and residence (rural versus urban white) to account for observed, known heterogeneity in underlying mortality risks (Preston and Haines, 1991).

In general, the results show that the direct replacement effects (IV[adj]) were quite modest in the United States around the turn of the century. Only about 10-30 percent of infant and child deaths were replaced. The replacement coefficients were shorter for younger women (not shown) who presumably had shorter birth intervals in the earlier stages of family building and hence had less latitude to make adjustments. The difference between the unadjusted IV estimate and the adjusted IV estimate is an approximate measure of hoarding (that is, gross replacement minus direct replacement) (Olsen, 1980:440-441). It was in the range of 0.3-0.5 of a child, generally between 0.4 and 0.5 of a child per woman. This results in a gross replacement effect (direct replacement plus hoarding) in the neighborhood of 60-80 percent. Finally, there did not appear to have been any clear differences in direct replacement of hoarding by race, nativity, or rural and urban residence across the census decade. If anything, the tendency toward direct replacement was smaller among older women in 1910 than in 1900, while the propensity to hoard changed little (not shown).

Overall, it must be concluded that direct replacement was relatively modest in the United States around 1900 and that there was still a substantial amount of hoarding. This was taking place during a period of both declining fertility and falling child mortality (see Table 7-2). Because both fertility and mortality were falling for a variety of reasons, there was little effect on natural increase from the declining death rate among children.[7] Also, results on replacement are not out of line with contemporary estimates for developing countries (Lloyd and Ivanov, 1988).

---

[6]Randall Olsen has kindly provided the author with a copy of his FORTRAN program to perform the estimations.

[7]Natural increase remained relatively constant at 12.8 per 1,000 from the 1890s to the decade of the 1900s (see Haines, in press, Table 1).

TABLE 7-6 Estimates of the Replacement Effect, United States, 1900 and 1910

	1900					1910				
Group	OLS	IV	IV[adj]	IV-IV[adj]	Sample Size	OLS	IV	IV-IV(adj)	IV[adj]	Sample Size
White	1.292	0.730	0.285	0.445	13,080	1.364	0.732	0.261	0.471	49,753
Black	1.186	0.532	0.241	0.291	1,373	1.268	0.580	0.284	0.296	5,118
Native white	1.354	0.712	0.277	0.435	9,892	1.413	0.693	0.252	0.442	37,822
Foreign white	1.162	0.695	0.290	0.404	3,171	1.255	0.769	0.303	0.466	11,916
Rural white (<2,500)	1.346	0.747	0.306	0.441	7,639	1.403	0.700	0.249	0.451	26,216
Urban white (>2,500)	1.262	0.759	0.276	0.483	5,441	1.327	0.782	0.275	0.507	23,537
Urban white(>8,000)	1.245	0.753	0.273	0.480	4,412	1.319	0.796	0.287	0.508	18,687
Total	1.273	0.711	0.280	0.431	14,513	1.340	0.722	0.263	0.459	55,230

NOTES: OLS, ordinary least-squares estimate. IV, instrumental variable estimate. IV [adj], corrected instrumental variable estimate, constructed using the Olsen (1980) method. Calculated for currently married women for whom children ever born and children surviving were known. Women with no births are naturally excluded.

SOURCE: Public use micro samples of the 1900 and 1910 U.S. censuses.

Some additional macro-level evidence is present in Table 7-7 in the form of regressions of fertility on lagged and current infant mortality, along with other variables. The upper panel uses the states of the United States in 1910. The dependent variable is the estimated adjusted gross reproduction rate for 1910, taken from the U.S. census of 1940 (Bureau of the Census, 1944). In the first regression, the gross reproduction rate for each state in 1910 is regressed on the child mortality index for that state in 1900, along with the proportions nonwhite, foreign born, and living in urban areas of 25,000 and over. Dummy variables for regions were also included. In this case, birth rates should be responding to previous levels of infant and child mortality; this was found. The sign was in the expected positive direction, but the coefficient was not statistically significant. The second equation substitutes the child mortality index in 1910 for that in 1900. Again, the sign is positive, although the coefficient can be expected to be biased because of simultaneous equations error (i.e., both the gross reproduction rate and child mortality are endogenous). This is corrected in the third equation, which is a two-stage least-squares estimation of the second equation. The instrument chosen is the body mass index (kilograms of body weight per meters of height squared) of World War I recruits for each state. This index is taken as an indicator of health conditions in the 30 years prior to 1917-1918 (Davenport and Love, 1921). The coefficient on the child mortality index in 1910 was increased but still remained statistically insignificant. The other independent variables show that urban residence and living in the Northeast were associated with lower fertility and that higher proportions of nonwhite and foreign born as well as residence in the South were related to higher birth rates.

The final set of regressions repeats this exercise for the towns of Massachusetts in 1860 and 1885 and for the 54 largest cities in 1915. (Infant mortality statistics ceased to be reported by town in 1890 and were published only for larger cities thereafter.) At all three dates, the general fertility ratio (births per 1,000 women aged 15-49) was regressed on the lagged infant mortality rate, urbanization, and the proportion of nonwhite and foreign born. (Proportion of foreign born was not available by town in 1860.) The city population size was used instead of the urban dummy variable used for 1860 and 1885 (equal to 1 if the town was greater than 5,000 persons in 1860 and greater than 10,000 persons in 1885). In all cases, a 3-year average of vital statistics around the census dates was used. The second equation at each date substituted the current for the lagged infant mortality rate. Finally, the last equation at each date reestimated the second equation with two-stage least-squares. The instrument selected was persons per dwelling, deemed to be an index of crowding and possible source of poor conditions for children.

For 1860, the coefficients on the infant mortality rate (lagged or current) were positive. They were significant in the lagged and two-stage least-squares specifications. The coefficient of infant mortality was again positive and significant in the lagged specification for 1885, but it became negative in the contemporaneous equation. It was not significant in the simultaneous specification equation. Finally, the lagged specification also exhibited a positive and significant effect of infant death rates on birth rates in 1915, although both the contemporaneous specifications yielded insignificant though positive effects.

Overall, these macro-level results support the idea that infant mortality did affect birth rates in the expected direction. For the Massachusetts results, the ordinary least-squares regressions with lagged infant mortality revealed the effect, and it was strongest in 1915.

CONCLUDING REMARKS

This chapter began with an effort to explore the relationship of infant (and early childhood) mortality to fertility in the United States over time. The pattern both in time series and from cross-sectional data indicates, however, that the United States is one of those complicated cases also observed by van de Walle (1986) for Europe. Much of the current interest in this issue has focused on recent experience of developing countries where infant and child mortality was high and for which, in many cases, there was a decline in mortality at young ages before, or concurrent with, the fertility transition. This was not the case for the United States. Fertility was in decline from the late 1700s or early 1800s. The overall sustained mortality transition of the modern era did not begin until about the 1870s. For the best documented case—Massachusetts—infant mortality did not begin a sustained decline until the 1890s, at a point when fertility had plateaued after a period of reduction.

Although the time series patterns did not tend to indicate that fertility and mortality were related in the nineteenth century, there is evidence that birth rates responded to changes in death rates by the late nineteenth and early twentieth centuries. Furthermore, the relationship strengthened over the early part of the twentieth century as the decline in infant mortality proceeded rapidly. There is also a suggestion of a lagged response of fertility to mortality change, indicating hoarding (or insurance) behavior. This is confirmed by some cross-sectional evidence for Massachusetts from the 1850s to the 1940s and for the country as a whole from the early twentieth century. Two historical studies (Bean et al., 1992; Woodbury, 1926) found evidence for a relationship for the American West in the nineteenth and early twentieth centuries and for eight American cities, 1911-1915. But the focus was largely on the link from fertility to infant mortality and not the reverse causal path. The lack of an apparent historical association between fertility and mortality may have led to the paucity of studies, since basic data had not suggested much to study.

Some new estimates of both direct replacement and hoarding from the 1900 and 1910 public use micro samples of the United States census also indicate that the link from infant and child mortality to fertility was present, but was relatively modest and in line with what has been observed in a number of developing countries in recent decades. Only about 10-30 percent of all child deaths were

TABLE 7-7 Regressions on Fertility, United States, 1910, and Massachusetts, 1860, 1885, 1915

	Mean	Methodology		
		OLS	OLS	TSLS
United States, 1910				
Dependent variable				
Gross reproduction rate	1.905			
Independent variables				
Constant		1.7510***	1.5447***	1.3120***
Mortality index 1900	0.998	0.0646	—	—
Mortality index 1910	1.013	—	0.2794	0.5081
Proportion urban 1910	0.232	−1.3691***	−1.3588***	−1.3680***
Proportion nonwhite 1910	0.141	0.5900	0.5141	0.4027
Proportion foreign born 1910	0.139	0.9175	0.9311	0.9905
(Northeast)				
Midwest		0.1299	0.1746	0.2274
Southeast		0.4943**	0.4955**	0.5201**
South Central		0.5760**	0.5157***	0.6106***
West		0.0068	0.0052	0.0117
Adjusted R^2		0.714	0.728	0.718
F ratio		15.71***	16.74***	16.08***
Sample size		48	48	48
Massachusetts, 1860				
Dependent variable				
General fertility ratio	98.1			
Independent variables				
Constant		69.7674***	99.6301***	46.3542***
Infant mortality rate 1855	102.1	0.0699***	—	—
Infant mortality rate 1860	106.7	—	0.0063	0.4897**
Town urban 1860	0.146	11.8796***	7.1200***	2.5420
Proportion nonwhite 1860	0.006	6.5002	−251.5500**	−171.5600

	Mean	(1)	(2)	(3)
Adjusted R^2		0.051	0.021	—
F ratio		6.87***	3.35**	4.26***
Sample size		328	332	332
Massachusetts, 1885				
Dependent variable				
General fertility ratio	75.9			
Independent variables				
Constant		53.6442***	61.2254***	46.3542***
Infant mortality rate 1880	118.0	0.0398***	—	—
Infant mortality rate 1885	122.6	—	-0.0477***	-0.3854
Town urban 1885	0.092	62.4616***	3.8879	6.8514
Proportion foreign born 1885	0.167	102.0477***	117.3809***	174.3831**
Proportion nonwhite 1885	0.012	6.5002	-251.5500**	60.6894***
Adjusted R^2		0.282	0.284	—
F ratio		34.45***	35.33**	15.73***
Sample size		342	347	347
Massachusetts, 1915				
Dependent variable				
General fertility ratio	90.4			
Independent variables				
Constant		26.6449**	31.3344***	33.1065***
Infant mortality rate 1910	113.1	0.1626**	0.1012	0.0074
Infant mortality rate 1915	92.2	—	-0.0177	-0.0166
City population 1915(1,000s)	52.988	-0.0214		
Proportion foreign born 1915	0.303	160.0214***	175.6258***	197.8413**
Proportion nonwhite 1915	0.008	-236.6930	-303.5979*	-294.0917
Adjusted R^2		0.454	0.414	0.401
F ratio		12.01***	10.37***	9.81***
Sample size		54	54	54

NOTES: OLS, ordinary least squares. TSLS, two-stage least squares. *, $p < 0.10$. **, $p < 0.05$. ***, $p < 0.01$. Instruments used: United States, 1910: Body mass index of World War I recruits; Massachusetts, 1860, 1885, 1915: persons per dwelling.

directly replaced by births, although hoarding seems to have been more considerable. Gross replacement was thus in the range of 60-80 percent. Reductions in infant and child mortality, such as were occurring in the twentieth century, would thus have had a direct offset in reduced birth rates by about 25 percent. But there would have likely been another indirect offset of up to 50 percent if hoarding declined over time when parents gained greater assurance of child survival.

The relationship between fertility and mortality strengthened during the early part of the twentieth century. The evidence for the United States from the 1850s to the 1940s supports the view that modest direct reductions in fertility can be expected from reductions in infant and childhood mortality, but that more might be expected as hoarding behavior diminishes. The United States is now at quite low levels of fertility and mortality compared both with the past and with contemporary developing countries, and it is not clear that the analysis of these effects for the contemporary United States would yield much of interest in this debate.

REFERENCES

Abbott, S.W.
   1897   The vital statistics of Massachusetts: A forty years' summary, 1856-1895. *Twenty-Eighth Annual Report of the Massachusetts State Board of Health.* Public Document No. 34. Boston, Mass.: State Board of Health.
Bean, L.L., G.P. Mineau, and D.L. Anderton
   1992   High-risk childbearing: Fertility and infant mortality on the American frontier. *Social Science History* 16(3):337-363.
Bureau of the Census
   1944   *Sixteenth Census of Population: 1940.* Washington, D.C.: U.S. Department of Commerce.
   1975   *Historical Statistics of the United States.* Washington, D.C.: U.S. Department of Commerce.
   1985   *Statistical Abstract of the United States, 1986.* Washington, D.C.: U.S. Department of Commerce.
   1994   *Statistical Abstract of the United States, 1994.* Washington, D.C.: U.S. Department of Commerce.
Coale, A.J., and N.W. Rives
   1973   A statistical reconstruction of the black population of the United States, 1880-1970. *Population Index* 39(1):3-36.
Coale, A.J., and M. Zelnick
   1963   *New Estimates of Fertility and Population in the United States.* Princeton, N.J.: Princeton University Press.
Davenport, C.B., and A.G. Love
   1921   Army anthropology based on observations made on draft recruits, 1917-18, and on veterans at demobilization, 1919. In *Anthropology. Medical Department of the United States Army in the World War*, Vol. 15, part 1. Washington, D.C.: U.S. Government Printing Office.

Fogel, R.W.
  1986 Nutrition and the decline in mortality since 1700: Some preliminary findings. Pp. 439-555 in S.L. Engerman and R.E. Gallman, eds., *Long-Term Factors in American Economic Growth*. Chicago: University of Chicago Press.

Forster, C., and G.S.L. Tucker
  1972 *Economic Opportunity and White American Fertility Ratios, 1800-1860*. New Haven, Conn.: Yale University Press.

Grabill, W.H., C. Kiser, P.K. Wheltpon
  1958 *The Fertility of American Women*. New York: Wiley.

Graham, S.N.
  1980 *1900 Public Use Sample User's Handbook*. Seattle: The Center for Studies in Demography and Ecology, University of Washington.

Haines, M.R.
  1979 The use of model life tables to estimate mortality for the United States in the late nineteenth century. *Demography* 16(2):289-312.

In press The American population, 1790-1920. In S. Engerman and R. Gallman, eds., *The Cambridge Economic History of the United States*, Vol. 2. Cambridge, England: Cambridge University Press.

Hobcraft, J.N., J.W. McDonald, and S.O. Rutstein
  1985 Demographic determinants of infant and early childhood mortality: A comparative analysis. *Population Studies* 39(3):363-385.

Knodel, J.
  1988 *Demographic Behavior in the Past: A Study of Fourteen German Village Populations in the Eighteenth and Nineteenth Centuries*. Cambridge, England: Cambridge University Press.

Komlos, J.
  1987 The height and weight of West Point cadets: Dietary change in antebellum America. *Journal of Economic History* 47(4):897-927.

Linder, F.E., and R.D. Grove
  1947 *Vital Statistics in the United States, 1900-1940*. Washington, D.C.: U.S. Government Printing Office.

Lloyd, C.B., and S. Ivanov
  1988 The effects of improved child survival on family planning practice and fertility. *Studies in Family Planning* 19(3):141-161.

Lynch, K.A., G.P. Mineau, and D.L. Anderton
  1985 Estimates of infant mortality on the western frontier: The use of genealogical data. *Historical Methods* 18(4):155-164.

MacMahon, B.
  1974 Infant mortality in the United States. Pp. 189-209 in C.L. Erhardt and J.E. Berlin, eds., *Mortality and Morbidity in the United States*. Cambridge, Mass.: Harvard University Press.

MacMahon, B., M.G. Kovar, and J.J. Feldman
  1973 *Infant Mortality Rates: Relationship with Mother's Reproductive History, United States*. National Center for Health Statistics. Vital and Health Statistics. Series 22, No. 15 (April).

Malthus, T.R.
  1830 *A Summary View of the Principle of Population*, 1970 ed. Antony Flew, ed. Baltimore, Md.: Penguin Books.

Mauskopf, J., and T.D. Wallace
  1984 Fertility and replacement: Some alternative stochastic models and results for Brazil. *Demography* 21(4):519-536.

Okun, B.
    1958   *Trends in Birth Rates in the United States since 1870.* Baltimore, Md.: Johns Hopkins University Press.
Olsen, R.J.
    1980   Estimating the effect of child mortality on the number of births. *Demography* 17(4):429-443.
Pampel, F.C., and V.K. Pillai
    1986   Patterns and determinants of infant mortality in developed nations, 1950-1975. *Demography* 23(4):525-542.
Pope, C.L.
    1992   Adult mortality in America before 1900: A view from family histories. Pp. 267-296 in C. Goldin and H. Rockoff, eds., *Strategic Factors in Nineteenth Century American Economic History: A Volume to Honor Robert W. Fogel.* Chicago, Ill.: University of Chicago Press.
Potter, J.E.
    1988   Birth spacing and child survival: A cautionary note regarding the evidence from the WFS. *Population Studies* 42(3):443-450.
Preston, S.H.
    1975   Health programs and population growth. *Population and Development Review* 1(2):189-199.
Preston, S.H., and M.R. Haines
    1991   *Fatal Years: Child Mortality in Late Nineteenth Century America.* Princeton, N.J.: Princeton University Press.
Preston, S.H., M.R. Haines, and E. Pamuk
    1981   Effect of industrialization and urbanization on mortality in developed countries. Pp. 223-254 in *International Population Conference: Manila, 1981*, Vol. 2. Liège, Belgium: International Union for the Scientific Study of Population.
Preston, S.H., D. Ewbank, and M. Hereward
    1994   Child mortality differences by ethnicity and race in the United States: 1900-1910. Pp. 35-82 in S.C. Watkins, ed., *After Ellis Island: Newcomers and Natives in the 1910 Census.* New York: Russell Sage Foundation.
Sanderson, W.C.
    1979   Quantitative aspects of marriage, fertility and family limitation in nineteenth century America: Another application of the Coale specifications. *Demography* 16(3):339-358.
Schapiro, M.O.
    1986   *Filling Up America: An Economic-Demographic Model of Population Growth and Distribution in the Nineteenth-Century United States.* Greenwich, Conn.: JAI Press.
Strong, M.A., S.H. Preston, A.R. Miller, M. Hereward, H.R. Lentzner, J.R. Seaman, and H.C. Williams
    1989   *User's Guide. Public Use Sample, 1900 United States Census of Population.* Philadelphia: Population Studies Center, University of Pennsylvania.
Thompson, W.S., and P.K. Whelpton
    1933   *Population Trends in the United States.* New York: McGraw-Hill.
Trussell, J., and R. Olsen
    1983   Evaluation of the Olsen technique for estimating the fertility response to child mortality. *Demography* 20(3):391-405.
Trussell, J., and S.H. Preston
    1982   Estimating the covariates of childhood mortality from retrospective reports of mothers. *Health Policy and Education* 3:1-43.

van de Walle, F.
   1986   Infant mortality and the European demographic transition. Pp. 201-233 in A.J. Coale and
          S.C. Watkins, eds., *The Decline of Fertility in Europe*. Princeton, N.J.: Princeton Uni-
          versity Press.
Woodbury, R.M.
   1926   *Infant Mortality and Its Causes*. Baltimore, Md.: The Williams and Wilkins Company.
Yasuba, Y.
   1962   *Birth Rates of the White Population of the United States, 1800-1860: An Economic Analy-
          sis*. Baltimore, Md.: Johns Hopkins University Press.

8

Fertility Response to Infant and Child Mortality in Africa with Special Reference to Cameroon

Barthélémy Kuate Defo

INTRODUCTION

Most demographic transition theorists would agree with the notion that current and future levels of infant mortality, combined with current stocks of children, are likely determinants of fertility, and many studies have shown a high correlation between infant and child mortality and fertility levels, both in their time trends and cross sectionally. Theoretical considerations, largely supported by empirical research findings, confirm the interdependence of child mortality and fertility. At a micro level, it has been found that the risk of a birth is significantly higher following the death of a child in the family (e.g., Ben-Porath, 1978; Olsen, 1980). However, the prevalent direction of causation, its mechanisms, timing, and strength differ among populations.

This study has two objectives: first, to provide an overview of the effects of infant and child mortality on fertility in African countries; and second, to assess the extent to which couples' reproductive behavior changes in response to child mortality using micro-data from Cameroon. These data contain information on the timing of all conceptions and infant mortality experiences of the respondents. They enable us to study the instantaneous and lagged effects of an infant death on the hazard of a conception and to derive replacement effects from hazard model estimates. These replacement effects provide insights into the contributions that declining infant and child mortality rates in Cameroon have had on the concurrent fertility reduction. The estimated parameters integrate aspects of life- cycle fertility that have previously been studied in isolation of each other: completed fertility, childlessness, and interbirth intervals.

In Cameroon the response to mortality involves volitional behavior in a high-fertility, high-mortality environment with very little modern contraceptive use. The case of Cameroon thus raises questions about the response to mortality in sub-Saharan Africa more generally where the levels of both mortality and fertility remain high in most countries (Hill, 1993; Cohen, 1993). In the virtual absence of effective means of contraception other than breastfeeding, the shortening of birth interval induced by a reduction in infant and child survivorship may signify a higher ultimate parity. Higher fertility may thus be largely a biological response to higher mortality. It is more likely that the behavioral response has a greater effect on the total number of children to whom a woman gives birth, or alternatively, on the parity of her last live birth since women entertain a rough idea of the number of surviving children they would like to have, even if they do not have a predetermined target (van de Walle, 1992). In this chapter, I do not estimate a tightly structural model of fertility because the main question—does child mortality matter for fertility behavior?—is still open. A positive answer to this question has been assumed in the demographic transition theory literature, but without much factual basis from developing countries. A central finding documented in this study is that current and past child mortality experiences play a strong role in reproductive behavior in Cameroon, even after correcting for measured and unmeasured heterogeneity.

EFFECTS OF INFANT AND CHILD MORTALITY ON REPRODUCTIVE BEHAVIOR IN AFRICA: WHAT DO WE KNOW?

Empirical studies of the effects of infant and child mortality on fertility in Africa fall into two broad categories: aggregate studies, which are based on samples consisting of national or subnational averages usually using censuses, cross-sectional surveys, or registration data; and individual-level studies, which are based on sample survey observations drawn from the reproductive experience of individual women. Table 8-1 presents an overview of published work that has attempted to measure the fertility response to infant and child mortality, using aggregate or individual data.

Aggregate Level

Studies based on aggregate data have one important advantage over individual data: the potential for measuring the overall implications of improvements in child survival for fertility and population growth. Because many of the hypothesized effects of changes in mortality on fertility work through changes in environmental conditions rather than through individual experience, studies based on individual data alone can only measure accurately the physiological and volitional replacement effects (United Nations, 1987). These effects are not expected to compensate fully for changes in mortality even if they operate jointly. Aggregate studies of the effects of infant and child mortality on fertility in Africa are

TABLE 8-1 Synopsis of Published Studies of the Effects of Infant and Child Mortality on Fertility in Africa: Aggregate and Individual Data

| Source | Characteristics of the Study | | | |
	Year/Period of Data Collection	Country/Strata	Study Design	Measure Mortality
Barbieri, 1994	1985-1989	10 sub-Saharan African countries[a]	DHS surveys	Probability of dying between 0-26 months
Bocquier, 1991	1986	Pikine, Senegal	Retrospective survey of 2,807 women aged 15-49 (and 7,632 births)	Child death
Brass, 1993	1969, 1978, 1989	Kenya	1969 census, 1977-1978 WFS and 1989 DHS surveys	$_5Q_{10}$ proportion of children died per woman
Brass and Jolly, 1993	1977-1978	Kenya and provinces and districts	WFS and DHS surveys	$_5Q_{10}$
Callum et al., 1988	1980	Egypt	Retrospective (WFS) survey	Child death
Cantrelle et al., 1978	1940-1972	12 sub-Saharan African countries[b]	Retrospective and prospective surveys	$_1Q_0, _2Q_1$ $_2Q_0$
Cantrelle and Leridon, 1971	1962-1968	Niakhar, rural Senegal	Longitudinal study of 8,456 live births	Child death
Coale, 1966	1940-1962	13 sub-Saharan African countries[c]	Retrospective surveys	$_1Q_0, _2Q_1$
Cochrane and Zachariah, 1984	1977-1978	Lesotho (1977) and Kenya (1977-1978) (in [WFS] a study of 25 LDCs)	Retrospective surveys	Child death
Farah, 1982	1975	Greater Khartoum, Sudan	Retrospective survey of 2,045 ever-married women aged 15-44	Child death

		Mortality Effects		Association Mortality-Fertility
Fertility	Type of Analysis	Replacement	Insurance	
TFR for women aged 15-40	Descriptive analysis and linear regression analysis (aggregate data)	Unclear	n.a.	Yes
Probability of a following conception	Nonparametric survival analysis (individual data)	Yes	n.a.	Yes
TFR	Descriptive analysis (aggregate data)	No	n.a.	No
TFR	Descriptive analysis (aggregate data)	No	n.a.	No
Percent of women with no additional births; mean number of children born	Descriptive and multivariate analyses (individual data)	Yes	Unclear	Yes
TFR, GFR	Correlation analysis (aggregate data)	n.a.	n.a.	Unclear
Mean birth interval	Descriptive analysis (aggregate data)	Yes	n.a.	Yes
TFR	Correlation analysis (aggregate data)	n.a.	n.a.	Unclear
Birth interval	Multivariate analysis (individual data)	Yes	n.a.	Yes
CEB	Simple classification analysis (individual data)	Yes	n.a.	Yes

continued on next page

TABLE 8-1 (*continued*)

Source	Year/Period of Data Collection	Country/Strata	Study Design	Measure Mortality
	Characteristics of the Study			
Folta and Deck, 1988	No date	Zimbabwe	Participant observation and in-depth interviews of 124 women	Child death
Heer and Wu, 1978	1966	Urban Morocco	Area probability sample of currently married women under age 50 who had experienced 3 or more live births	Number of the first three children that survived either to age 10 or to the time of interview
Jensen, 1993	1988, 1990	Bungoma and Kwale, Kenya	Cross-sectional interviews with 132 women aged 18-78	Number of children deceased
Jensen, 1996	1988-1989	Kenya, Zimbabwe, Botswana	DHS surveys	Infant & child death
Livenais, 1984	1973, 1978	Rural Mossi, Burkina-Faso	Cross-sectional surveys	$_1Q_0$
Okojie, 1991	1985	Bendel state, Nigeria	Retrospective survey of 1,895 ever-married women aged 15-50	Proportion of surviving children
Sembajwe, 1981	1973	Western Nigeria	Retrospective survey	Proportion of children dead

NOTES: TFR, total fertility rate; GFR, general fertility rate; $_1Q_0$, infant mortality rate; $_2Q_1$ = second-year mortality rate; $_2Q_0$, first two years mortality rate; $_5Q_0$, first five years mortality rate; CEB, children ever born; n.a., not applicable; WFS, World Fertility Survey; DHS, Demographic and Health Survey; LDC, less-developed countries.

[a]The 10 sub-Saharan African countries are Botswana (1988), Burundi (1987), Ghana (1988), Kenya (1989), Liberia (1986), Mali (1987), Senegal (1986), Togo (1988), Uganda (1988-1989), and Zimbabwe (1988-1989).

Fertility	Type of Analysis	Mortality Effects		Association Mortality- Fertility
		Replacement	Insurance	
Fertility following a child death	Qualitative analysis (individual data)	Yes	n.a.	Yes
Number of life births subsequent to the third	Multiple classification analysis (individual and aggregate data)	Yes	Unclear	Yes
CEB	Multiple classification analysis (individual data)	Yes	n.a.	Yes
Hazard of a following birth	Event history analysis (individual data)	Yes	n.a.	Yes
TFR	Descriptive analysis (aggregate data)	No	n.a.	No
CEB	Two-stage ordinary least squares (individual data)	Yes	n.a.	Yes
CEB	Regression (individual analysis)	Yes	n.a.	Yes

[b]The 12 countries are Benin (1961), Guinea (1954-1955), Burkina-Faso (1960-1961), Niger (1960), Angola (1940, 1950), Zaire (1955-1957), Cameroon (1960), Kenya (1962), Mozambique (1950), Rwanda (1952-1957), Tanzania (1957), and Uganda (1956).

[c]The 13 countries are Benin (1961), Guinea (1954-1955), Burkina-Faso (1960-1961), Niger (1960), Angola (1940, 1950), Zaire (1955-1957), Cameroon (1960), Kenya (1962), Mozambique (1950), Rwanda (1952-1957), Tanzania (1957), Uganda (1956), and Senegal (1963-1970, 1972).

either cross-sectional studies based on national aggregates using data drawn from several African countries (e.g., Coale, 1966; Cantrelle et al., 1978; Barbieri, 1994) or from a specific country, subregion, or province within a country (e.g., Heer and Wu, 1978; Livenais, 1984; Brass, 1993; Brass and Jolly, 1993).

The general finding from these aggregate-level studies is that in Africa mortality decline has had either no effects or unclear effects on fertility. Thus, the evidence from these studies is inconclusive. The absence of a demonstrable link between childhood mortality and fertility at the aggregate level apparently may stem from the fact that intermediate variables, which act more directly on these rates, are obscuring the strong positive relationship at work at the individual level (Cantrelle et al., 1978). In Kenya, for example, Brass (Brass, 1993; Brass and Jolly, 1993), analyzing previous child mortality declines, and their effect on recent fertility declines, argues that "the observations supply no evidence of any consistent relation between the falls in fertility and the preceding (and continuing) child mortality trends" (Brass, 1993:78). Coale (1966) and Cantrelle et al. (1978) found that the zero-order correlations for the 47 subregions of countries for which data were available between aggregate fertility and mortality rates were –0.38 and –0.37, respectively, thus failing to support the widely observed positive association between childhood mortality and fertility.

Individual Level

In recent years, most of the published research on the mortality-fertility relationships has been based on survey data, such as the World Fertility Surveys (WFS) and the Demographic and Health Surveys (DHS). The individual-level studies reviewed in Table 8-1 consistently show that the death of an infant leads to a shorter interval between that birth and the next, and therefore provides a clear indication that, at the individual level, there is a significant fertility response to child loss. For example, a detailed study of the Sine region of Senegal (Cantrelle and Leridon, 1971) shows that the death of an infant (which is equivalent to weaning) affects fertility. Cochrane and Zachariah (1984) use data from the WFS of Kenya and Lesotho (among other countries studied) to measure the influence of neonatal (0-1 month) and postneonatal (2-11 months) deaths of first, third, and fifth children on the length of subsequent birth interval. They find that birth intervals are reduced following the death of a child. They also show that breastfeeding is an important factor affecting differences in birth intervals. Furthermore, they found that the reduction in birth intervals is significantly greater for neonatal deaths than postneonatal deaths for the interval between the first and second birth but not for the other parities. This finding suggests that the mortality-induced reduction in birth interval may vary across parity. Analyzing the possible effects of mortality on fertility among the Yoruba in Nigeria, Sembajwe (1981) observes that the proportion of children dead increases as the number of children ever born alive increases. In this society, however, the answer "up to

God" to the question about the family size does not seem to be influenced by the experience of child loss.

The study by Callum et al. (1988) uses individual- and community-level data from the Egypt WFS to attempt to assess both replacement and insurance effects of child mortality through an examination of actual fertility outcomes according to the number of children who have died for women of equal parity and family size. Their fertility outcomes during the 5 years preceding the survey were related to the number of children ever born and living and the number of children who had died during the 5 years prior to the date of interview. As regards the replacement effects, they found that (1) an infant death is associated with a reduction of about 6 months (roughly 15-20 percent) in the interval to the next live birth; (2) there is a significantly lower likelihood of contraceptive use in the event of an infant death, which persists after controlling for parity and socioeconomic status; and (3) most of the reduction in interval length among nonusers of contraception is accounted for by the biological effect of the reduction in the anovulatory period. Regarding the insurance effect, there was some evidence of an individual insurance response to the experience of child loss, especially in Cairo, Alexandria, and urban lower Egypt. The authors speculate that, in the context of relatively high mortality, common in Africa, an insurance strategy is more likely to be adopted in response to generally perceived rather than individually experienced mortality risks, and that, therefore, measurement at the individual level fails to capture the full effect of the insurance response.

The fertility response to child loss in Kenya deserves special attention for two reasons. First, it is the only African country for which there have been several studies of the mortality effects on fertility both at the aggregate and individual levels. Second, there are sharp discrepancies between findings at the aggregate level and at the individual level: All aggregate-level studies find either no effects or unclear effects of child mortality on fertility (Coale, 1966; Cantrelle et al., 1978; Brass, 1993; Brass and Jolly, 1993; Barbieri, 1994), whereas all individual-level studies (Cochrane and Zachariah, 1984; Jensen, 1993, 1996) find strong evidence of fertility response to child loss. This raises important population policy and substantive questions regarding the weight to give to the evidence of mortality effects on fertility at the aggregate level versus individual level in Africa more generally. Contraceptive use seems to have played a role in the strength of the relationship between mortality and fertility in Kenya. Indeed, child mortality was one of the main factors used to explain the high fertility rate in Kenya during the late 1970s, and child survival programs were estimated to be more cost effective than family planning programs in terms of lowering fertility (Cochrane and Zachariah, 1984). Looking at the linkage between child mortality and contraceptive use, Njogu (1992) identified in the late 1970s a strong and negative effect on contraceptive use among women who had experienced child loss. Ten years later the overall level of child mortality had declined and the effect of contraceptive use had lessened. Kelley and Nobbe (1990) point to the high correlation between infant mortality and family planning use at the regional level, the highest use of contraceptives being found in areas with low infant mortality. Jensen's study (1996) uses data from two areas in Kenya (the Muslim Kwale in Coast Province and the Christian Bungoma in Western Province) and finds a strong influence of child mortality on fertility and contraceptive use, suggestive of hoarding behavior. In both areas child mortality is associated with high fertility and constitutes the strongest barrier toward using modern contraceptives.

There are virtually no good ethnographic studies of relevance to the fertility response to child loss in Africa. The only published work to our knowledge is the study by Folta and Deck (1988) in Zimbabwe. This study uses participant observation and in-depth interviews of 124 Shona women in Zimbabwe to show that social pressure to replace a dead child can lead to immediate pregnancy with poor nutrition, poor infant health, and thus a recurring cycle of infant death. In this setting, the death of a child (especially the first child) potentially undermines the stability of the family, its social relationships, women's health and status, economic security, and marital longevity.

HYPOTHESES

Fertility is inextricably bound up with many aspects of economic and social behavior. At both the micro and the macro level, it is useful to think of fertility as mediated by a set of variables defining exposure to intercourse, the probability of conception, and the probability of successful gestation and parturition. These intermediate variables constitute components of a conceptual framework of the determinants of fertility, which, by definition, must stand between fertility and any type of social or economic explanation. All elements of choice or social behavior work through the intermediate variables to influence fertility.

The relationships between infant mortality and fertility are exceedingly complex, and many of the factors involved are poorly understood. A joint decline of infant mortality and fertility rates in recent years as observed in Cameroon is typical for a number of African countries (for reviews, see Locoh and Hertrich, 1994; Hill, 1993; Cohen, 1993) and non-African countries (United Nations, 1987) over the past decade. The sources of this correlation may be categorized according to the direction of the effect.

First, infant mortality and fertility may be positively correlated if both investments in child health and demand for children are functions of the same prevailing influential variables (Preston, 1978; Panis and Lillard, 1993).

Second, a rapid pace of childbearing may cause high mortality. The overwhelming evidence is that short birth intervals have strong effects on infant and child mortality; such a result has been reported in Cameroon (Kuate Defo and Palloni, 1996) and elsewhere (for a review, see Hobcraft, 1994). This effect of fertility on mortality can occur because of (1) increased sibling competition for resources (including child care, family assets, and income); (2) increased opportunities for transmission of infectious diseases as a result of overcrowding, which has been shown to be an important determinant of infant and child mortality in Cameroon; or (3) the maternal depletion syndrome, in which a rapid pace of fertility may imply that the mother has not had sufficient time to regain her health or nutritional status to adequately host a fetus and facilitate its normal growth.

Finally, high child mortality may induce high fertility (Preston, 1978). This may happen as a result of several mechanisms. The death of the child initiating the birth interval may trigger the rapid closure of the interval either through a physiological replacement mechanism whereby the death of the child leads to cessation of breastfeeding and the consequent shortening of postpartum amenorrhea; through a volitional replacement mechanism (that is, the responsiveness of pregnancy decisions to the occurrence of the death of infants who either never breastfed or stopped breastfeeding before death); or through a generalized survival uncertainty (that is, as the probability of survival falls, there is also a tendency to have children earlier and thus closely spaced).

In assessing the effects of infant mortality on fertility, I depart from previous studies on Africa (and reviewed above) and other parts of the world that have shown that, over the course of the family life cycle, couples learn about childbearing and child mortality (e.g., Preston, 1978; Ben-Porath, 1978; Mensch, 1985; United Nations, 1987). These experiences may well lead them to revise and adjust their desired number of children and possibly diminish or increase their propensity to replace deceased children. Because we do not explicitly model breastfeeding and contraceptive behavior (since these variables may be endogenous to the fertility decision), we cannot empirically distinguish these two causal mechanisms directly for the short-term replacement effects. (That is, we cannot separate the physiological from the volitional replacement effects of the death of child of parity i who opens the interval $[i, i + 1)$ and dies within the first year and before the conception of the child of parity $i + 1$.) In this case we group these two physiological and volitional replacement mechanisms of increased risks following conception under the term "replacement behavior." Moreover, it has been shown that, in many parts of sub-Saharan Africa where prolonged breastfeeding is prescribed and sexual intercourse during lactation is forbidden, the physiological effect is culturally built into behavior patterns (Ware, 1977). For the long-term replacement effects in the subsequent intervals, significant effects of the death of a child of parity i on the hazards of conceiving children of parity $i + 2$, $i + 3$, $i + 4$, and so forth cannot be ascribed to a biological/physiological mechanism but only to a volitional (behavioral) mechanism, as discussed below. Furthermore, because the level of contraceptive use is low in Cameroon (the level of use of efficient contraceptive methods was 2 percent in 1978 and only 16 percent in 1991 of which one-fourth was accounted for by modern methods) and there has been no marked increase in contraceptive use between the two surveys (DSCN, 1983; Balepa et al., 1992), the probability of using contraception in a particular period would change marginally. This is tantamount to confining our analysis to women who did not use any form of contraception during the waiting time to succeeding conception. Thus, the very nature of the data (mostly noncontracepting women) allows us to isolate to a greater extent the mediating effect of breastfeeding alone on conception rates in response to mortality. This is a "natural" sample and there is no bias since women who do not use contraception are not self-selected for lower fertility. There is as yet little evidence of conscious limitation of family size in most sub-Saharan African societies (Caldwell and Caldwell, 1981; van de Walle, 1992). Evidence indicates that, in most sub-Saharan African societies, postpartum abstinence is practiced specifically to ensure that the supply and quality of breast milk are adequate and to enhance child survival (Page and Lesthaeghe, 1981). Knowledge and use of indigenous contraceptive practices usually seem to be aimed at preventing conception at certain times (thus affecting the waiting time to the next conception and birth) or from certain unions that are undesirable, rather than at limiting the ultimate size of the family. Hence, the potential effect of a child death on birth spacing is at its maximum in this setting.

In this chapter, I test three hypotheses regarding the fertility responses to child death:

Hypothesis 1: A child death has both instantaneous (short-term) and lagged (long-term) effects on conception risks (or birth-to-conception intervals).

The instantaneous effect is likely to be more important in a setting where there is little conscious decision to space births or to limit fertility, and couples practice little or no contraception, as in Cameroon until the late 1980s (Balepa et al., 1992).

Hypothesis 2: The fertility response to child loss is stronger for the death of first-parity births (and eventually second-parity births) than for the death of higher-parity births.

Many African societies attach special cultural values to the first offspring. This may affect the way the survival of the first born is perceived by the couple and the community, and a loss of a first child by death is often interpreted as the failure of the mother to fulfill her proper role in society. In most African societies, women are expected to become pregnant shortly after marriage, and the pressure on these women is often high to produce living children so as to secure their status with the husband's family. For example, Folta and Deck (1988) note that among the Shona in Zimbabwe, it is after the birth of the first child that women are provided with their own dwellings, and it is critical that certain rituals be followed properly to prevent illness and death of this child.

The eagerness with which African unions are stabilized is reflected in the quantum and tempo for the first birth: First-birth intervals are typically shorter than other intervals. For the new mother, the firstborn is a sign of belonging to a new family and confers the status of a full family member for her in her husband's family. Thus, a number of rituals are associated with the birth of the first child. The new mother must fulfill these rituals to ensure her progeny. Pregnancy, for example, calls into play a series of rituals that are required to assure the continued fertility of the woman and protection of her children. Hence, the death of the firstborn (or second births) may have a large effect on both short- and long-term fertility responses, far exceeding the simple replacement effect.

Hypothesis 3: The fertility response to a child loss (and the importance of mechanisms discussed above) varies by parity.

Most previous studies of the effects of child mortality on fertility have assumed that those effects were the same across parities. Preston (1978:7) points out that

> in populations where conscious limitation of family size is negligibly important, completed family size can be viewed simply as the cumulative outcome of uncorrelated birth intervals spanning a woman's reproductive life. In such populations, it is legitimate to regard intervals and completed family size as simultaneously determined: hence interval effects translate immediately into fertility effects.

This argument is consistent with observations from a number of studies on Africa. We allow the fertility response to infant and child mortality as well as the effects of all other measured and unmeasured variables to vary both by parity and duration of exposure.

DATA SOURCES

In the empirical analysis in this chapter, I use data from the 1978 Cameroon World Fertility Survey (CWFS) and the 1991 Cameroon Demographic and Health Survey (CDHS). The core questionnaires were very similar, making it easy to undertake comparative studies. Given the differences in behavior that may be expected between ever-married and never-married women, I restrict my data to fertility of ever-married women who did not have a premarital birth.[1]

The CWFS was conducted from January to October 1978 under the auspices

---

[1]Premarital births were dropped from the analyses because of the imprecision about the beginning of exposure and the duration of exposure to the risk of bearing a child and because it is not known the extent to which the survival status of the premarital birth may be related to fertility behavior of the women later in marriage. In general, premarital births are not identified as belonging to the girl in rural areas where there is a strong sense that a premarital birth is a shameful experience, bringing dishonor, disgrace, and embarrassment on the family of the woman, and parents will generally claim the birth as their own to avoid this. However, in trial analyses including women with premarital births, none of my inferences are altered and the conclusions from this study remain robust.

of the Cameroon Ministry of Planning and Regional Development in collaboration with the WFS. The CWFS is a large in-depth survey and the first that is nationally representative of Cameroon. A total of 8,219 women aged 15-54 years answered questions about their fertility, marriage histories, and other characteristics. Of these women, 1,253 were excluded from the analysis because they were aged 50-54, never married, or had had premarital births.

The CDHS is a nationally representative sample of 3,871 women aged 15-49 years. Of these women, 835 were excluded because they were never married and 432 were excluded because they had premarital births. The final sample is comprised of 2,604 ever-married women with no premarital births. A preliminary inspection of the data revealed that the sample does not differ in terms of mortality statistics from the original sample, and differences in fertility patterns between the two samples are quite marginal.

One drawback of the WFS- and DHS-type data sets is that the characteristics of parents are documented only at the time of the survey and not at the time that each child under study was exposed to the risk of mortality or each woman was exposed to the risk of a new conception. These characteristics may have changed during the reproductive life of the women and differed at the time of birth or death of their children. In most studies based on these data, the analysis is based on the assumption that those characteristics remain the same for a sufficiently long period into the past. Because I do not have such background variables that follow the sequence of exposure and occurrence, I make that assumption here as well. The selected variables are defined in Table 8-2.

By construction, the estimated intervals measure the period from a birth to the conception of the next live birth. They are based on data for month and year of birth of children reported retrospectively in 1978 (for the CWFS) and 1991 (for the CDHS). In the CWFS, from the birth history data involving all births, both the year and month were reported for 41 percent of all births, the calendar year (but no month) was given for 48 percent, whereas for 11 percent of all births dates were reported in terms of "years ago" or age at event (Kuate Defo, 1996). This implies that some dates of births (in months) were imputed. The imputation procedure in the WFS used other information reported by the respondent from which a logical period within which the birth probably occurred and then randomly assigned a date within that period. This situation can create problems in the analysis of birth intervals. For example, in the case of a following conception, the problem may arise from the fact that the timing of the following conception (or birth) is unspecified, and there may also be the possibility of reverse causation, misclassification of exposure, or selection bias. Strategies for dealing with these problems are considered in the Appendix.

These data also provide the opportunity to relate the length of interbirth intervals to the survival status of previous children. Obviously, any variations between women in interbirth intervals that can be attributed to differences in child death experience give only a partial measure of the replacement effect

TABLE 8-2 Definition of Variables Used in the Multistate Hazards Analysis

Variable Definition	Specification
Duration (DUR) measures	Number of months/100 spent in the current spell
Exposure since first marriage (DUR1)	Length of the first conception interval, measured in months/100
Exposure since first birth (DUR2)	Length of the second conception interval, measured in months/100
Exposure since second birth (DUR3)	Length of the third conception interval, measured in months/100
Exposure since third birth (DUR4)	Length of the fourth conception interval, measured in months/100
Exposure since fourth birth (DUR5)	Length of the fifth conception interval, measured in months/100
Exposure since fifth birth (DUR6)	Length of the sixth conception interval, measured in months/100
Child mortality measures (CMM)	Series of time-varying dummy variables capturing the sequencing of an infant death and couple's future reproductive behavior
The child who opens the birth-to-conception interval $[i, i + 1)$ dies in his first year of life and at least 1 month before the conception of the child of parity $i + 1$ (i.e., the child closing the interval) (CMM1)	A dummy time-varying variable = 1 if a mother lost her child who opens the birth-to-conception interval $[i, i + 1)$ in his first year of life and at least 1 month before the conception of the index child (i.e., the child of parity $i + 1$) (N.B.: this measure confounds the physiological and volitional replacement effects)
The child who opens the birth-to-conception interval $[i, i + 1)$ dies at least 1 month before the conception of the child who closes the future intervals $[i + 2, i + 3)$ or higher (CMM2)	A dummy time-varying variable = 1 if a mother lost her child who opens the birth-to-conception interval $[i, i + 1)$ in his first year of life and at least 1 month before the conception of the child of rank $i + 2$, $i + 3$, $i + 4$, and so forth (N.B.: captures both infant and child mortality)
The first (second) birth dies in the first year of life and at least 1 month before the conception of children of higher parities (CMM3)	A dummy time-varying variable = 1 if a mother lost her first (alternatively second) birth in his first year of life and at least 1 month before the conception of child of rank 2, 3, 4, 5, and 6 (alternatively rank 3, 4, 5, and 6)

continued on next page

TABLE 8-2   (*continued*)

Variable Definition	Specification
Mother has some education	A dummy time-invariant variable = 1 if a mother has attended primary level education or higher, and 0 otherwise
Low-fertility ethnic groups	A dummy time-invariant variable = 1 if a mother is affiliated with the ethnic groups of the Grand North and the East regions
Muslim religion	A dummy time-invariant variable = 1 if the mother is a Muslim, and 0 otherwise
Employed before first marriage	A dummy time-invariant variable = 1 if the woman was employed outside the home before her first marriage, and 0 otherwise
Sex composition of previous living children	A dummy time-varying variable = 1 if a mother has more previous living boys than girls, and 0 otherwise
Changes in marital status	A dummy time-varying variable = 1 if a marriage or remarriage was dissolved (e.g., by divorce, separation, or death of the spouse), and 0 otherwise
Time trend	A dummy time-invariant variable = 1 if the conception occurred within the last 10 calendar years preceding the survey date

because replacement of lost children can be accomplished not only through changes in birth intervals but also through prolonging the reproductive period. In addition, those aspects of the intentional replacement effect that influence timing will be mixed with the physiological effect, particularly in populations where family planning is practiced.

FORMULATION AND ESTIMATION OF FERTILITY RESPONSE TO CHILD LOSS

I formulate and implement a multistate duration hazard model as a framework for estimation of the effects of child mortality on fertility (for details, see the Appendix). My model assumes that experienced child mortality is exogenous to fertility behavior and that there is no other source of correlation between mortality and fertility. This assumption excludes the possibility of hoarding behavior and ignores any other trade-off. This simplification is justified to some extent because there is apparently little evidence of either hoarding behavior or selectivity of child mortality in the fertility process in Cameroon, in part given the high incidence of sterility and strikingly low levels of contraceptive use in this setting. My empirical specification models fertility as a sequential decision-making process with a stochastic component whereby, at each moment in time, the couple decides on behaviors that affect the risk of conception. Life-cycle fertility is only one aspect of female life-cycle behavior. In this chapter, I focus on fertility histories, ignoring possible interrelationships between fertility and other life-cycle behavior such as labor supply, education, and marital decisions. My approach aims to estimate parameters of hazards for times to conceptions. Estimated parameters measure direct (given other decisions) and indirect (through other decisions) effects of infant mortality on fertility transitions.

My unit of observation is a woman's entire fertility history, with a hazard equation for each birth-to-conception interval. The timing of a conception may depend on the duration since the wedding date (i.e., the age of the woman at first marriage), the duration since the last birth, the birth order, and the duration since a child died. I limit the analysis to fertility of ever-married women (thereafter referred to as marital fertility), that is, the woman first becomes at risk of a conception at the wedding date. Each subsequent conception interval starts at the date of termination of the previous pregnancy, which is the birth date of the previous child. I limit the analysis to conceptions ending in live births because, in most developing countries, reporting and dating of miscarriage, stillbirths, and induced abortions are known to be heavily flawed. Furthermore, much of this information was either not recorded in my data sets or the timing of events was unknown or the duration variables were heavily distorted. I account for these unmeasured characteristics in fertility outcomes by entering in the estimation equations woman-specific and parity-specific unobserved components. I do not account for a period of postpartum anovulation beyond the first month infertile period following a birth because the duration of this period can be influenced by the mother through the duration and intensity of breastfeeding. As such, breast-feeding is a form of contraception and endogenous to the fertility process. Larsen (1994) found that contraception has only a minor effect on estimates of sterility and fertility in countries such as Cameroon in which modern methods are currently used by 6 percent or fewer of the female population of reproductive age.

My analysis places fertility behavior within a life-cycle perspective. A common way of characterizing the timing of births is in terms of the probability of a woman's first birth at different ages (or duration of exposure) and spacing between subsequent birth parities (Hotz et al., in press). My modeling strategy of the effects of infant death on fertility starts with the premise that fertility is usually indicated by birth spacing, parity, and maternal age at maternity. I incorporate these three dimensions of fertility by estimating dynamic models of the timing and spacing of births, while allowing those effects to vary by parity. I estimate the joint probability of first, second, third, fourth, fifth, and sixth conceptions, respectively, conditional on reaching the beginning of each subsequent interval without having had a conception of the next rank. Thus, I estimate dynamically the effects of infant mortality on fertility intervals. This approach is analogous to a piecewise hazard analysis of birth intervals (which would have involved as many separate likelihood functions as there are pieces of intervals) (e.g., Rodriguez et al., 1984; Mensch, 1985), except that it enriches this strategy by jointly estimating all birth intervals so that there is only one likelihood function to be computed (Heckman and Walker, 1991; see also the Appendix). I model the duration of exposure to the risk of conceiving the jth child using a Weibull model (Lancaster, 1985; Heckman and Walker, 1991).[2] I model this by estimating the conditional fertility function: conditional on the number of children a woman has, what is the likelihood that she will bear another child given her mortality experience since a given prior time. Clearly, a young woman of high parity must of necessity have had closely spaced births, whereas an older woman of lower parity may well have had long intervals between her children. I allow for this time-varying covariate by estimating jointly the effects of covariates within distinct time-to-conception intervals (parities). Thus, the effects of each covariate are allowed to vary over a woman's reproductive career through interactions with each period of exposure to the risk of conception. For example, the effects of mother's education are evaluated jointly for the following intervals: (1) from marriage date (or age at first marriage) to first conception, (2) between date of first birth and conception of second birth, (3) between date of second birth and conception of third birth, (4) between date of third birth and conception of fourth birth, (5) between date of fourth birth and conception of fifth birth, and (6) between date of fifth birth and conception of sixth birth. Thus, at a given parity, I have the cumulative reproductive history of the woman until that parity.

Duration Dependencies Dur(*t*)

In the absence of infant mortality, the baseline hazard function duration dependence Dur(*t*) consists of the duration of exposure to the risk of conception (i.e., the duration since the woman became at risk of conceiving the jth child). It includes, respectively, a general function of the age of the woman that corresponds to the wedding date (or maternal age at first union) for first conceptions and a general function of the duration since the last birth (or the birth date of the child initiating the birth-to-conception/censoring interval) for subsequent intervals.

---

[2]I also experimented with alternative specifications of the fertility response to changes in infant and child mortality by formulating hazards models assuming both the piecewise exponential (proportional hazard) and a Gompertz hazard model for the risk of a subsequent conception starting with the first birth, but none of my conclusions was altered with these alternative specifications.

Child Mortality Measures *Z(t)* and Replacement Effects

In this chapter, I am especially interested in the timing of replacement and the relationship between replacement strategy and family size. This is because little attention appears to have been paid in studies of the fertility response to child loss, to the possibility that such fertility behavior may be linked to achieved parity. Replacement behavior is detected by the inclusion of a series of measures of experienced child mortality. I explicitly account for the possibility that the effect of a child death on fertility may vary over time through the woman's reproductive life cycle. The replacement behavior is specified as a time-dependent variable. The death of a child is assumed to have both an instantaneous and lagged effect. I assume that the replacement effects may be parity dependent and may differ by such characteristics as religion, ethnicity, time period, and the sex composition of the surviving children.

My formulation departs from previous procedures in the way I define the time-varying variables that capture the effects of the death of the child who opens the birth interval. I first estimate a series of models with infant mortality time-dependent covariates as dummy variables, each indicating whether the child who opens a given birth-to-conception interval has died: at least 1 month before the conception of the child who closes that interval; before the conception of the child who closes the immediately succeeding birth-to-conception interval; and so forth. For example, when assessing the effects of child mortality on the birth interval $[i, i + 1)$, I examine whether the death of the child of rank i antedated the conception of child of rank $i + 1$. I also assume a normal conception period of 9 months plus an extra month of postpartum infertility following birth; I recognize that—in the absence of good data on gestational length from most surveys— premature births are a particular case in which there may be confusion of cause and effect. A premature birth of rank $i + 1$ is associated with a shorter birth-to-conception interval $[i, i + 1)$ because the duration of gestation is less than a full-term birth of 9 months. Also, prematurity increases the risk of stillbirth or infant death (Bakketeig et al., 1979; Hoffman and Bakketeig, 1984). To purge for this potential bias, I assess both jointly and sequentially the effects of the death of child of rank, say i, on the birth-to-conception of live birth intervals $[i, i + 1)$, $[i + 1, i + 2)$, $[i + 2, i + 3)$, $[i + 3, i + 4)$, and so forth.

To assess the short-term effects of a child death, I measure the extent to which the death of a child of parity i (the child who opens the birth-to-conception interval $[i, i + 1)$) occurring in the first year of life and at least 1 month before the next conception of a child of parity $i + 1$ (the child who closes the birth-to-conception interval $[i, i + 1)$) significantly increases the risks of conceiving the child of parity $i + 1$. The fertility effects of an infant death in its first year of life and before the next conception is a mixture of the physiological effects (having to do with the curtailment of breastfeeding) and volitional replacement effects. The mean duration of breastfeeding in Cameroon has changed little over time (19.3 months in the 1978 survey and 19.8 months in the 1991 survey).

To assess the long-term effects of a child death, I use two measures of child mortality. The first captures the extent to which the death of a preceding child of parity i (i.e., the child who opens the birth-to-conception interval $[i, i + 1)$) at least 1 month before the conception of a child of parity $i + 2$, $i + 3$, $i + 4$, and so forth (i.e., the child who closes the birth-to-conception interval $[i + 1, i + 2)$, $[i + 2, i + 3)$, $[i + 3, i + 4)$, and so forth, respectively), significantly increases the risk of conceiving a child of parity $i + 2$, $i + 3$, $i + 4$, and so on, respectively. In this case, the estimated causal effects of child loss on fertility will be termed "long-term" mortality effects since they operate in future subsequent intervals for which the child whose death is of interest is not the child who opens that birth-to-conception interval. Furthermore, available evidence from Africa and elsewhere (for reviews, see Page and Lesthaeghe, 1981; Hull and Simpson, 1985; Winikoff et al., 1988; Popkin et al., 1993) has established that a major determinant of breast-feeding cessation is a new pregnancy, in that women stop breastfeeding once they realize they are pregnant. Thus, if I find, for example, that the death of child i significantly increases the risk of conception of child $i + 2$, $i + 3$, $i + 4$, and so on, I am then certain that such effects cannot be contaminated by prematurity or be ascribed to the physiological effect of lactation. Hence, the long-term mortality effects will be essentially attributable to behavioral (volitional) replacement effects. The second measure examines the effect of the death of the first (or the second) child in its first year of life and at least one month before the conception of subsequent siblings, as the risk of conceiving a child of a higher birth order.

Exogenous Time-Invariant Factors X and Time-Varying Regressors $Y(t)$

The time-invariant exogenous variables include maternal education, ethnicity, religion, and employment before first marriage. These variables were selected for analyses because they have been shown to covary with child survival and reproductive behavior in Cameroon (Kuate Defo, 1996; Kuate Defo and Palloni, 1996; Larsen, 1994, 1995). The time-varying exogenous variables include the sex composition of the previous surviving siblings and marital dissolution. I do not directly control for breastfeeding and contraception since these variables may be endogenous.

Maternal Education

Education, especially female education, has been seen theoretically as influencing fertility in several possible ways. Female education potentially raises the value of her time through the labor market, which means that the opportunity cost of her time forgone in child care is greater. This means that maternal education is likely to have effects on fertility independent of its economic implications

(Rodriguez and Cleland, 1981), and some have argued that it is the cognitive shifts that education brings which are important in explaining its link to lower fertility and higher contraceptive use (Cleland and Wilson, 1987). Following Ben-Porath (1978), I treat mother's schooling as reflecting the long-term desired family size, given the evidence on the fertility-education link in Africa (Acsadi et al., 1990).

Ethnicity

In countries with considerable ethnic diversity, such as Cameroon, mortality and fertility levels have often been found to vary significantly with ethnicity, even when other factors correlated with ethnicity are held constant (United Nations, 1991; Kuate Defo, 1996). I distinguish the lower than national average fertility ethnic groups (the Foulbe-Fulani and the Kaka-Baya from the northern and eastern provinces) from the other ethnic groups from the rest of the country. Each ethnic group has its set of customs, rituals, and practices associated with major life events (e.g., childbirth, marriages, deaths) that may influence the couple's fertility responses to their children's mortality. Such practices and rituals may include: (1) obstetric methods used by traditional birth attendants, especially in the eastern and northern provinces; and (2) traditions affecting the initiation, type, and duration of breastfeeding, particularly in the northern province where inappropriate weaning practices have been identified as the major cause of malnutrition (Kuate Defo, 1996). Therefore, I expect ethnic affiliation to capture behavioral differences across population groups that are not ascribed to other unobservables.

Religion

The main religions in Cameroon are traditional, Muslim, Protestant, and Catholic. Religious differentials in demographic measures may reflect differences in female education, contraceptive use, or beliefs about the length of the postpartum taboo. The Islamic canon prescribes a postpartum taboo only for as long as the bleeding lasts, which is considered to be 40 days. As a result, the 40-day rule appears frequently in the anthropological literature dealing with Islamic populations of the Sahel (Schoenmaeckers et al., 1981). Many Muslim populations, however, are quite clearly in transition from the traditional to the Islamic rule, whereas others seem to continue to adhere to the traditionally African pattern.

Employment Before First Marriage

In most developing countries, a woman's employment before marriage is a marker for higher socioeconomic status, higher level of education, and aspirations for modernity. To the extent that a woman's exposure to the outside world gives her more choices and opportunities to make life-cycle decisions (e.g., timing of marriage, timing and pace of childbearing), I would expect women who were employed before their first marriage to differ from others with respect to fertility and fertility responses to an eventual child death.

Sex Composition of Living Children

The sex of living children may influence the effects of infant mortality on fertility if the couple wants more boys or more girls. Because of the patriarchal nature of most lineages of the Cameroonian society, it is possible that the fertility response to an infant death may depend on the sex of surviving siblings. At least among the Muslims, the Arabic expression *Abu-Elbanat* (the father of daughters) is used widely as a derogatory description of fathers without sons, thus suggesting male preference among the Muslim populations of Cameroon. Moreover, in a number of studies, one of the latent forces in the stated desires of women who want additional children is the sex composition of their living children (e.g., Farah, 1982; Acsadi et al., 1990). Finally, using data from urban Sahel, Trussell et al. (1989) found that girls were less intensively breastfed than boys and that, as a result, the postpartum infertile period was shorter when the previous birth was a girl than a boy.

Changes in Marital Status

In Cameroon, marriage continues to offer women security and social support. Thus, disruption of social ties and community contexts can be a highly stressful experience. In Africa, it is widely believed that it is a man's right to have offspring and that infertility is a woman's problem. Furthermore, it is considered legitimate for a man to abandon a childless or subfertile wife. Therefore, infertile women tend to experience greater marital instability and are more likely to have been married more than once. If such unobserved heterogeneity in fertility has a causal influence on marital status, then marital status cannot be strictly exogenous. However, since such unobserved variation will mostly affect early childbearing (the first or second births at best), I assume in this chapter that marital status is predetermined for most of the fertility process in Cameroon.

Time Trend

The time trend corresponds to the year in which the duration of exposure to the risk of conceiving a child begins. I explore the robustness of the estimated birth process models to the inclusion of this time trend variable. Traditional duration models abstract from life-cycle and period phenomena and focus on durations between events irrespective of their occurrence in either calendar time or in the life cycle of the individuals. I test for the importance of period effects by adding a dummy variable for conceptions occurring during the 10 years prior to each survey as a covariate to the baseline set of regressors. Restricting the analyses to the intervals, say beginning 2 and 10 years before the survey, may reduce recall error for intervals that began very long ago and reduce selection biases for very recent intervals, but this may lead to a downward bias in conception rates (the key dependent variable here) since the inclusion, for example, of the closed birth intervals beginning as long as 10 years before the survey may overrepresent women with low fecundity (Guz and Hobcraft, 1991) and may not capture the significant reductions in the levels of sterility in Cameroon over the past two decades and the induced increase in fertility (Larsen and Menken, 1991; Larsen, 1995).

Accounting for Unobserved Heterogeneity

In any given society at a given time, even though no conscious effort is made by individual families to limit fertility, actual fertility will fall short of reproductive potential because of physiological conditions limiting fertility, such as malnutrition, or because of cultural circumstances such as breastfeeding practices or an intercourse taboo, which have the unintended effect of lowering fertility. This suggests that a number of unmeasured factors either specific to each woman (woman-specific unobserved heterogeneity) or specific to attained parity for a given woman (parity-specific unobserved heterogeneity) may have an influential role on her reproductive behavior and outcome.

Perhaps the most important factors underlying the relationship between infant and child mortality and fertility in developing countries are the effects of nutrition and lactation. These factors are, however, unmeasured for the woman's entire reproductive career in most survey data, including the DHS or WFS data; although both surveys measured lactation for the last and penultimate children (WFS) or the children born within the preceding 5 years of the survey date (DHS), only the DHS has recently collected some anthropometric indicators for women at the time of the survey in selected countries, including Cameroon. Thus, the information on breastfeeding available in the WFS or DHS data does not allow us to tease out the role of lactation as a mediating mechanism in the relationship between child mortality and fertility over more than 5 years of the survey. Indeed, 5 years is a very short period for most demographic processes to capture changes in one phenomenon (e.g., fertility) in response to another (e.g., child mortality) in a way as to assess whether there are lagged effects. These unmeasured characteristics are particularly important for most African countries where an economic crisis has subjected the majority of families to a dramatic shift in purchasing power since the 1980s.

Woman-Specific Unobserved Heterogeneity

Woman-specific unobserved characteristics include factors such as her preferences, fecundity, genetic effects on fecundity, individual adjustments in desired family size, perceived mortality risks from past and present experiences, and various social customs or events that inadvertently affect coital frequency, fecundity, or fetal mortality. Indeed, the long postpartum taboo has been a basic element in producing the child-spacing pattern in tropical Africa, although there are considerable differences with respect to its observance.

Among unmeasured woman-specific factors that separately or jointly determine child mortality and fertility are pathological factors. Their influence is particularly important in tropical Africa where they are usually either infections or malnutrition (Cantrelle et al., 1978). I follow the demographic tradition (e.g., Bongaarts, 1981; Lesthaeghe, 1989). Conception is followed by gestation which is followed by a period of postpartum infecundity before a woman becomes at risk of the next conception. The time to first conception is a convolution of the time from menarche to marriage or cohabitation and the waiting time to pregnancy given exposure. I estimate models with nonparametric woman-specific unobserved heterogeneity. Several unmeasured strategies can be employed to attempt replacement, such as resumption of sexual intercourse or interruption of contraceptive use, all of which leave an imprint in the length of a birth interval. Most of these characteristics are unmeasured in most survey data available to date. Thus, I control for such parity-specific unobserved characteristics in our models (see the Appendix).

Parity-Specific Unobserved Heterogeneity

Parity-specific unobserved heterogeneity captures the limiting behavior and the biological sterility at a given parity. The question of interest here hinges on how the limiting behavior is effected. Some women may not have another child even if they experience a child death; this may be the case if limiting behavior is due to medical reasons. Second, the social norm in most African societies is that when a woman's own daughter begins bearing children, her status of grandmother may preclude her bearing children so that she can oversee the rearing of her grandchildren (Caldwell and Caldwell, 1981; Acsadi et al., 1990). The extent to which such norms might be violated and the limiting behavior reversible if a child death should occur is unknown and deserves investigation.

Evidence from the 1991 survey suggests that, in Cameroon, only 12.4 percent of women have a stated limiting behavior (no desire for additional children); this percentage increases with increases in the number of surviving children, from 0.2 percent among women with no surviving child to 35.5 percent among women with six or more surviving children (Balepa et al., 1992). Thus, it is possible that some women may reverse their limiting behavior in the aftermath of a child death. These are unobserved factors that may affect the fertility behavior at a given parity and that I attempt to capture by specifying a parity-specific random component in my models (see the Appendix). The evidence regarding insurance strategy in Africa is scanty and at best conjectural, in part because of a lack of good data. On a world scale, most of the observed variations in natural fertility levels within marriage are probably due to variations in the length of the intervals between successive births, resulting mainly from variations in the length of the postpartum nonsusceptible period and from variations in fecundity. In some parts of Africa, high levels of sterility also play an important role in that a sizable number of women either remain childless (Larsen and Menken, 1991; Larsen, 1994, 1995) because of primary sterility or cease childbearing relatively early because of secondary sterility. Primary sterility normally results in no more than 5-6 percent of married women remaining permanently childless, although for several African populations, the figure ranges from 10 to 40 percent (Lesthaeghe et al., 1981). In most previous studies of fertility, the assumption has been that all women eventually give birth; that is, there is no sterility or limiting behavior. This is an unrealistic assumption in the context of Cameroon, where infertility is quite high and well recognized. Clearly, in many societies, a certain fraction of couples cannot conceive any children because of reproductive deficiencies. Indeed, Larsen and Menken (1991) found that during the 1970s the prevalence of sterility was relatively high in Cameroon. Sterility is an important proximate determinant of fertility in Africa and in Cameroon. At the age of 34, the proportion of sterile women reached 40 percent in the CWFS of 1978 and 31 percent in the CDHS of 1991 (Larsen, 1994). If efforts aimed at lowering sterility in Cameroon were to prove successful, an increase in fertility and population growth might follow.

EMPIRICAL FINDINGS

Table 8-3 assesses the effects of neonatal (first month of life) and postneonatal (1-11 completed months) deaths of the first, second, third, and fourth parity children on the length of subsequent birth intervals, controlling for maternal parity. It shows the median birth intervals according to the survival status of the child initiating the interval at the time of the conception of the index child or at the time of censoring, as well as the reduction in the time elapsed to the time of the conception of the next birth that is associated with the death of the child who starts the interval. These median birth intervals were obtained by life table procedures to account for censoring of exposure to the risk of a following conception.

At the national level, the two data sets show a steady increase in median interval length with survivorship of the child, ranging from 22 months in the case of a death in the first month of life (in the CDHS) to 31 months in the case of a child who survives at least a year. The effect of infant mortality on birth spacing

TABLE 8-3 Median Birth Intervals Between Parity i and Parity $i + 1$

| Selected Variables | Child Survives the First Year of Life | | Child Dies in the First Year of Life and before the Conception of the Index Child | | | |
| | | | 0 Months | | 1-11 Months | |
	CWFS (1)	CDHS (2)	CWFS (3)	CDHS (4)	CWFS (5)	CDHS (6)
Overall length	30	31	24	22	26	25
Parity-specific pattern						
Parity						
1 - 2	30	28	23	21	26	23
2 - 3	29	29	24	21	24	27
3 - 4	30	29	23	28	26	26
4 - 5	30	30	24	22	27	25
Pattern by other selected characteristics						
Age at maternity						
<20 years	29	25	23	17	26	21
20+	30	31	22	26	28	29
Education						
None	30	30	24	21	27	25
Some	30	31	24	23	24	25
Religion						
Catholic	29	31	24	21	25	26
Protestant	30	31	23	23	26	24
Muslim	29	29	26	23	28	26

may be appreciated more easily with the differences between intervals in which the child survived infancy and those intervals in which the infant died. In the top half of the table I examine the parity-specific pattern of variation in median birth interval associated with an infant death, whereas in the lower half of the table I examine the pattern of variation in median birth interval ascribed to an infant death by selected comparable characteristics in the two data sets.

The overall pattern is that the reduction in median birth-to-conception interval for a child who dies in the first year of life compared with a child who survives through the first year of life is 5 months (or 17 percent reduction) and 7 months (or 22 percent reduction) in the CWFS and CDHS, respectively. When the analysis is fine-tuned by age, the reduction in median birth-to-conception interval for a child who dies compared with a child who survives is 6 months (or 20 percent reduction) and 9 months (or 29 percent reduction) in the neonatal period and 4 months (or 13 percent reduction) and 6 months (or 19 percent reduction) in the postneonatal period in the CWFS and CDHS, respectively.

0-11 Months		CWFS			CDHS		
CWFS (7)	CDHS (8)	(1)-(3)	(1)-(5)	(1)-(7)	(2)-(4)	(2)-(6)	(2)-(8)
25	24	6	4	5	9	6	7
25	23	7	4	5	7	5	5
24	24	5	5	5	8	2	5
25	26	7	4	5	4	3	3
25	24	6	3	5	8	5	6
24	19	6	3	5	7	4	6
25	28	8	2	5	5	2	2
26	24	6	3	4	9	5	6
23	24	6	6	7	8	6	7
24	24	5	4	5	9	4	7
25	24	7	4	5	8	7	7
27	25	3	1	2	6	3	6

Table title: Reductions in Median Birth Interval Associated with the Death of the Child Initiating the Birth Interval

These results consistently show that the reduction in median birth-to-conception interval associated with an infant death in the two data sets is larger in the neonatal period than in the postneonatal period, the difference being 3 months in the more recent data set (the CDHS data). These results support my hypothesis that the earlier a child death occurs the more quickly childbearing will be resumed.

When the samples are stratified by selected characteristics such as parity, maternal age, female education, and religion, the emerging patterns show some strong similarities among certain subgroups of the population. For example, the results consistently show that in both data sets, the reduction in birth-to-conception interval associated with an infant death occurring in the first year of life is again larger in the neonatal period than the postneonatal period. The largest difference in reduction (of 6 months, from 8 months to 2 months) between the neonatal and postneonatal is noted among older women. The pace of closure of a birth-to-conception interval is quicker among teenagers than among older women, both in the neonatal and postneonatal period.

In general, at the same parity, median birth intervals are shorter for women with child mortality experience, varying from around 30 months when the child survives the first year of life to 21 months when the child initiating the interval dies in the first month of life and before the conception of the second child (index child). For the first year as a whole, the average reduction in median birth interval between parities when the child who initiates the interval dies before the conception of the second (index child) is invariably 5 months in the two data sets, which suggests a robust finding. The pace of childbearing is much more rapid when the child dies in the neonatal period than in the postneonatal period. In particular, there is a shorter duration of the postpartum infertile period following a child death at first parity. These relationships between infant loss and pace of childbearing hold at all parities and are statistically significant in both data sets. Furthermore, in the two data sets, the difference in reduction between the neonatal and the postneonatal period is about 3 months (or about 10 percent reduction), thus suggesting that the replacement of a lost child is approximately 3 months sooner when the child dies in the neonatal period than when it dies in the postneonatal period.

Multistate and Multivariate Hazard Estimates

In this section, I examine the sign and magnitude of the effects of child loss on the timing and spacing of births with and without controlling for observed and unobserved covariates so as to test the hypotheses enunciated above. Such effects address questions of how fertility behavior responds to exogenous variations in the child mortality experience and other observed and unobserved variations in a woman's characteristics that affect her fertility decisions and preferences. Knowledge of such measured and unmeasured effects may provide good approximations to the consequences of policy interventions (e.g., to reduce infant and child mortality) for fertility control and may provide important benchmarks against which to compare findings from other settings in Africa. The short-term mortality effects are termed "replacement behavior" effects and for them I distinguish between the physiological and volitional replacement effects. The long-term mortality effects evoke mainly volitional replacement effects.

Tables 8-4 through 8-10 present the parameter estimates of a six-equation joint hazard model of mortality effects on fertility. The analyses are restricted to the first six transitions, as discussed in the Appendix. These tables identify the birth-to-conception intervals during which there are statistically and demographically significant effects of child mortality or other covariates on fertility behavior. The effect estimates for hazard models indicate the influence of a particular variable on the probability of a birth, net of the other variables. Where an effect estimate is positive, women in that category are more likely to give birth than women in the category with a negative effect estimate. The greater the difference in effects estimated between the highest and lowest values for categories of a particular covariate, the greater the impact of that covariate on the estimated risk of birth.

Short-Term Mortality Effects on the Timing and Spacing of Births

Tables 8-4 through 8-9 present the findings as they relate to short-term replacement effects of mortality on fertility. These tables show the results from a model with one measure of child mortality (abbreviated CMM1 in Table 8-2). This measure captures the extent to which the death—of the child who opens the birth-to-conception interval $[i, i + 1)$—in its first year of life and at least 1 month before the conception of the $(i + 1)^{th}$ child increases the risk of that following conception. Such a measure of the fertility response to a child death in its first year of life is a mixture of volitional replacement effects and physiological effects having to do with the cessation of breastfeeding. Mortality effects attributable to volitional replacement effects alone are presented below.

Table 8-4 shows the results from a six-equation joint hazard model with only the child mortality measure (CMM1) and the duration measures.

As expected, the death of a child significantly increases the risk of the immediately following conception. For example, such risk is increased by 83 percent according to the CWFS data and 80 percent according to the CDHS data for the conception of the second child (when the first child dies in its first year of life and at least 1 month before the conception of the second child).

Overall, the relative risks of a subsequent conception caused by the death of the child who starts the birth-to-conception interval vary between a low of 1.61 (for the transition to a third birth in the CWFS) to a high of 2.31 (for the transition to a sixth birth in the CDHS). Thus, the death of a child in the family leads to significantly lower probabilities of stopping childbearing, but there is no linear trend across parities. As hypothesized, the operation of the physiological replacement mechanism (by breastfeeding cessation) links mortality in infancy with the length of birth intervals, and the stronger the mechanism, the shorter the length of birth-to-conception interval caused by a child death. This mechanism appears to be in operation here. Also, if the volitional replacement strategy is at work, an improvement in child mortality can never result in a fully compensatory reduction in births because fertility control is always imperfect; if couples replace births through a compression of birth-to-conception intervals, the fertility response to child loss will be fairly immediate, and the results here lend support to the operation of this mechanism (see also discussion on long-term replacement effects, below). The relatively large demographic impact of these physiological and volitional replacement effects is expected to occur in a country such as

TABLE 8-4 Six-Equation Joint Hazard Model of Short-Term Mortality Effects on Fertility Without Controlling for Measured Covariates and Unobserved Heterogenity

| Variable | CWFS, 1978: Transition to Conception | | | |
	First Birth	Second Birth	Third Birth	Fourth Birth
Intercept	0.673**	0.945**	−0.938**	−0.909
	(0.023)	(0.026)	(0.031)	(0.034)
ln duration	0.262**	0.230**	0.188**	0.419**
	(0.019)	(0.008)	(0.0135)	(0.013)
Shift of the conception hazard upon infant death (CMM1)^a		0.604**	0.478**	0.541**
		(0.045)	(0.044)	(0.053)
Negative log-likelihood		24,555		

NOTES: Standard errors are in parentheses below the estimated coefficients. Significance level: **, 1 percent; *, 5 percent (two-tailed)

Cameroon with high infant mortality, prolonged intense breastfeeding, and natural fertility.

Because women with a child death are likely to have had greater exposure to the risk of conception than those without, exposure must be controlled in the analysis as done here (for further detail, see the Appendix). In the absence of such control, the measured effects will exaggerate the replacement effect. The results show that the length of time to various conceptions is shorter in the CWFS than in the CDHS. For example, the relative risks of the logarithm of the duration of exposure to the risk of conceiving the first birth since first marriage is 1.30 in the CWFS and 1.90 in the CDHS. These results imply that the waiting times to conceptions is shorter in the CDHS (the 1991 data) than in the CWFS, thus suggesting a quicker pace of childbearing in the former than the latter data set.

In Table 8-5, I assess the extent to which the short-term mortality effects on birth-to-conception intervals could be spurious owing to lack of controls for measured factors affecting mortality, fertility, or both. Thus, both fertility and mortality experience should be related to common factors such as education, socioeconomic status, and cultural factors.

Holding the exogenous regressors constant, a child loss in infancy continues to accelerate significantly the times to the next conception and increases the fertility transition rates at all parities.

CDHS, 1991: Transition to Conception

Fifth Birth	Sixth Birth	First Birth	Second Birth	Third Birth	Fourth Birth	Fifth Birth	Sixth Birth
−0.985**	0.959**	−0.429**	−0.735**	−0.804**	−0.885**	−0.797	−1.048**
(0.041)	(0.044)	(0.031)	(0.031)	(0.043)	(0.050)	(0.052)	(0.061)
0.418**	0.428**	0.646**	0.934**	0.938**	1.086**	1.101**	1.128**
(0.017)	(0.016)	(0.029)	(0.0253)	(0.029)	(0.031)	(0.039)	(0.045)
0.629**	0.496**		0.589**	0.694**	0.767	0.631**	0.838**
(0.062)	(0.070)		(0.054)	(0.057)	(0.063)	(0.068)	(0.081)

10,772

[a]Death of the immediately preceding child in the first year of life and 1 month before the conception of the index child.

The relative risks of a subsequent conception caused by a child death appear to change rather trivially for all transitions, with a small reduction of 6 percent in the relative risk of conceiving the second birth (from 1.83 to 1.77 in the CWFS, and from 1.80 to 1.74 in the CDHS) reflecting the highest impact of controlling for measured covariates that, not surprisingly, affect fertility independently of the mortality effects.

Although female education has been shown elsewhere to influence fertility behavior, the two data sets from Cameroon fail to show significant effects of education. This finding is not surprising, because the pronatalist ethic in Cameroon until recently means that most women tend to aspire to high fertility. There are significant ethnic differences in fertility. The low-fertility ethnic groups are less likely to bear a conception at each transition compared with the high-fertility ethnic groups. This is especially the case for the transition from first marriage to the conception of the first birth and the transition from the first birth to the conception of the second birth. Women who are employed before their first marriage have lower conception risks and are likely to postpone their first three conceptions. The data fail to detect any significant differences at higher parities. In fact, after correcting for unobserved heterogeneity (see Tables 8-6 and 8-7 below), these women tend to have higher conception hazards for parity five (for woman-specific unobserved heterogeneity) and for parity four (for par-

TABLE 8-5 Six-Equation Joint Hazard Model of Short-Term Mortality Effects on Fertility Controlling for Measured Covariates

	CWFS, 1978: Transition to Conception			
Variable	First Birth	Second Birth	Third Birth	Fourth Birth
Intercept	−0.486**	−0.466**	−0.472**	−0.442**
	(0.030)	(0.044)	(0.048)	(0.057)
ln duration	0.313**	0.357**	0.349**	0.589**
	(0.018)	(0.010)	(0.011)	(0.014)
Shift of the conception hazard upon infant death (CMM1)[a]		0.574** (0.047)	0.475** (0.050)	0.539** (0.055)
Mother is educated˙	0.013	−0.076	0.009	−0.037
	(0.059)	(0.061)	(0.077)	(0.073)
Low-fertility ethnic groups	−0.322**	−0.195**	−0.056	−0.152**
	(0.059)	(0.061)	(0.077)	(0.073)
Muslim religion	0.076*	−0.043	0.001	−0.019
	(0.033)	(0.041)	(0.044)	(0.050)
Shift of the conception hazard upon marital dissolution[b]	−0.247** (0.043)	−0.333** (0.063)	−0.245** (0.063)	−0.392** (0.065)
Employed before first marriage	−0.259**	−0.065	−0.142*	0.033
Mother has more previous living boys than girls		−0.637** (0.043)	−0.765** (0.049)	−0.699** (0.056)
Time trend[c]	−0.765**	−1.174**	−0.799**	−0.982**
	(0.101)	(0.133)	(0.134)	(0.115)
Negative log-likelihood		23,657		

NOTES: Standard errors are in parentheses below the estimated coefficients. Significance level: **, 1 percent; *, 5 percent (two-tailed).

CDHS, 1991: Transition to Conception

Fifth Birth	Sixth Birth	First Birth	Second Birth	Third Birth	Fourth Birth	Fifth Birth	Sixth Birth
−0.467**	−0.607**	−0.423**	−0.254**	−0.311**	−0.437**	−0.269**	−0.433**
(0.062)	(0.075)	(0.033)	(0.057)	(0.067)	(0.080)	(0.090)	(0.110)
0.570**	0.528**	0.670**	1.148**	1.226**	1.254**	1.335**	1.324**
(0.018)	(0.018)	(0.023)	(0.026)	(0.029)	(0.032)	(0.038)	(0.041)
0.626**	0.475**		0.556**	0.694**	0.756**	0.637**	0.818**
(0.065)	(0.072)		(0.055)	(0.059)	(0.066)	(0.070)	(0.085)
−0.009	−0.071	0.015	−0.004	0.042	−0.073	−0.085	−0.011
(0.076)	(0.088)	(0.039)	(0.037)	(0.043)	(0.045)	(0.064)	(0.063)
−0.128*	−0.079						
(0.052)	(0.068)						
−0.128*	0.126*	0.076*	−0.046	0.125*	−0.094*	0.047	−0.121*
(0.052)	(0.066)	(0.037)	(0.038)	(0.050)	(0.046)	(0.064)	(0.068)
−0.442**	−0.020						
(0.081)	(0.115)						
0.089	−0.009						
−0.697**	0.600**		−0.787**	−0.900**	−0.694**	−0.859**	−0.789**
(0.065)	(0.075)		(0.063)	(0.068)	(0.078)	(0.086)	(0.112)
−0.914**	−1.180**	−0.463**	−0.470**	−0.286**	0.121**	0.304*	−0.249
(0.181)	(0.280)	(0.063)	(0.062)	(0.096)	(0.130)	(0.129)	(0.158)

10,371

aDeath of the immediately preceding child in the first year of life and 1 month before the conception of the index child.

bMonth before the conception of the index child.

cTen-year period preceding survey.

ity-specific unobserved heterogeneity) than other women, perhaps indicating a catching-up behavior.

There are also significant religious differences in the transition to the conception of the first birth and to higher (five or more) conceptions. In both the CWFS and CDHS, the hazard of first conception is significantly higher among Muslim women than among others. At higher parities, there is no consistent pattern of shift of the conception hazard by religious affiliation. The CWFS for which the information is available suggests negative (and significant at least for the first birth) effects of maternal employment outside the home and fertility; this finding is consistent with earlier studies that have found a negative association between female labor force participation and fertility. As regards changes in marital status, marital dissolution shifts downward the conception hazard at all transitions, although no significant effect of marital dissolution is found for the sixth transition after controlling for parity-specific unobserved heterogeneity (Tables 8-6 and 8-7). In essence, married women are more likely to have children than are unmarried women.

The sex composition of previous surviving children shows significant differences in subsequent fertility behavior. When the couple has more surviving boys than girls, there are significant decreases in the conception hazard at all parities and in both data sets. This result is robust to controls for both woman-specific unobserved heterogeneity and parity-specific unobserved heterogeneity (Tables 8-6 through 8-8). Basically, the relative risks of a subsequent conception associated with the sex of previous children favoring boys range between 0.45 and 0.55 in both data sets, which corresponds to a reduction in the risks of conception varying between 45 and 65 percent. Thus, the sex of the previous children appears to affect subsequent fertility behavior, but this has no bearing on the mortality effects of the child who opens the index birth-to-conception interval (i.e., the birth-to-conception interval under study). Indeed, I also investigate the interaction between the sex of the previous children and the death of the child who starts the index birth-to-conception interval, but both data sets fail to show any significant interaction effects (results not shown).

In my analysis, I explore the robustness of the estimated birth process model to the inclusion of a time trend variable. I test for the importance of period effects by adding a dummy variable for conceptions occurring during the 10 years before each of the surveys as a covariate to the baseline set of regressors. In all of the specifications and in both data sets, I find a consistent and negative effect of the calendar period (fertility behavior of the last 10 years preceding the survey date) on all transition rates, suggesting a decline in fertility levels in Cameroon. More recent births are less likely to be followed by another conception than births that occurred further in the past. These results suggest that the intervals between successive parities have lengthened over time (for more recent parity cohorts). Consistent with the negative relationship between time trend and hazard of the following conception, the hazard rates for all parities and both data sets have declined at all parities over time. Indeed, the decline reaches 26 percent for the conditional probability of first, second, and third births and 24 percent for the hazard of a fourth birth (see Table 8-8 below).

Controlling for period effects has little influence on the estimates of other regressors, although the negative time trend estimates are statistically significant. In particular, corrections for woman-specific unobserved heterogeneity and parity-specific unobserved characteristics do not weaken this effect (Tables 8-6 through 8-8). During the 1980s, infertility declined significantly among women less than 40 years old, and women's expected numbers of infertile years between the ages of 20 and 39 fell from 7.3 to 6.0 years between the 1978 WFS and the DHS of 1991 (Larsen, 1995). But I find no evidence that declining sterility (captured in the unobserved components introduced in my models) could explain the observed trend in declining conception hazards in recent periods. It is possible that the economic crisis that Cameroon, just as most African countries, has undergone since the mid-1980s may have affected the fertility behavior of couples in recent years.

Table 8-6 displays the short-term replacement effects after correcting for woman-specific unobserved heterogeneity (while holding exogenous covariates constant). The nonparametric maximum likelihood estimator for the mixing distribution involves a two point-of-support distribution for the unobserved heterogeneity (no additional points could be estimated because of convergence problems).[3]

In Table 8-6 I consider the possibility that woman-specific unobserved characteristics may influence the robustness of the replacement effects. Although there are significant unobserved characteristics of the woman affecting her conception risks, these unobservables are empirically unimportant in explaining the fertility responses to child loss in both the CWFS and the CDHS. In particular, a comparison of the estimated relative risks of a following conception caused by the death of the child who starts the index birth-to-conception interval in the gross effects model (i.e., Table 8-4) and in Table 8-6 shows that those risks change little after correcting for woman-specific unobserved factors. For example, the relative risk of conceiving the second child is 1.83 and 1.78 before and after such correction in the CWFS and hardly changes for the subsequent intervals; similarly, whereas the relative risks of conceiving the second child decrease by nearly 25 percent after such correction in the CDHS, there is no change after such correction worthy of notice for the other transitions in the CDHS.

---

[3]However, it has been shown that the result for a two point-of-support model are quite similar to those for a three point-of-support distribution for the unobserved heterogeneity (Popkin et al., 1993). Note that for all estimated models using the CDHS, my models could not converge beyond the fourth parity once I introduce unobserved components in the estimation equations. Thus, the results with the CDHS are restricted only to the first four transitions in all models with woman-specific or parity-specific unobserved heterogeneities.

TABLE 8-6 Six-Equation Joint Hazard Model of Short-Term Mortality Effects on Fertility Controlling for Measured Covariates and Woman-Specific Unobserved Heterogeneity

Variable	CWFS, 1978: Transition to Conception			
	First Birth	Second Birth	Third Birth	Fourth Birth
Intercept	−7.481**	0.016**	−0.362**	−1.073**
	(0.204)	(0.136)	(0.145)	(0.119)
ln duration	2.324**	0.363**	0.349**	0.612**
	(0.070)	(0.009)	(0.011)	(0.020)
Shift of the conception hazard upon infant death (CMM1)^a		0.575**	0.475**	0.547**
		(0.047)	(0.049)	(0.055)
Mother is educated	0.014	−0.075	0.009	−0.037
	(0.059)	(0.060)	(0.077)	(0.073)
Low-fertility ethnic groups	−0.096**	−0.196**	0.057	−0.153**
	(0.028)	(0.044)	(0.049)	(0.052)
Muslim religion	0.005	−0.043	0.002	−0.019
	(0.025)	(0.041)	(0.044)	(0.049)
Employed before first marriage	−0.448**	−0.070	−0.144*	0.054
	(0.036)	(0.060)	(0.059)	(0.058)
Mother has more previous living boys than girls		−0.693**	−0.768**	−0.707**
		(0.043)	(0.049)	(0.056)
Shift of the conception hazard upon marital dissolution^b	0.006	−0.339**	−0.244**	−0.376**
	(0.037)	(0.064)	(0.063)	(0.063)
Time trends^c	−0.502**	−1.182**	−0.800**	−1.011**
	(0.106)	(0.133)	(0.135)	(0.120)
Woman-specific unobserved heterogeneity	7.766**	−0.485**	−0.111	0.635**
	(0.185)	(0.130)	(0.138)	(0.095)
Negative log-likelihood		21,759		

NOTES: Standard errors are in parentheses below the estimated coefficients. Significance level: **, 1 percent; *, 5 percent (two-tailed).

CDHS, 1991: Transition to Conception

Fifth Birth	Sixth Birth	First Birth	Second Birth	Third Birth	Fourth Birth	
−5.086**	4.779	−4.917**	−4.212**	−3.472**	−5.209**	
(0.408)	(0.795)	(0.156)	(0.158)	(0.213)	(0.665)	
0.982**	0.682**	2.122**	2.069**	1.711**	1.738**	
(0.031)	(0.029)	(0.084)	(0.074)	(0.047)	(0.052)	
0.610**	0.483**		0.295**	0.656**	0.706**	
(0.054)	(0.070)		(0.039)	(0.050)	(0.056)	
−0.008	−0.071	0.014	−0.004	−0.042	−0.075	
(0.076)	(0.087)	(0.039)	(0.037)	(0.045)	(0.045)	
−0.051	0.083					
(0.056)	(0.058)					
−0.118*	0.083	0.195**	−0.041	0.047	−0.074	
(0.048)	(0.058)	(0.039)	(0.044)	(0.047)	(0.050)	
0.192**	−0.017					
(0.068)	(0.087)					
−0.878**	−0.688**		−0.913**	−1.083**	−0.855**	
(0.055)	(0.073)		(0.042)	(0.057)	(0.064)	
−0.349**	−0.048					
(0.077)	(0.103)					
−1.103**	−1.245**	−0.312**	−0.079	−0.359**	−0.033	
(0.147)	(0.256)	(0.085)	(0.094)	(0.105)	(0.097)	
4.706**	4.222**	5.055**	4.271**	3.362**	4.926**	
(0.405)	(0.791)	(0.144)	(0.152)	(0.209)	(0.662)	

7,293

aDeath of the immediately preceding child in the first year of life and 1 month before the conception of the index child.

bOne month before the conception of the index child.

cTen-year period preceding the survey.

The effects of woman-specific unobserved factors appear to be most important for the transition from first marriage to first birth in both data sets and to fluctuate somewhat for subsequent transitions. The strikingly high relative risks of conceiving the first child associated with woman-specific unobserved characteristics may be capturing the woman's inherent fecundity following intensive exposure to the risk of conception after first marriage, since motherhood is the normal expectation for a new bride in most African societies. Note that in the CWFS, the coefficients for the woman-specific unobserved heterogeneity are negative for the transition to the conception of the second and third births (and negative and statistically significant for the transition from first birth to the conception of the second birth). By contrast, results from the more recent CDHS survey consistently show all the coefficients for woman-specific unobserved heterogeneity to be positive and statistically significant, thus suggesting a positive relationship between those unmeasured characteristics and the probabilities of a following conception. Recall that the CWFS was fielded in 1978 and that until the late 1970s, there was little sign of reduction in the incidence of primary and secondary sterility in Cameroon (David and Voaz, 1981; Larsen and Menken, 1991; World Health Organization, 1991; Larsen, 1994, 1995). These results seem to capture the incidence of secondary sterility among women in Cameroon until the late 1970s and the changing trends in the incidence of sterility over time in Cameroon, which seem to have increased women's fertility desires and to have reduced their waiting time to conceptions.

Table 8-7 presents the short-term replacement effects after correcting for parity-specific unobserved heterogeneity (while holding constant the measured factors).

In both data sets, correcting for parity-specific unobserved factors slightly lowers the relative risks of a subsequent conception in the aftermath of a child death. The reduction in relative risks ranges between 10 percent (for the transition to the conception of the third birth) to around 16 percent (for all other transitions) in the CWFS and between 10 percent (for the transition to the conception of the third birth) and 23 percent (for the transition from first marriage to the conception of the first birth) in the CDHS. However, the explanatory power of the mortality effects remains unchanged after such correction. The estimated replacement effects remain statistically significant for all transitions and for both data sets.

Net of the measured covariates, the implied stopping probabilities associated with parity-specific unobserved heterogeneity show no consistent pattern and essentially fluctuate from one parity to the next, but the magnitude of the differential diminishes at higher birth orders in both data sets. It is possible, for example, that in families with many children there is a greater likelihood that some of the children were not wanted or were expected to die. In such a case the death of a child would not call for replacement, and this will affect the pattern of effects of parity-specific unobserved factors.

In Table 8-8, I jointly account for woman-specific and parity-specific unobserved heterogeneities in the hazards of conception and the associated mortality effects. Again, it is found that for all parities, the fertility responses to child mortality are indeed robust to controls for unobservables.

There are significant fertility differences by parity-specific unobserved heterogeneity: The higher fertility of women is reflected in their lower stopping probability at any birth order, although there is a tendency to increase when woman-specific heterogeneity is accounted for. The relative risks of a subsequent conception of the second and third births are 1.78 and for the fourth birth are 1.93, which are quite similar to the relative risks obtained from the previous models for the same transitions (see Tables 8-6 and 8-7). Overall, the short-term replacement behavior is indeed robust.

Long-Term Mortality Effects on the Timing and Spacing of Births

Tables 8-9 and 8-10 examine the long-term mortality effects on fertility. Two measures of mortality are used. The first measure captures the long-term mortality effects of a child who opens the birth-to-conception interval $[i, i + 1)$ and dies at least 1 month before the conception of children of parities $i + 2$, $i + 3$, $i + 4$, and so forth (abbreviated CMM2 in Table 8-2). The second measure focuses on the mortality of the first (and the second) birth and explores the effects of the death of the first child (or the second child) in its first year of life and at least 1 month before the conception of the second, third, fourth, fifth, and sixth births (or the third, fourth, fifth, and sixth births in the case where the death of the second birth is of interest) (abbreviated CMM3 in Table 8-2). Table 8-9 presents the results for the survival status of the preceding siblings prior to the conception of the index child, whether or not the mortality experienced was within the first year of life. In Table 8-9 I evaluate the net effects of the mortality of the first, second, third, fourth, and fifth birth on future fertility behavior while controlling for the survival of other children. I find that the mortality of the first children (in the CWFS) and the first and second children (in the CDHS) have significant positive effects on the probabilities of conceiving children of higher birth orders. I pursue the extent to which the death of the first and second child significantly increases the risks of conceiving children of higher birth orders in Table 8-10, restricted to the CDHS data for which such effects emerge strongly and consistently. Much of the replacement effect may not show up in terms of differences in birth interval length but rather in additional subsequent births. To capture fully the volitional replacement effect, child deaths before some specific parity must be related to subsequent fertility. This also avoids the confounding effects of fertility on mortality.

A common approach in previous studies has been to compare the additional children born subsequent to a specific parity between women who have experienced a child death up until that point and those who had not. In Tables 8-9 and

TABLE 8-7 Six-Equation Joint Hazard Model of Short-Term Mortality Effects on Fertility Controlling for Measured Covariates and Parity-Specific Unobserved Heterogeneity

	CWFS, 1978: Transition to Conception			
Variable	First Birth	Second Birth	Third Birth	Fourth Birth
Intercept	0.132**	−0.186**	−0.182**	−0.192**
	(0.024)	(0.037)	(0.045)	(0.053)
ln duration	1.298**	1.046**	1.025**	1.160**
	(0.014)	(0.011)	(0.014)	(0.023)
Shift of the conception hazard upon infant death (CMM1)[a]		0.426** (0.032)	0.375** (0.041)	0.370** (0.043)
Mother is educated	0.016	−0.065	0.008	−0.037
	(0.059)	(0.060)	(0.077)	(0.073)
Low-fertility ethnic groups	−0.052	−0.130**	0.068	−0.201**
	(0.028)	(0.039)	(0.051)	(0.059)
Muslim religion	0.167**	−0.035	−0.041	0.005
	(0.028)	(0.035)	(0.044)	(0.049)
Employed before first marriage	−0.293**	−0.075	−0.348**	0.252**
	(0.026)	(0.052)	(0.057)	(0.056)
Mother has more previous living boys than girls		−0.809** (0.034)	−0.455** (0.046)	−0.750** (0.052)
Shift of the conception hazard upon marital dissolution[b]	−0.099** (0.027)	−0.225** (0.053)	−0.279** (0.061)	−0.592** (0.069)
Time trends[c]	−0.594**	−1.401**	−1.095**	−0.640**
	(0.102)	(0.117)	(0.155)	(0.157)
Parity-specific stopping unobserved heterogeneity	Parity 0	Parity 1	Parity 2	Parity 3
Estimates	−1.710**	−2.639**	−1.806**	−2.621**
	(0.043)	(0.083)	(0.063)	(0.116)
Implied probabilities	0.153	0.067	0.141	0.068
Negative log-likelihood		21,213		

NOTES: Standard errors are in parentheses below the estimated coefficients. Significance level: **, 1 percent; *, 5 percent (two-tailed).

		CDHS, 1991: Transition to Conception			
Fifth Birth	Sixth Birth	First Birth	Second Birth	Third Birth	Fourth Birth
−0.247**	−0.401**	−0.014	0.030	0.016	0.139*
(0.057)	(0.071)	(0.027)	(0.043)	(0.047)	(0.057)
1.363**	1.074**	1.929**	2.192**	2.363**	2.335**
(0.030)	(0.040)	(0.024)	(0.045)	(0.056)	(0.101)
0.453**	0.344**		0.328**	0.588**	0.605**
(0.043)	(0.057)		(0.039)	(0.041)	(0.050)
−0.008	−0.071	0.014	−0.004	0.042	−0.074
(0.076)	(0.087)	(0.039)	(0.037)	(0.045)	(0.045)
0.040					
(0.057)	(0.064)				
−0.126*	0.075	0.203**	−0.085*	−0.004	−0.151*
(0.048)	(0.059)	(0.027)	(0.039)	(0.045)	(0.052)
0.098	0.044				
(0.070)	(0.083)				
−0.762**	−0.712**		−0.712**	−0.783**	−0.598**
(0.052)	(0.067)		(0.047)	(0.049)	(0.056)
−0.231*	0.003				
(0.082)	(0.098)				
−0.857**	−1.534**	−0.246**	0.002	−0.385**	−0.210*
(0.164)	(0.223)	(0.056)	(0.092)	(0.106)	(0.110)
Parity 4	Parity 5	Parity 0	Parity 1	Parity 2	Parity 3
−2.488**	−2.853**	−1.997**	−2.459**	−2.093**	−2.170**
(0.126)	(0.191)	(0.068)	(0.121)	(0.113)	(0.141)
0.077	0.054	0.119	0.079	0.110	0.102
		6,787			

[a]Death of the immediately preceding child in the first year of life and 1 month before the conception of the index child.

[b]One month before the conception of the index child.

[c]Ten-year period preceding the survey.

TABLE 8-8 Six-Equation Joint Hazard Model of Short-Term Mortality Effects on Fertility Controlling for Measured Covariates and Woman-Specific and Parity-Specific Unobserved Heterogeneities

	CDHS, 1991: Transition to Conception			
Variable	First Birth	Second Birth	Third Birth	Fourth Birth
Intercept	−11.242**	1.089**	0.872**	0.222*
	(0.210)	(0.066)	(0.073)	(0.090)
ln duration	9.643**	2.637**	2.664**	2.449**
	(0.144)	(0.041)	(0.055)	(0.105)
Shift of the conception hazard upon infant death (CMM1)[a]		0.582**	0.581**	0.656**
		(0.038)	(0.042)	(0.054)
Mother is educated	0.016	−0.005	0.043	−0.076
	(0.039)	(0.037)	(0.046)	(0.044)
Muslim religion	0.181**	−0.177**	0.085	−0.049
	(0.028)	(0.037)	(0.047)	(0.056)
Mother has more previous living boys than girls		−0.747**	−0.909**	−0.854**
		(0.047)	(0.057)	(0.065)
Time trend[b]	−0.298**	−0.312**	−0.305*	−0.267*
	(0.056)	(0.092)	(0.107)	(0.120)
Woman-specific unobserved heterogeneity	16.126**	−1.414*	−1.197*	−0.546**
	(0.398)	(0.056)	(0.056)	(0.074)
Parity-specific stopping unobserved heterogeneity	Parity 0	Parity 1	Parity 2	Parity 3
Estimates	−1.953**	−2.248**	−1.879**	−1.744**
	(0.106)	(0.108)	(0.107)	(0.138)
Implied probabilities	0.124	0.095	0.132	0.149
Negative log-likelihood	125			

NOTES: Standard errors are in parentheses below the estimated coefficients. Significance level: **, 1 percent; *, 5 percent (two-tailed).

[a]Death of the immediately preceding child in the first year of life and 1 month before the conception of the index child.

[b]Ten-year period preceding the survey.

8-10, I find that there are indeed strong volitional replacement effects, at least as regards the death of the first child in both data sets and the second child in the CDHS. In either case, the death of the first (or second) child is shown to significantly increase the hazard of conceiving children of parity 2, 3, 4, 5, and 6 (for the death of the first child) and children of parity 3, 4, 5, and 6 (for the death of the second child).

Table 8-9 presents the mortality effects using the first measure (CMM2) of the long-term effects. I find that in both data sets, the death of the first child is significantly associated with increased relative risks of conceiving the second, third, fourth, fifth, and sixth children. These relative risks are at least 20 percent higher than the baseline risks (the risks of conception following a surviving child) in both data sets and range from 1.18 to 1.39. As regards the death of the second child, the CWFS data are consistent only with the short-term mortality effects, but fail to show significant long-term effects. The CDHS data, on the other hand, show consistently that the death of the second child has both short-term and long-term mortality effects on birth spacing. Indeed, the relative risks of the conception of the third, fourth, fifth, and sixth children associated with the death of the second at least 1 month before the conception of each of these children range from 1.33 (for the transition to the conception of the third birth) to 2.07 (for the transition to the conception of the sixth birth), although the increase in such risks is not monotonic. The CWFS data further suggest that the death of the third child increases significantly the relative risks of conceiving the fifth child, but not the fourth or the sixth, whereas the death of the fourth child tends to significantly reduce the risks of conceiving the fifth child once previous mortality experience within the family is taken into account. Similarly, the CDHS data suggest that the death of the third child significantly reduces the risks of conceiving the fifth birth. Because the more widely spaced pattern is the pattern of childbearing that most couples choose in most African societies because of postpartum taboos and practices and longer breastfeeding durations, it will be easier to replace a child death with an additional birth through a compression of interbirth intervals. On the other hand, if couples plan closely spaced births, they will have to replace any child deaths later in a woman's reproductive span when fecundity may have declined. This may explain some of the insignificance of the higher-parity effects of the mortality of previous children. These results are somewhat consistent with Ben-Porath's (1978) study in which most of the coefficients of previous death of a child were not statistically significant: They tended to be positive and smaller in absolute size than the generally negative coefficients of the older siblings who died. These findings would indicate that, when a death occurs and the next birth occurs earlier, subsequent births may not be shifted back by full change in birth intervals, which is another way of saying that replacement is partial as many previous studies have shown (e.g., Preston, 1978).

TABLE 8-9 Six-Equation Joint Hazard Model of Long-Term Mortality Effects on Fertility: The Child Who Opens the Birth-to-Conception Interval [i, $i + 1$) Dies at Least 1 Month Before the Conception of Children of Higher Parities (CMM2)

| Variable | CWFS, 1978: Transition to Conception | | | |
	First Birth	Second Birth	Third Birth	Fourth Birth
Intercept	−0.672**	−0.724**	−0.788**	−0.747**
	(0.022)	(0.022)	(0.026)	(0.030)
ln duration	0.261**	0.169**	0.142**	0.360**
	(0.018)	(0.009)	(0.014)	(0.012)
Shift of the conception hazard upon death				
First child		0.201**	0.327**	0.292**
		(0.048)	(0.060)	(0.066)
Second child			0.204**	0.157
			(0.069)	(0.110)
Third child				0.101
				(0.085)
Fourth child				
Fifth child				
Negative log-likelihood	24,873			

NOTES: Standard errors are in parentheses below the estimated coefficients. Significance level: **, 1 percent; *, 5 percent (two-tailed).

CDHS, 1991: Transition to Conception

Fifth Birth	Sixth Birth	First Birth	Second Birth	Third Birth	Fourth Birth	Fifth Birth	Sixth Birth
−0.763	−0.758**	−0.429**	−0.501**	−0.556**	−0.570**	−0.558**	−0.858**
(0.035)	(0.040)	(0.031)	(0.031)	(0.034)	(0.038)	(0.043)	(0.049)
0.347**	0.389**	0.646**	0.831**	0.859**	0.943**	0.990**	10.014**
(0.019)	(0.028)	(0.022)	(0.022)	(0.0262)	(0.0275)	(0.042)	(0.046)
0.253	0.162*		0.330**	0.332**	0.278**	0.240*	0.319*
(0.060)	(0.079)		(0.058)	(0.061)	(0.073)	(0.097)	(0.125)
−0.193	−0.269			0.284*	0.605**	0.304*	0.726**
(0.167)	(0.139)			(0.124)	(0.195)	(0.149)	(0.216)
0.381*	0.094				−0.020	−0.055	−0.363**
(0.145)	(0.117)				(0.090)	(0.098)	(0.113)
−0.104*	−0.018					−0.016	−0.080
(0.051)	(0.068)					(0.066)	(0.081)
	−0.045						−0.005
	(0.072)						(0.053)

11,062

TABLE 8-10 Six-Equation Joint Hazard Model of Long-Term Mortality Effects on Fertility: The First (or Second) Child Who Opens the Birth-to-Conception Interval [i, $i + 1$) Dies in Its First Year of Life and at Least 1 Month before the Conception of Children of Higher Parities (CMM3)

Variable	CDHS, 1991: Transition to Conception					
	First Birth	Second Birth	Third Birth	Fourth Birth	Fifth Birth	Sixth Birth
Intercept	−0.429**	−0.969**	−1.402**	−1.713**	−1.012**	−1.668**
	(0.030)	(0.082)	(0.459)	(0.392)	(0.240)	(0.207)
ln duration	0.645**	0.844**	0.868**	0.937**	0.981**	0.982**
	(0.023)	(0.022)	(0.025)	(0.026)	(0.037)	(0.042)
Shift of the conception hazard upon death in the first year of life						
First child		0.517**	0.947**	1.258**	0.559*	1.100**
		(0.080)	(0.459)	(0.393)	(0.243)	(0.216)
Second child			0.494	1.030*	0.431	0.995**
			(0.463)	(0.395)	(0.232)	(0.210)
Negative log-likelihood	11,020					

NOTES: Standard errors are in parentheses below the estimated coefficients. Significance level: **, 1 percent; *, 5 percent (two-tailed).

Effects of the First Child's Death on Long-Term Fertility Behavior

Tables 8-9 and 8-10 show the effects of the survival status of preceding siblings on the hazards of conception of the subsequent births. Table 8-10 fine-tunes the indicator of the mortality experience of preceding siblings by focusing on the survival of the first two siblings in the first year of life at the time of the conception of the index child who is the third, fourth, fifth, and sixth child (when assessing the effects of the first child's death), while controlling for the survival status of the second birth. These indicators are designed to test my second hypothesis regarding the distinctive role played by the survival status of the first (and to some extent the second birth) on the fertility decision process of couples as they go through their life-cycle fertility.

Before having children, couples have little knowledge on which to base expectations of the future health and survival of their offspring. As they begin to have children and develop or revise family-building strategies, it is plausible that their perceptions of their "luck" with children—the probability of survival and their inherent frailty—are, in large part, based on their experience with the first born. Moreover, as discussed above, in most African cultures in general and in Cameroon in particular, the first child has special meaning in a social context where specific rituals and values are attached to the first born, and on which the prestige, social integration, and family recognition of the new mother is founded.

As in Table 8-9, in Table 8-10 I assess the distribution of the effects of the death of the first and second births on subsequent birth intervals. Such estimates clearly separate the physiological mechanism from the purely behavioral mechanism of child replacement. Indeed, since breastfeeding does not extend beyond a given birth interval for the child initiating the interval, the effects of the death of child of parity j on the probability of conceiving child of rank say $j + 3$ is independent of the breastfeeding status of child j.

Table 8-10 shows the matrix of transition to higher parities given the survival status of the first and second births. In all transitions, the death of the first child significantly shifts upward the hazard of conceptions of higher-order births. This result is robust across the two data sets. I find that, even when the first child survival status is considered only in the first year of life at the time of the conception of the subsequent births, there are still robust fertility responses to that mortality experience. In contrast, deaths of higher-order children are less associated with increased hazards of subsequent conception. These results suggest that the death of the first child may be more crucial for life-cycle fertility behavior than the death of higher-parity siblings. The long-term response suggests that volitional replacement or insurance behavior is occurring. It is, however, surprising that the survival experience of subsequent children is so much less important. Mensch (1985) suggests that if the timing of the volitional response depends on the level of fertility, then it can be expected that, in a setting where fertility and desired family size are high, a conscious response to mortality will appear only at later parities. My results suggest that this conjecture is not confirmed by the Cameroon data.

As discussed, the social context of reproduction in most African societies is likely to make the couple have a complete lack of "security" as regards their chances to have progeny following the first child's death. Hence, the death of the first born (or second births) may have a large effect on both short- and long-term fertility responses, far exceeding the simple replacement effect. Therefore, the fertility behavior of a woman may be more influenced over time by the sense of "insurance" derived from the survival status of her first birth rather than a set target family size. Thus, the empirical implication of the long-term replacement strategy caused by the death of a first birth may be evidence of hoarding behavior. Indeed, Ben-Porath (1978) notes that hoarding and replacement behavior are substitutes in that families may learn to expect high mortality and respond to it by hoarding. This argument is especially pertinent in the African context because many African women find it difficult to understand that the number of their offspring is, to a large extent, within human control (van de Walle, 1992). Childlessness and infertility are often ascribed to supernatural forces rather than to the outcome of impaired reproductive health (Larsen, 1995).

Parity-Specific Effects of the Fertility Response to Child Loss

As noted above, most previous studies of the effects of child mortality on fertility have assumed that those effects were the same across parities. Essentially, such studies preclude the reproductive life-cycle perspective in assessing the effects of child death on the hazards of closing the birth interval. That is, the effects of all variables are constrained to be equal across parities. This assumption may have undesirable effects on the life-cycle perspective to reproductive behavior since it assumes, among other things, that the process is homogeneous across parities when, in fact, the effects of many variables, including mortality, are parity specific. In fact, countless demographic, epidemiologic, and medical studies have consistently shown that firstborns had higher mortality risks than subsequent births and that above parity 4 or so, the mortality risks increase with parity.

Previous analyses of the effects of child mortality on birth intervals raise a number of problems. Couples with many children are more likely than couples with few children to have shorter intervals on the one hand and more experience of child deaths on the other. This may create a spurious negative correlation between child mortality and closed birth intervals and exaggerate the effect of prior mortality on the birth intervals. My specification of the time sequence of child mortality and subsequent conception eliminates such bias. The two data sets show that the magnitude of the relative risks of a subsequent conception due to a child death vary across parity, as expected. Furthermore, the effects of a number of measured covariates, as well as unobserved factors (particularly woman-specific unobserved heterogeneity), tend to vary greatly by parity.

I also attempted a number of interaction effects between mortality measures and selected covariates. But none of them was statistically significant in the final models. In particular, I test the hypothesis that the death of a child of the preferable sex may result in a different pattern of fertility response than the death of a less preferable one by interacting the preceding child mortality experience with sex of the deceased child.

SUMMARY AND DISCUSSION

In this chapter I formulate and estimate a system of hazard models as a reduced-form approach to dynamic models of fertility response to child loss. In both data sets used and for all estimated transitions, child deaths reduce the length of birth intervals and increase the probability of conceiving a subsequent child.

Basically, a child death in the family leads to significantly lower probabilities of stopping at a given parity, particularly at lower parities. Thus, replacement behavior is a significant phenomenon, occurs fairly quickly, and has long-term effects (particularly following the death of the first child). In both data sets, an infant death is shown to be associated with a reduction of the median birth interval of 5 months. Several studies summarized by Preston (1978) suggest a maximum of 13 months, whereas the evidence from Cameroon (where there is still full adherence to the practice of breastfeeding) points to values between 4 and 9 months at the national level. Estimates obtained by Grummer-Strawn et al. (in this volume) are approximately 6 months for the African countries studied, 4 months for Asia, and 3 months for Latin America. I also find that the reduction in birth intervals is greater for neonatal deaths than postneonatal deaths. Basically, the earlier a child death, the more quickly childbearing would resume and the shorter the subsequent interbirth interval. The average interval between births increased steadily from 14.8 months following a stillbirth to 15.9 months if the first baby of two died within 1 month, to 35.1 months if the firstborn survived at least 2 years. This is almost certainly true for other African societies, particularly those where long periods of postnatal abstinence are traditionally practiced.

Controlling for a series of measured covariates has negligible influence on these results. Furthermore, there is little evidence that unobservables correlated across observations (women) or across parities for the same woman, which have received much attention in the demographic literature, are empirically important in explaining fertility responses to a child death once woman-specific and parity-specific stopping behavior has been accounted for. The estimated effects of other variables in the regressions are found to be very similar both in the presence and absence of controls for unobserved heterogeneity, suggesting that these controls—although significantly associated with the hazards of conception—are not critical for studying the effects of infant and child mortality on fertility.

The effects of the death of the first birth on fertility in the future (transitions from the third birth to the conception of the fourth birth, from the fourth birth to the conception of the fifth birth, and from the fifth birth to the conception of the sixth birth) are indicative of strong lagged fertility responses to child death, in addition to robust instantaneous fertility responses to the first child loss (transition from the first birth to the conception of the second birth). The most likely situation may be one in which couples' replacement strategy and reaction to the first child's death is swift and their attempts to accelerate a conception will follow shortly after the death of a wanted child. Furthermore, response with longer lags is also possible and appears to significantly matter. Ben-Porath (1978) notes that there might be a learning process in a sequential framework when experienced mortality affects expected mortality. This learning process seems consistent with my findings that the death of the first two children (and especially the firstborn) shift upward the conception hazards for the subsequent births, thereby reducing the average birth intervals among women who have lost their first children compared with those who have not (even after controlling for the mortality of higher-order births).

My finding that an infant death has both short-term and long-term effects on fertility behavior is consistent with the evidence generated elsewhere in Africa (e.g., Bocquier, 1991). I had hypothesized that the behavioral replacement effect could be accomplished by compressing interbirth intervals, as my results across parities show. Furthermore, I note as expected that the empirical implication of the behavioral replacement mechanism is a lagged fertility response to changes in mortality, as shown by the robust findings regarding the mortality effects of the first and second births on future reproductive behavior.

In comparing the increases in conception risks in the short-term upon infant death (when the child who opens the birth-to-conception interval dies in the first year of life and at least 1 month before the conception of the index child) (e.g., Table 8-8) and the increases in conception risks in the long-term upon death of infants of successive parities (when a child who opens the birth-to-conception interval $[i, i + 1)$ dies in the first year of life and at least 1 month before the conception of the child of parity $i + 2, i + 3, i + 4$, and so forth) (Table 8-10), my results demonstrate that the volitional replacement mechanism is generally less powerful than the physiological replacement effect working through breast-feeding, since all the estimated risks in the model confounding the physiological and volitional replacement effects are higher than those of the models of volitional replacement effects alone.

Despite an ever-growing body of data on African demography and a range of theories of demographic change, much is still unclear about the relationships between mortality and fertility in this region, especially the insurance strategy of fertility response to child loss. Furthermore, much more empirical research has been devoted to the replacement-type fertility response to infant and child mortality and to the physiological effect than to the extent to which surrounding mortality conditions affect individual fertility, as in the case involving the insurance effect. Any empirical studies of the insurance effect require some measure of couples' perceptions of child death risks (see Montgomery, in this volume). The ideal data for such analysis would be from prospective surveys that provide direct before and after comparisons of stated intentions as well as actual behavior. There is a need to combine quantitative and qualitative research methodologies to address these links, because the knowledge and understanding of the sociocultural context of the fertility and mortality processes in Africa is still limited.

Aggregate data reviewed here indicate a fairly sluggish response of fertility to infant mortality in the studies in African countries, in contrast to a few studies carried out elsewhere using aggregate time series data that have looked at the effects of infant and child mortality on fertility over time (Yamada, 1984; Schultz, 1985) and have found significant effects. The lack of significant effects in Africa may be due at least in part to left-out variables (possibly operating simultaneously on fertility and mortality) that may operate in one context and not in the other, or to the nature of the data and its quality, or to measurements and estimation problems, or a combination of the above.

It is likely that the way in which fertility responds to improvements in child survival in Africa will depend not only on the age pattern of declines but also on changes in the distribution of causes of death. In this respect, an emerging issue in the link between child mortality and fertility is the impact of the HIV epidemic on fertility (Cohen and Trussell, 1996). In areas where AIDS deaths are concentrated, it is possible that there is a desire to increase fertility to replace lost adults (Ainsworth et al., in this volume). At the same time, Gregson (1994) suggests that the prevalence of HIV and AIDS may reduce fertility, principally through an increased and more effective use of condoms. At the present, however, evidence is not sufficient to cast further light on the potential relationships (Cohen and Trussell, 1996).

APPENDIX:
HAZARD MODELS AS A REDUCED-FORM APPROACH TO DYNAMIC (LIFE-CYCLE) MODELS OF FERTILITY RESPONSE TO CHILD MORTALITY

This appendix presents my implementation of a system of hazard models for the estimation of the effects of mortality on times to conception. The framework is derived from a general framework for estimation of flexibly parameterized competing risks and multistate duration models (Lancaster, 1985; Heckman and Singer, 1985). Leung (1988) critically evaluates standard assessment methods and favors the use of hazard models in which right-censored conception intervals and time-varying covariates can be handled. My model follows that specification and also controls not only for woman-specific unobserved heterogeneity as several previous studies have done (e.g., Newman and McCulloch, 1984; Leung, 1988; Panis and Lillard, 1993), but also for parity-specific stopping unobserved heterogeneity (as in Heckman and Walker, 1990, 1991). This system consists of a six-equation joint equation model in which each equation represents the hazard of making a particular transition to a birth of parity j, caused by the death of a child of lower parity. My measures of mortality (described in the text) are designed to establish the time sequence between the timing of a child death and the timing of subsequent conceptions, a necessary exposure-occurrence condition to make causal inferences between the occurrence of a child death and the shift in risks of a following conception.

I describe the essential features of this six-equation joint equation hazard models as a reduced-form approach to the life-cycle models of fertility that have been developed in the literature, and I apply this system of hazard models to fertility response to infant and child mortality. Such a system of hazard models within a life-cycle perspective is important for several reasons. First, introducing a decision-making process within a life-cycle framework (i.e., couples essentially update their decisions regarding childbearing over their reproductive career) makes explicit the existence of other life-cycle options among which couples may choose to substitute their fertility at different ages over the life cycle. As such, changes in mortality experience over the life cycle may result in changes in the timing of fertility demand (thus implying parity-specific decision making), even if they do not cause lifetime fertility to change. Second, the life-cycle context is also the appropriate setting within which to consider the consequences of the stochastic nature of human reproduction and reproductive behavior. Third, the dynamic setting provides a more appropriate context within which to examine the relationships between infant and child mortality and fertility. Finally, modeling human reproduction as a stochastic process has a long tradition in population biology and mathematical demography (Sheps and Menken, 1973).

My empirical specification follows the econometric approaches to life-cycle models of fertility. I pay attention to the timing of first birth and the spacing between births, and I argue that the spacing of births is influenced by the past and recent infant mortality experience of couples. Thus, since biological constraints would prevent most couples from having all desired births at once, it is of interest to ask, once the first birth occurs, what mechanisms lead to longer or shorter birth intervals? Two considerations suggest examining explicitly dynamic fertility models. The first is the inherently multiperiod nature of the data. The second is that, from both theoretical and policy perspectives, the age at first birth, the spacing between births, and the joint timing of fertility with other life-cycle choices have important ramifications, in part because the fertility decision is inherently discrete and there is considerable heterogeneity in completed family size. Thus, any single equation approach inherently runs into the problem of how to treat the women who never experienced the event (e.g., a woman who never had a birth in regressions on age at first birth) or women who never (up to the interview date) had a subsequent birth in regressions on birth spacing.

One approach to this problem is standard hazard modeling (Lancaster, 1990). In that approach, instead of directly modeling the timing of the event, one models the probability of the occurrence of the event in each period (Newman and McCulloch, 1984). That is, the probability of the jth birth in period (or by exposure) i, conditional on it not having occurred through period $i - 1$. This hazard approach provides a natural way to model incomplete histories, nonoccurrence of the event (a subsequent birth), and a set of covariates. Such an approach has been attempted in a few previous studies (e.g., Mensch, 1985). In her study, Mensch examines the timing of replacement hypothesis by carrying out separately the analysis for specific birth intervals (or parities). It, however, does not solve several other problems (for a review, see Hotz et al., in press). First, it provides little insight into how to summarize the information in past and future covariates. Second, it does not solve the dynamic selection problem. To be in the sample of individuals on which one estimates the time between the first and second birth, one must have had a first birth. This is a selected sample. This simple hazard model provides no insight into the effects of that selection. Finally, this model has the unfortunate characteristic of mixing the parameters for the speed with which the event occurs with the parameters for whether or not the event occurs. No such restriction follows from economic theory. A dynamic econometric strategy that addresses these problems has been formulated by Heckman (Heckman and Singer, 1985; Heckman and Walker, 1991). Heckman's formulation is in continuous time and consists of applying systems of hazard models (Heckman and Walker, 1991). Life-cycle fertility is naturally analyzed using the standard birth process of the stochastic processes literature (Hoel et al., 1987; Sheps and Menken, 1973) where completed fertility is viewed as the result of separate processes governing the transition to each parity. In its most general form, the model posits that current period fertility is a function of age, time since last birth, the woman's time-invariant (observed and unobserved) characteristics, and all the time-varying covariates (both observed and unobserved). Thus, one has a system of hazard models (one for each parity) linked by woman-specific common observed and unobserved covariates. Newman and McCulloch (1984) and Heckman and Singer (1985) developed a refinement (in continuous time) of this system of hazards approach, and their model suggests some natural simplifications of this general (inestimable) specification. In Heckman's feasible estimation in continuous time (and applied in this study), the current period hazard is modeled as a linear index function that includes a general function of the age of the woman and a general function of the duration since the last birth.

A woman's birth history is assumed to evolve in the following way. The woman becomes at risk of conceiving the first birth at calendar time $\tau = 0$ (here assumed to be the date of first marriage). I define a finite-state continuous-time birth process $B(\tau)$, $\tau > 0$, $B(\tau) \ \varepsilon \ \Omega$, where the set of possible attained birth states (parities) is finite $[\Omega = (0,1,2,...,N), N < \infty]$. Ω defines the number of children born. $B(\tau)$ is parity attained at time τ. Transition occurs on or after $\tau = 0$. I assume that all durations $T_1,...,TN$ conditional on the appropriate history H have absolutely continuous distributions. In my specification, and following Heckman's formulation in continuous-time of the system of hazards approach to fertility behavior (Heckman and Singer, 1985; Heckman and Walker, 1991), I implement a continuous-time approach to the system of hazard models of fertility response to infant and child mortality. Within the framework of this system of hazards, if a woman becomes at risk for the conception of the jth birth at time $\tau(j - 1)$, the conditional hazard at duration tj is

$$\mu_j\{t_j \ | \ H[\tau(j-1) + t_j]\} = \mu_{0j}\{t_j \ | \ H[\tau(j-1) + t_j]\} \ \exp[\lambda_j \mathrm{Dur}(t) \qquad (1)$$
$$+ \ \beta_j X + \eta_j Y(t) + \delta_j Z(t)],$$

where t is the waiting time to conception (that is, the birth-to-conception interval t) for a given woman. $Z(t)$ captures the mortality effects, X represents a vector of time-invariant covariates, $Y(t)$ represents a vector of time-varying covariates, and

Dur(t) is a vector of duration dependencies. If no child dies, $Z(t)$ is set to zero. These variables are described in greater detail in the text. The baseline hazard μ_{0j} $\{t_j \mid H[\tau(j-1) + t_j]\}$ is a risk shared by all women. Under the assumption that all durations $T_1,...,T_N$ are absolutely continuous given H, equation (1) can be integrated to obtain the survivor function:

$$S\{t_j \mid H[\tau(j-1) + t_j]\} = \exp[-\int I \, (\mu_j\{u \mid H[\tau(j-1) + u]\} \, du)], \qquad (2)$$
$$I = 0, 1, ..., t_j.$$

Under this function of survivorship, the birth process evolves as follows. A woman at risk for a first birth at $\tau = 0$ continues childless a random length of time t_1 governed by the survivor function

$$S\{t_1 \mid H[\tau(0) + t_1]\} = \exp[-\int_I (\mu_1\{u \mid H[\tau(0) + u]\} \, du)], \qquad (3)$$
$$I = 0, ..., t_1.$$

At calendar time $T_1 = \tau(1)$, the woman conceives and moves to the state $B(\tau)$ = 1. In the general case where $B(\tau) = k - 1$ for $\tau(k-1) \le T < t(k)$, and $T_k = \tau(k)$ $- t(k-1)$ is governed by the conditional survivor function:

$$S\{t_k \mid H[\tau(k-1) + t_k]\} = \exp[-\int_I (\mu_k\{u \mid H[\tau(k-1) + u]\} \, du)], \qquad (4)$$
$$I = 0, 1, ..., t_k.$$

Thus, the conditional density function of duration $T_k = t_k$ is

$$(\mu_k\{t_k \mid H[\tau(k-1) + t_k]\} \,)(S\{t_k \mid H[\tau(k-1) + t_k]\} \,). \qquad (5)$$

If H includes all relevant conditioning information of the entire birth process, the conditional hazard function of $(T_1, ..., T_N)$ given $H[\tau(0) + \Sigma_i t_i]$, $(i = 1, ..., N)$ is therefore

$$\mu\{t_1 ,..., t_N \mid H[\tau(0) + \Sigma_i t_i]\} = \Pi_k \mu_k\{t_k \mid H[\tau(k-1) + t_k]\}, \qquad (6)$$

where $k = 1, ..., N$ and $i = 1, ..., N$. To simplify the notation, denoting μ_t the conditional hazard function of the birth process in equation (6), I obtain from equation (1):

$$\mu_T = \Pi_k \mu_{0k} \{t_k \mid H[\tau(k-1) + t_k]\} \, \exp[\lambda_k \text{Dur}(t) + \beta_k X + \eta_k Y(t)$$
$$+ \delta_k Z(t)]. \qquad (7)$$

Parity dependence is incorporated by allowing coefficients to vary with parity. One important feature of this system of hazard model formulation is that it provides a natural way to allow time-varying covariates to affect the timing of the transition to each parity separately from how they affect completed family size (for a review, see Hotz et al., in press).

Estimation of the joint hazard function defined in equation (7) proceeds under the assumption that the baseline hazard function can be efficiently represented by a Weibull hazard model defined as

$$\mu_T = \Pi_k \exp[\gamma_k + \beta_k X + \eta_k Y(t) + \delta_k Z(t)]t^{\vartheta}_k \, , \tag{8}$$

where γ_k and ϑ_k are the intercept and the slope of the Weibull hazard for the risk of the conception of the kth birth at time $\tau(k-1)$, respectively. Note that

$$\mu_{0k} \{t_k \mid H[\tau(k-1) + t_k]\} = \exp[\gamma_k + \gamma_k \log(t)] = \exp(\gamma_k)t^{\vartheta}_k \tag{9}$$

specifies the Weibull hazard rate. The Weibull hazard model is used because previous studies from various settings within the framework of dynamic models of fertility behavior (e.g., Lancaster, 1985; Heckman and Walker, 1987, 1990, 1991; Popkin et al., 1993) have shown that the duration structure of life-cycle fertility is well represented by a Weibull. Furthermore, the Weibull distribution is an important generalization of the exponential distribution and allows for a power dependence of the hazard on time. Finally, the Weibull model is, to some extent, preferable to other models because of the larger maximized log likelihood (Kalbfleisch and Prentice, 1980).

In the models specified so far, I have assumed that all covariates that might confound the association between child mortality and fertility are measured. This is unlikely to be the case if unobserved population heterogeneity is present. Indeed, Heckman et al. (1985) have shown the empirical importance of accounting for unobservables in the analysis of timing and spacing of births, both on policy and interpretive grounds. Accounting for them is often necessary so as to produce estimates that isolate genuine behavioral effects of covariates (such as child mortality) on fertility, and the existence of unobservables provides a motivation and interpretation for the presence of statistically significant lagged birth intervals in fitted survival rates for birth parities beyond the first parity (Heckman and Walker, 1991). Hence, although the methods for dealing with unobserved heterogeneity in demographic research are still undeveloped (Trussell and Rodriguez, 1990), it is possible to assess the sensitivity of my estimates to unobserved heterogeneity. Almost always, whenever unobserved heterogeneity has been introduced in waiting-time models, a random-effects structure has been assumed; I follow that tradition. At the individual level, fertility regressions are generally subject to the standard unobserved individual characteristics concern of the labor supply literature (for a review, see Hotz et al., in press). In my specification, I distinguish two forms of heterogeneity in life-cycle fertility: woman-specific unobserved characteristics that are known to the woman and affect her reproductive behavior and parity-specific unobserved characteristics that are not known to the woman but that may produce their own dynamics if the woman learns about her unobservables over the life cycle, as discussed in the text. My concern for parity-specific unobserved characteristics in fertility analysis follows a long-standing demographic tradition that postulates changing female fecundity across parities as an important determinant of fertility (Gini, 1924; Sheps, 1965; Sheps and Menken, 1973). Fecundity differences among women undoubtedly contribute to declining parity-specific hazards that are a universal feature of fertility data, but it is difficult to obtain good measures of fecundity (Bongaarts, 1981; Acsadi et al., 1990). Heckman and Walker (1991:11-15) show that, under most conditions, if there is persistent heterogeneity across parities, estimates of the parameters of the hazards obtained by estimating the model separately will be biased. Cameroon is a quasi-non-contracepting (natural fertility) society through the late 1980s. In such a setting, my dynamic formulation of the fertility behavior models implies that woman-specific (approximately) time-invariant population heterogeneity in the unobserved component of preferences (including coital fre-quency assumed to be time-invariant within each period or interval) and response to child mortality experience will not always have similar effects on interbirth timing as it has on first-birth timing. Such differences in effects is implicit in my dynamic formulation that treats timing of first birth separately from birth spacing. The assumption that the unobserved component of the model is time invariant underlies the classical demographic model of fecundity of Gini (1924), Sheps (1965), and Sheps and Menken (1973). These unobserved characteristics are assumed independent of the initial state of the birth process. Thus, consistent with Heckman's general formulation (Heckman and Singer, 1985; Heckman and Walker, 1987, 1990, 1991), my specification of the heterogeneity detaches the interval until the first birth from subsequent interbirth intervals. Such an ap-proach is more appealing in developing countries in general than in developed countries, because the modal family size (around five children per woman in Cameroon) in the former is considerably higher than in the latter (it stands at about two children per woman). This implies that in developed countries, there will be generally one interbirth interval (as in the Heckman and Walker's (1990) study in Sweden where third births are not common and fourth births are rare), making estimation of the correlation in unobservables between interbirth inter-vals impossible; this is in contrast to the situation in sub-Saharan African coun-tries (and in Cameroon in particular) where the average family size is five or higher. Strongly peaked preferences for a given number of children will be fitted through nondefective hazards for parities below the desired fertility size and essentially zero hazards thereafter. This was the case, for example, in Heckman and Walker (1987, 1990, 1991), who use this characteristic of the model to focus on the decision to have a third child in Sweden, and in the present study where I use this feature of the model to focus on the decision to have a sixth child in Cameroon. I account for woman-specific and parity-specific unobserved heterogeneities by augmenting the conditional hazard in equation (8) to obtain the following form:

$$\mu\{t_1,...., t_N \mid H[\tau(0) + \Sigma_i t_i]; \Theta, \Phi\} \tag{10}$$
$$= \Pi_k \exp [\gamma_k + \beta_k X + \eta_k Y(t) + \delta_k Z(t) + \zeta_k \Theta + \alpha_k \Phi] t^{\vartheta}_k ,$$

where Θ represents the unobserved characteristics of the woman, and Φ captures the parity-specific stopping unobserved characteristics. In my empirical implementation of the system of hazards described here, I estimate the distribution of unobservables by the nonparametric maximum likelihood estimator (NPMLE) procedure described in Heckman and Singer (1984). This procedure approximates any distribution function of unmeasured covariates with a finite mixture distribution. The approximation is designed to maximize sample likelihood. Each of the parameters (including the factor loading on the random effect) is allowed to vary with parity. Because equation (10) produces estimators obtained from exponential models based on a maximum likelihood approach, those estimators are generally more efficient than those obtained from nonexponential waiting-time distribution models (Olsen and Wolpin, 1983; Wolpin, 1984). A useful feature of the Heckman and Singer (1984) NPMLE used here is that it allows for the possibility of point mass $\Phi = -\infty$, a value that sets hazard (10) to zero to allow a distinction between limiting behavior and the biological sterility discussed in the text. The only model in the literature similar to the Heckman's formulation is that of Newman and McCulloch (1984) who estimate a birth process with duration dependence modeled as a three-point spline and assume a parametric distribution of the unobserved heterogeneity, which excludes parity-specific unobserved heterogeneity. Basically, they take the random effect to be person-specific and time invariant. In my empirical implementation of the specification of the woman-specific time-invariant random effect, I use Heckman and Singer's (1984) NPMLE for the mixing distribution of the heterogeneity component, since, when parametric models are used, the results are sensitive to the distribution imposed on the unmeasured covariates.

Following Heckman and Walker (1987, 1991), I generalize this system of hazard models to include previous durations; that is, for the transition to second birth, I have as covariates the duration between first marriage and first birth, in addition to the time of exposure to the risk of conceiving a second birth since the birth of the first birth; for the transition to the third birth, I have as covariates the duration between first marriage and first birth, between first and second births, in addition to the time of exposure to the risk of conceiving a third birth since the birth of the second birth, and so on. Clearly, women who experience a first birth learn something about their Φ, and this information might enter their information set and affect fertility decisions (e.g., coital frequency, contraceptive decisions) for the second birth. In particular, I model the probability of no birth within interval t of the jth birth (the survivor function) as

$$S_j\{t_j \mid H[\tau(j-1) + t_j], \Phi\} = P^{(j-1)} + [1 - P^{(j-1)}] \Pi_k [1 - h(k)], \qquad (11)$$
$$k = 1, 2, ..., N,$$

where $h(k)$ is the probability of the jth birth in interval t, conditional on the jth birth not having occurred through interval $t - 1$. In other words, this survivor function is the probability of parity-specific stopping behavior after the $(j - 1)^{th}$ birth, plus the probability that there is not parity-specific stopping behavior, but that the birth has not occurred yet. Because the fertility process only runs for a finite time (in the WFS and DHS surveys and in the CWFS and CDHS in particular, the fertility process is truncated at age 49), some of the $(1 - P)$ women who do not exhibit parity-specific stopping behavior will nevertheless never have the jth birth, eventually under some time path of covariates according to the specification of the model.

Uncorrected heterogeneity leads to biased estimates of duration variables. Unobserved variables are permitted to be functions of time since marriage (for the transition to the first conception) and since the last birth (for the transition to subsequent a conception). For example, the fertility level and schedule of women who experience a child death at a given point in time is a biased estimate of the fertility level and schedule that women with similar observed characteristics would have had had they not experienced a child death. Thus, the fertility responses to a child death may not be only a function of other measured characteristics of the woman, but may also be related to unmeasured characteristics associated with each woman and each parity of a particular woman.

This system of hazards formulation in continuous time suggests natural restrictions on how the covariates enter the model. As in the static models, my models are implemented including only current period (interval) covariates in the current period (interval) hazard. The model thus summarizes the values of past and current covariates through its dependence on parity, time since first marriage, time since last birth, and the dynamic selection of the time-invariant random effect (or unobserved heterogeneity). A general multistate computer program, CTM, is used to estimate the model (Yi et al., 1987).

ACKNOWLEDGMENTS

This research was supported by a grant from the Subvention Générale du Conseil de Recherche en Sciences Humanes of Canada to the University of Montreal. Thanks are due to Joel Tokindang for his research assistance, and to Mark Montgomery, Tom LeGrand, Julie DaVanzo, Alberto Palloni, Barney Cohen, and two anonymous referees for their insightful comments on an earlier draft of this manuscript.

REFERENCES

Acsadi, G., G. Johnson-Acsadi, and R. Bulatao
  1990   *Population Growth and Reproduction in Sub-Saharan Africa: Technical Analyses of Fertility and Its Consequences.* Washington, D.C.: The World Bank.
Bakketeig, L., H. Hoffman, and E. Harley
  1979   The tendency to repeat gestational age and birth weight in successive births. *American Journal of Obstetrics and Gynecology* 195:1086-1103.
Balepa, M., M. Fotso, and B. Barrère
  1992   *Enquête Démographique et de Santé Cameroun 1991.* Yaoundé: Direction Nationale du Deuxième Recensement Général de la Population.
Barbieri, M.
  1994   Is the current decline in infant and child mortality in sub-Saharan Africa a sign of future fertility changes? Pp. 21-42 in T. Locoh and V. Hertich, eds., *The Onset of Fertility Transition in Sub-Saharan Africa.* Liège, Belgium: Ordina Editions.
Ben-Porath, Y.
  1978   Fertility response to child mortality: Microdata from Israel. Pp. 161-180 in S. Preston, ed., *The Effects of Infant and Child Mortality on Fertility.* New York: Academic Press.
Bocquier, P.
  1991   Les relations entre mortalité des enfants et espacement des naissances dans la Banlieue de Dakar (Sénégal). *Population* 46:813-831.
Bongaarts, J.
  1981   The impact on fertility of traditional and changing child-spacing practices. Pp. 111-129 in H. Page and R. Lesthaeghe, eds., *Child-Spacing in Tropical Africa: Traditions and Change.* New York: Academic Press.
Brass, W.
  1993   Child mortality improvement and the initiation of fertility falls in Kenya. *International Population Conference* 1:73-80.
Brass, W., and C. Jolly, eds.
  1993   *Population Dynamics of Kenya.* Committee on Population, National Research Council. Washington, D.C.: National Academy Press.
Caldwell, J., and P. Caldwell
  1981   The function of child-spacing in traditional societies and the direction of change. Pp. 73-92 in H. Page and R. Lesthaeghe, eds., *Child Spacing in Tropical Africa: Traditions and Change.* New York: Academic Press.
Callum, C., S. Farid, and M. Moussa
  1988   Child loss and its impact on fertility. Pp. 239-278 in A. Hallouda, S. Farid, and S. Cochrane, eds., *Egypt: Demographic Responses to Modernization.* Cairo: Central Agency for Public Mobilization and Statistics.
Cantrelle, P., and H. Leridon
  1971   Breast-feeding, mortality in childhood and fertility in a rural zone of Senegal. *Population Studies* 25:505-533.
Cantrelle, P., B. Ferry, and J. Mondot
  1978   Relationships between fertility and mortality in Tropical Africa. Pp. 181-205 in S. Preston, ed., *The Effects of Infant and Child Mortality on Fertility.* New York: Academic Press.
Cleland, J., and C. Wilson
  1987   Demand theories of the fertility transition: An iconoclastic view. *Population Studies* 41:5-30.
Coale, A.
  1966   Estimates of fertility and mortality in Tropical Africa. *Population Index* 32.

Cochrane, S., and K. Zachariah
  1984   Infant and Child Mortality as a Determinant of Fertility: The Policy Implications. World
           Bank Staff Papers no. 556. Washington, D.C.: The World Bank.
Cohen, B.
  1993   Fertility levels, differentials and trends. Pp. 8-67 in K. Foote, K. Hill, and L. Martin, eds.,
           Demographic Change in Sub-Saharan Africa. Committee on Population, National Re-
           search Council. Washington, D.C.: National Academy Press.
Cohen, B., and J. Trussell, eds.
  1996   *Preventing and Mitigating AIDS in Sub-Saharan Africa.* Committee on Population, Na-
           tional Research Council. Washington, D.C.: National Academy Press.
David, N., and D. Voaz
  1981   Societal causes of infertility and population decline among the settled Fulani of North
           Cameroon. *Man* 16:644-664.
DSCN (Direction de la Statistique et de la Comptabilité Nationale)
  1983   *Enquête Nationale sur la Fécondité du Cameroun 1978, Rapport Principal.* Yaoundé:
           Ministère de l'Economie et du Plan.
Farah, A.
  1982   The influence of child mortality on fertility related attitudes and behavior in Greater
           Khartoum. *Cairo Demographic Centre Research Monograph Series* 10:227-261.
Folta, J., and E. Deck
  1988   The impact of children's death on Shona mothers and families. *Journal of Comparative
           Family Studies* 19:433-451.
Gini, C.
  1924   Premières recherches sur la fécondabilité de la femme. *Proceedings of International
           Mathematics Congress* 2:889-892.
Gregson, S.
  1994   Will HIV become a major determinant of fertility in sub-Saharan Africa? *Journal of
           Development Studies* 30(3):650-679.
Guz, D., and J. Hobcraft
  1991   Breast-feeding and fertility: A comparative analysis. *Population Studies* 45:91-108.
Heckman, J., and B. Singer
  1984   A method for minimizing the impact of distributional assumptions in econometric models
           for duration data. *Econometrica* 52:271-320.
  1985   Social science duration analysis. In J. Heckman and B. Singer, eds., *Longitudinal Analy-
           sis of Labor Market Data.* Cambridge, England: Cambridge University Press.
Heckman, J., and J. Walker
  1987   Using goodness of fit and other criteria to choose among competing duration models: A
           case study of the Hutterite data. In C. Clogg, ed., *Sociological Methodology.* Washing-
           ton, D.C.: American Sociological Association.
  1990   The relationships between wages and income and the timing and spacing of births: Evi-
           dence from Swedish longitudinal data. *Econometrica* 58:1411-1441.
  1991   Economic models of fertility dynamics: A study of Swedish fertility. *Research in Popu-
           lation Economics* 7:3-91.
Heckman, J., J. Hotz, and J. Walker
  1985   New evidence on the timing and spacing of births. *American Economic Review* 75:179-
           184.
Heer, D., and J. Wu
  1978   Effects in rural Taiwan and urban Morocco: Combining individual and aggregate data.
           Pp. 135-159 in S.H. Preston, ed., *The Effects of Infant and Child Mortality on Fertility.*
           New York: Academic Press.

Hill, A.
  1993   Trends in childhood mortality. Pp. 153-217 in K.A. Foote, K. Hill, and L. Martin, eds., *Demographic Change in Sub-Saharan Africa.* Washington, D.C.: National Academy Press.
Hobcraft, J.
  1994   *The Health Rationale for Family Planning: Timing of Births and Child Survival.* New York: United Nations.
Hoel, P., S. Port, and C. Stone
  1987   *Introduction to Stochastic Processes.* Prospect Heights, Ill.: Waveland Press.
Hoffman, H., and L. Bakketeig
  1984   Heterogeneity of intrauterine growth retardation and recurrence risks. *Seminars in Perinatology* 8:15-24.
Hotz, J., J. Klerman, and R. Willis
  in   The economics of fertility in developed countries: A survey. In M. Rosenzweig and O. Stark, eds., *Handbook of Population and Family Economics.* Amsterdam, Holland: North-Holland.
Hull, V., and M. Simpson
  1985   *Breast-feeding, Child Health and Child Spacing: Cross-Cultural Perspectives.* London:
  press   Croom Helm.
Jensen, A.
  1993   Child Survival and Fertility in Kenya. Paper presented at the XXIIIrd IUSSP International Population Conference, Montréal, Canada, August.
  1996   The Impact of Child Mortality on Fertility in Kenya, Zimbabwe and Botswana: Reexamining the Links. Unpublished manuscript, Norwegian Institute for Urban and Regional Research, Oslo, Norway.
Kalbfleisch, J.D., and R.L. Prentice
  1980   *The Statistical Analysis of Failure Time Data.* New York: John Wiley & Sons.
Kelley, A., and C. Nobbe
  1990   Kenya at the Demographic Turning Point? Hypotheses and a Proposed Research Agenda. World Bank Discussion Papers no. 107. Washington, D.C.: The World Bank.
Kuate Defo, B.
  1996   Areal and socioeconomic differentials in infant and child mortality in Cameroon. *Social Science and Medicine* 42:399-420.
Kuate Defo, B., and A. Palloni
  1996   Determinants of mortality among Cameroonian children: Are the effects of breast-feeding and pace of childbearing artifacts? *Genus* LI:69-96.
Lancaster, T.
  1985   Generalized residuals and heterogeneous duration models with applications to the Weibull models. *Journal of Econometrics* 28:54.
  1990   *The Econometric Analysis of Transition Data.* New York: Cambridge University Press.
Larsen, U.
  1994   Sterility in sub-Saharan Africa. *Population Studies* 48(3):459-474.
  1995   Differentials in infertility in Cameroon and Nigeria. *Population Studies* 49:329-346.
Larsen, U., and J. Menken
  1991   Individual level sterility. A new method of estimation with application to sub-Saharan Africa. *Demography* 28:229-249.
Lesthaeghe, R.
  1989   *Reproduction and Social Organisation in Sub-Saharan Africa.* Berkeley: University of California Press.

Lesthaeghe, R., P. Ohadike, J. Kocker, and H. Page
    1981   Child-spacing and fertility in sub-Saharan Africa: An overview of issues. Pp. 3-23 in H.
            Page and R. Lesthaeghe, eds., *Child Spacing in Tropical Africa: Traditions and Change.*
            New York: Academic Press.
Leung, S.
    1988   A test for sex preferences. *Journal of Population Economics* 1:95-114.
Livenais, P.
    1984   Déclin de la mortalité dans l'enfance et stabilité de la fécondité dans une zone rurale
            Mossi (Haute-Volta). *Cahiers ORSTOM* XX(2):273-282.
Locoh, T., and V. Hertrich, eds.
    1994   *The Onset of Fertility Transition in Sub-Saharan Africa.* Liège, Belgium: Ordina Edi-
            tions.
Mensch, B.
    1985   The effect of child mortality on contraceptive use and fertility in Colombia, Costa Rica,
            and Korea. *Population Studies* 39(2):309-327.
Newman, J., and C. McCulloch
    1984   A hazard rate approach to the timing of births. *Econometrica* 52:939-961.
Njogu, W.
    1992   Trends and determinants of contraceptive use in Kenya. *Demography* 28:83-99.
Okojie, C.
    1991   Fertility response to child survival in Nigeria: An analysis of microdata from Bendel
            State. *Research in Population Economics* 7:93-112.
Olsen, R.
    1980   Estimating the effect of child mortality on the number of births. *Demography* 17:429-
            443.
Olsen, R., and K. Wolpin
    1983   The impact of exogenous child mortality on fertility: A waiting time regression with
            dynamic regressors. *Econometrica* 51:731-749.
Page, H., and R. Lesthaeghe, eds.
    1981   *Child Spacing in Tropical Africa: Traditions and Change.* New York: Academic Press.
Panis, C., and L. Lillard
    1993   Timing of Child Replacement Effects on Fertility in Malaysia. Labor and Population
            Program Working Paper Series 93-13. Santa Monica, Calif.: RAND.
Popkin, B., D. Guilkey, J. Akin, L. Adair, and R. Udry
    1993   Nutrition, lactation and birth spacing in Filipino women. *Demography* 30:333-352.
Preston, S.H., ed.
    1978   *The Effects of Infant and Child Mortality on Fertility.* New York: Academic Press.
Rodriguez, G., and J. Cleland
    1981   Socio-economic determinants of marital fertility in twenty countries: A multivariate
            analysis. In *World Fertility Survey Conference 1980: Record of Proceedings 2.*
            Voorburg, Netherlands: International Statistical Institute.
Rodriguez, G., J. Hobcraft, J. Menken, and J. Trussell
    1984   A comparative analysis of the determinants of birth intervals. *WFS Comparative Studies*
            30:1-30.
Schoenmaeckers, R., I. Shah, R. Lesthaeghe, and O. Tambashe
    1981   The child-spacing tradition and the postpartum taboo in tropical Africa: Anthropological
            evidence. Pp. 25-71 in H. Page and R. Lesthaeghe, eds., *Child Spacing in Tropical
            Africa: Traditions and Change.* New York: Academic Press.
Schultz, T.P.
    1985   Changing world prices, women's wages, and the fertility transition: Sweden, 1860-1910.
            Journal of Political Economy 93(6):1126-1154.

Sembajwe, I.
1981   Fertility and Infant Mortality Amongst the Yoruba in Western Nigeria. Changing Family Project Series Monograph no. 6. Canberra, Australia: Department of Demography.
Sheps, M.
1965   An analysis of reproductive patterns in an American isolate. *Population Studies* 19:65-80.
Sheps, M., and J. Menken
1973   *Mathematical Models of Conception and Birth.* Chicago, Ill.: University of Chicago Press.
Trussell, J., and G. Rodriguez
1990   Heterogeneity in demographic research. Pp. 111-132 in J. Adams, D. Lam, A. Hermalin, and P. Smouse, eds., *Convergent Issues in Genetics and Demography.* Oxford, England: Oxford University Press.
Trussell, J., E. van de Walle, and F. van de Walle
1989   Norms and behavior in Burkinabe fertility. *Population Studies* 43(3):429-454.
United Nations
1987   *Family Building by Fate or Design.* New York: United Nations.
1991   *Child Mortality in Developing Countries: Socio-Economic Differentials, Trends and Implications.* New York: United Nations.
van de Walle, E.
1992   Fertility, conscious choice and numeracy. *Demography* 29:487-502.
Ware, H.
1977   The relationship between infant mortality and fertility: Replacement and insurance effects. Pp. 205-222 in *International Population Conference*, Vol. I. Mexico. Liège, Belgium: IUSSP.
Winikoff, B., M. Castle, and V.H. Laukaran
1988   *Feeding Infants in Four Societies: Causes and Consequences of Mothers' Choices.* New York: Greenwood Press.
Wolpin, K.
1984   An estimable dynamic stochastic model of fertility and child mortality. *Journal of Political Economy* 92(5):852-874.
World Health Organization
1991   *Infertility.* Geneva: World Health Organization.
Yamada, T.
1984   Causal Relationships between Infant Mortality and Fertility in Developed and Less Developed Countries. National Bureau of Economic Research (NBER) Working Paper no. 1528. NBER, Cambridge, Mass.
Yi, K., J. Walker, and B. Honoré
1987   CTM: A User's Guide. Unpublished manuscript, National Opinion Research Center, University of Chicago.

9

The Relationship Between Infant and Child Mortality and Subsequent Fertility in Indonesia: 1971-1991

Elizabeth Frankenberg

The relationship between infant and child mortality and subsequent fertility at both the aggregate and the familial level has long interested demographers, sociologists, and economists. The idea that mortality decline precipitates fertility decline has its origins in the historical demography of Europe and is a linchpin of demographic transition theory. At the aggregate level two questions have focused on the demographic future of developing countries:

(1) Would fertility declines accompany the mortality declines observed in developing countries in the mid-1900s?

(2) How would population growth rates change as mortality declined?

Underlying these questions and stimulating interest at the family level is the notion that a couple's fertility is in part a product of the mortality environment in which they are building a family. Actual or expected child deaths prompt a fertility response, so as child deaths become more rare, fertility patterns change.

Work on the link between mortality and fertility has sought to answer a variety of questions, some only tangentially related to the "bottom line" of how fertility levels and population growth rates change as mortality declines. Most theoretical models of fertility response make predictions about conscious behavioral responses to actual or expected child deaths, given assumptions about couples' family formation goals. A number of authors recognize the potential complexity of those goals when preferences for family size, sex composition, and timing are entertained (Preston, 1978; Ben-Porath, 1976; Wolpin, 1984). The theoretical literature draws a distinction between strategies of hoarding and replacement. Both strategies involve the attempt to achieve some target number of surviving children. Hoarding is described as a fertility response to expected mortality, where women give birth to a larger number of children than they ultimately desire in expectation that some will die. Replacement is described as the strategy of having an additional child only in the event that a previous child dies. Other theoretical models are more concerned with how the biological processes surrounding childbearing are affected by a death in ways that in turn affect fertility (Preston, 1978).

Empirical work has focused both on identifying the types of responses to mortality and on quantifying the ultimate effect of child death on completed family size (Olsen, 1980; Mauskopf and Wallace, 1984; Mensch, 1985; Heer and Wu, 1978). Fertility-related outcomes of interest include completed family size, parity progression ratios, interbirth intervals, and contraceptive use. The increasing availability of birth history data, which record the sequence and timing of a woman's births and the survival status of each birth, have fundamentally altered the scope for empirical work on the topic. In this chapter I focus on relationships at the family level in Indonesia, using data from the 1987 and 1991 Demographic and Health Surveys (DHSs).

INDONESIA: A DEMOGRAPHIC AND SOCIOECONOMIC OVERVIEW

Indonesia, with almost 200 million people inhabiting an equatorial belt of more than 15,000 islands, is the fourth most populous country in the world. The archipelago is home to a diverse group of cultures and ethnicities, including more than 300 distinct language groups. Indonesia has experienced rapid economic growth in the past 25 years, with per capita income rising at an annual rate of about 4.5 percent, from $50 in the late 1960s to $650 in 1992 (World Bank, 1994). Accompanying this economic growth have been increases in access to schools and health services and, in turn, improvements in measures of human resources. For example, the number of people per physician declined from over 100,000 in the 1950s to around 13,000 in the 1980s (Hugo et al., 1987), while life expectancy at birth increased from 32 to around 53 over this period. Adult illiteracy declined from 61 percent in 1960 to 23 percent in 1990 as the number of primary, junior secondary, and senior secondary schools rose (World Bank, 1994; Hugo et al., 1987; World Bank, 1984).

Of more importance for this chapter than general socioeconomic trends are changes in demographic characteristics in Indonesia over time. Numbers for Indonesia as a whole are not available until the late 1960s, but some information about earlier periods is available for subregions. This discussion is taken from Nitisastro's comprehensive effort to document population change in Indonesia in the 1900s (Nitisastro, 1970). Estimates of vital rates for Java in the 1930s are available from registration systems for some areas (predominantly urban), as well as from small-scale studies of infant mortality. Nitisastro assembles available information and concludes that in the 1930s crude birth rates for Java were higher than 40 per 1,000, while life expectancy at birth was between 30 and 35 years, and infant mortality was between 225 and 250 per 1,000. Estimates of infant mortality rates on Sumatran plantations (where recording of births and deaths was believed to be relatively accurate) yield rates of 160-370 per 1,000. As early as the 1930s, programs relating to hygiene and malaria control began on Java, perhaps reducing mortality in some areas (Hull, 1989).

The 1940s were a period of extreme hardship throughout Indonesia, but especially on Java. The Japanese occupied Indonesia from 1942 to 1945. Between 1945 and 1949 Indonesia fought a war of independence against the Dutch. The decade was characterized by severe population dislocations, food shortages, decreasing fertility, and increasing mortality. Examination of the age structure of the population recorded in a 1958 labor force survey and the 1961 census indicates that the number of survivors from births in the 1940s was much smaller than the number of survivors from births in the preceding and subsequent periods (Nitisastro, 1970). During the 1950s, the early years of independence, crude birth rates returned to their prewar levels of more than 40 per 1,000. Simultaneously, a fairly intensive public health campaign began and mortality declined. Estimates of infant mortality rates from Jakarta, Surabaya, and Wonosobo (a region of central Java) range from 148 to 178 per 1,000—a considerable decline relative to estimated rates of the 1930s.

The 1971 census marks the beginning of the period for which estimates of fertility and mortality patterns are available for Indonesia as a whole, although differences across data sources in sample and content thwart precise documentation of trends. Since the late 1960s both mortality and fertility levels have declined considerably in Indonesia. Scholars believe that in most of Indonesia, the mortality decline began in the 1950s, while fertility did not start to fall until the mid-1960s. Efforts to promote family planning in Indonesia began as early as the 1950s (Hugo et al., 1987). In 1957 various local groups combined to form the Indonesian Planned Parenthood Organization, which sold contraceptives, invited family planning advisors from abroad to visit Indonesia, and in 1963 conducted a series of seminars on contraception for health professionals from Java and Bali (Hugo et al., 1987). The activities of the organization were disrupted by the political events of the mid-1960s, but in 1970 the National Family Planning Coordinating Board (BKKBN) was formed with orders to report directly to President Soeharto.

Estimates of total fertility and infant mortality rates between 1967 and 1991 are summarized in Table 9-1. The table documents a decline in total fertility from 5.61 in the late 1960s to around 3.0 in 1991—a decline that began slowly but accelerated over time. Infant mortality has fallen from 143 per 1,000 in the late 1960s to around 70 per 1,000 in the early 1990s, but the pace of the decline is more erratic than the decline in fertility. The mid-1970s and the mid-1980s appear to be periods of little change in mortality.

TABLE 9-1 Estimated Fertility and Infant Mortality Rates Post-1965

Source	Period	Total Fertility Rate	Period	Infant Mortality Rate
1971 census	1967-1970	5.61	1968-1996	143
1976 SUPAS	1971-1975	5.20	1972-1973	112
1980 census	1976-1979	4.68	1977-1978	112
1985 SUPAS	1980-1985	4.06	1982-1983	71
1991 DHS	1984-1987	3.73		
1990 census	1986-1989	3.31	1987-1988	70
1991 DHS	1988-1991	3.02	1988-1991	68
1994 DHS	1991-1994	2.85	1991-1994	57

NOTE: SUPAS, intercensal population survey.

In reviewing the demographic trends in Indonesia, some evidence supports the contention that mortality decline preceded fertility decline. It appears that mortality began to fall during the 1950s, partially in response to increases in food availability and in public health services, but that fertility did not decline until the mid-1960s. Once the fertility decline began, however, it did so at an accelerating pace, independent of the more erratic pattern of mortality decline. A similar pattern is observed in the historical data on Europe, where the most rapid declines in mortality and fertility appear to have occurred simultaneously (Matthiessen and McCann, 1978).

DATA

In the past several decades Indonesia has made demographic and socioeconomic data collection a priority. The Indonesian Central Bureau of Statistics has implemented numerous special topic surveys, as well as conducting diennial censuses of the population and of levels of village infrastructure.

Data for this chapter are drawn from the 1987 and 1991 Demographic and Health Surveys of Indonesia. These surveys are joint efforts of the Central Bureau of Statistics and Demographic and Health Surveys, with input from the Ministry of Health and from the BKKBN. The 1987 DHS collected information from 11,884 ever-married women between the ages of 15 and 49, living in 20 of Indonesia's 27 provinces. These data put the total fertility rate at 3.4 per woman and the infant mortality rate at 70.2 per 1,000 births for the 1982-1987 period (Central Bureau of Statistics et al., 1989). The 1991 DHS collected information from 22,909 ever-married women between the ages of 15 and 49. The 1991 survey, which covered all 27 of Indonesia's provinces, documents a fertility rate

TABLE 9-2 Vital Rates, 1984-1986

Vital Rate	1987	Standard Error	1991	Standard Error	Ratio	z Score
Fertility rates						
15-19	74	10	95	8	0.82	3.15
20-24	180	15	193	12	0.99	1.45
25-29	167	16	179	12	1.03	1.28
30-34	126	16	134	12	0.97	0.85
35-39	70	13	81	11	0.97	1.21
40-44	30					
45-49	10					
TFR to 39	3.09		3.41		0.91	
Mortality rates						
Infant mortality	66.8	7.6	75.7	6.4	0.88	1.86
Neonatal mortality	24.5	4.6	32.7	4.2	0.75	2.60
Postneonatal mortality	43.4	6.2	44.5	5.0	0.98	0.26

NOTE: TFR, total fertility rate.

SOURCE: 1987 and 1991 Demographic and Health Surveys.

of 3.02 and an infant mortality rate of 68 per 1,000 in 5 years before the survey (Central Bureau of Statistics et al., 1992).[1]

DHS data sets are almost uniformly regarded as of high quality, and the Indonesian data are no exception. Table 9-2 demonstrates the comparability of the 1987 and 1991 data. Estimates of age-specific and total fertility rates (up to age 39) are calculated for women in the 20 provinces surveyed in the 1987 data for the period 1984-1986. The 1991 data were reweighted to match the geographic and age distributions prevailing in 1987 in the 20 provinces surveyed as part of the 1987 DHS. I also calculated standard errors, the ratio of the two estimates, and z-scores testing for significant differences between the estimates. These data provide an indication of the magnitude of the differences.

The two surveys generate reasonably consistent estimates of age-specific fertility rates for the 1984-1986 period, although the total fertility rate from the 1991 data is higher than that from the 1987 data, in part because the 1991 estimates of fertility among those aged 15-19 is considerably higher than the estimates from the 1987 data (the z score indicates a significant difference between the two numbers). I also compared mortality rates estimated from the two sur-

---

[1]The 1994 DHS Final Report became available as this chapter was being written. The 1994 DHS data put Indonesia's fertility rate at 2.85 for the 1991-1994 period and the infant mortality rate at 57 per 1,000 (Central Bureau of Statistics et al., 1995).

veys. Estimates of infant mortality for the 1984-1986 period are higher in the 1991 data (75.7 per 1,000) than in the 1987 data (66.8 per 1,000), although the difference is not significant. The difference stems from discrepancies in estimated neonatal mortality (a difference that is statistically significant). Postneonatal mortality rates for the 1984-1986 period are very similar (43.4 per 1,000 from the 1987 data, 44.5 per 1,000 from the 1991 data).

The DHS data contain birth histories, in which respondents provided information on the dates of birth and death for all their children. Considerable attention has focused on how reliably these dates are reported and the extent to which missing data that require imputation procedures could bias estimates of demographic parameters (Boerma et al., 1994; Sullivan et al., 1990). The general conclusion of analyses of World Fertility Survey (WFS) and DHS data quality is that estimates of mortality, fertility, and durations of interbirth intervals, particularly within 15 years of the survey date, are not seriously biased by date misreporting (Sullivan et al., 1990; Lantz et al., 1992; Potter, 1988). The Indonesia data contain cases in which children's month of birth is not reported by the mother. Failure to report a birthdate is more common when the child died than when the child survived. In the 1987 data, month of birth was imputed for 17.2 percent of the births in the 15 years before the survey. In the 1991 data, month of birth was imputed for 13.6 percent of births occurring in the 15 years before the interview.

DESCRIPTIVE STATISTICS

Initial efforts to link infant and child mortality to fertility were based on comparisons of the number of children ever born (and children surviving) among women with different child mortality experiences (Olsen, 1980; Mauskopf and Wallace, 1984). These comparisons were made in part because demographic data were often limited to a woman's report of the number of children ever born and number of children who died. Typically, correlations are positive for several reasons. These reasons highlight the statistical pitfalls associated with analyses of links between child mortality and subsequent fertility. Some of the reasons also explain positive correlations between child mortality and other aspects of reproductive patterns.

First, the larger the number of children ever born, the more children who are exposed to the risk of death. Women who give birth to more children will on average have more children die, simply because of a binomial association (the larger the number of trials, the larger the number of deaths) (Olsen, 1980).

Second, if babies die before they are weaned, the cessation of breastfeeding may hasten the return of ovulation after a birth and thus hasten the conception of a subsequent infant (van Ginneken, 1974). This phenomenon, sometimes referred to as the physiological effect, has been recognized for more than a century

(Knodel, 1978): This mechanism has the most scope for effect in settings where average breastfeeding durations are long.

Third, women who have given birth to a large number of children are likely to have experienced reproductive patterns (e.g., teenage childbearing, late child-bearing, short birth intervals) that have been shown to be associated with in-creased risks of child mortality in a voluminous number of analyses. In other words, reproductive patterns that generate large numbers of births imply height-ened risk of death (Rinehart and Kols, 1984; Ross and Frankenberg, 1993).

Fourth, some women may have characteristics that predispose them to both high fertility and high mortality. For example, some women may be fatalistic about their ability to control their fertility and the health of their children, whereas others may actively seek out the technologies that change their fertility and their children's health. This difference in level of initiative may well drive differences in fertility and in child health outcomes and is likely to be correlated with charac-teristics such as education. In fact, some would argue that women are not predis-posed to high fertility and mortality, but rather that their allocation of resources reflects a choice of high fertility and mortality. This type of argument appears throughout the demographic and economic literature. Rodriguez et al. (1984) discuss the strong correlation among birth intervals for a given woman, indepen-dent of parity. Trussell et al. (1985) show that this correlation can be only partly explained by factors such as propensity to breastfeed or to use contraception. Pebley and Stupp (1987) discuss the fact that many of the factors associated with risk of child mortality are also associated with birth intervals.

Fifth, women who experience child deaths may intentionally bear additional children in an effort to attain their fertility goals. The possibility that women consciously change their fertility patterns in response to actual or anticipated child mortality is of primary interest. Would a particular woman choose a differ-ent number of births or space her births differently if her perceptions of the mortality risks of her children were different or if one of her children died? Designing a statistical test that isolates a conscious response to actual or per-ceived risk of mortality is extremely difficult because of the reasons detailed above that contribute to positive associations between mortality and fertility.

Data limitations also pose difficulties for empirical assessments of the de-gree to which the number of children ever born varies by mortality experience. The women of greatest interest are those who have completed their families and stopped having children. But fertility surveys typically collect data from women currently able to reproduce, who may or may not have finished bearing children. In addition, women who have finished having children tend to be older and may not reliably document births and deaths that occurred in the distant past.

Differences in completed family size by mortality experience are one of several potential indicators of a fertility response to child mortality. Other mea-sures that are easier to work with, given the existence of surveys of women of reproductive age, are parity progression ratios and birth intervals. Parity progression ratios are defined as the proportion of women at parity x who go on to have an $x + 1$ birth within a specified time period. Birth intervals are simply the time that elapses between two adjacent births. Because these indicators can be computed for women regardless of whether they have finished childbearing, they are well suited for use with demographic data. Comparison of parity progression ratios or birth intervals for women with differing child mortality experiences can indicate the degree to which very specific components of reproductive patterns vary by survival status, but say little about how levels of completed fertility are likely to change as mortality declines.

In this section I present cross tabulations and graphs describing the relationship between infant and child mortality experience and fertility levels and patterns for three periods: 1971-1977, 1978-1984, and 1985-1991. The DHS data from Indonesia appear to be of relatively high quality with respect to the completeness of reporting births, deaths, and associated dates. However, to the extent that dates are misreported or events are omitted in ways that are systematically related to the timing of fertility, the results in my descriptive tables could be affected.

I begin with a graph evaluating the effect of an early child death on completed family size in terms of the number children ever born and the number of surviving children. This graph derives from a method described by Wolpin (in this volume) in a recent review of the literature. The method was developed as a means of calculating directly the number of excess births that arise from a death. The method focuses on women at the end of their reproductive span, comparing numbers of children ever born with the number who survived for women whose reproductive histories are nearly identical to a point in time save for the survival status of one child. Any number of reproductive sequences can be compared. I focus on two simple patterns. First I identify women between the ages of 41 and 46 (in 1984 and 1991) who had a first child within the first 2 years of marriage. I stratify these women by the survival status of this first child at 2 years of marriage and compare the number of children ever born with the number of children surviving. The second comparison is based on a subset of women from the first comparison: those whose first child was still alive 2 years after the marriage and who had a second child between the second and fourth year of marriage. Women whose second child was alive 4 years after the marriage are compared with women whose second child did not survive to 4 years after the marriage. These comparisons are presented in Figure 9-1 and Figure 9-2.

Figure 9-1 contains the statistics described above for women 41-46 years of age at two points: 1984 and 1991. Several points emerge from the graph. First, family sizes for these women have clearly declined over time. Among older women whose first child was alive after 2 years of marriage, the average number of children ever born is 6.05 in 1984. By 1991 mean children ever born has declined by 0.76 children, to 5.31. Declines of a similar magnitude are observed for women whose second child was alive after 4 years of marriage (see Figure 9-

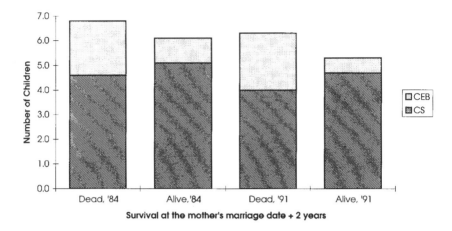

FIGURE 9-1 Children ever born (CEB) and children surviving (CS) by survival status of the first child for women aged 41-46 with a birth in the first 2 years of marriage.

2). Fertility declines over time are steeper for women whose first child survived to the date of interest than for women whose first child died. When the first or second child survived, the number of children ever born drops by 26 percent over the period. When the first or second child died the decline is around 19 percent.

Second, the number of children ever born is always greater for women whose first or second child died by the requisite date than for women whose first or second child was still alive. The differences in children ever born by survival status of the first or second child actually grow over time. In 1984 women whose first child died have around 0.75 more children ever born than women whose first or second child survived. The difference is 1.04 for women whose second child died compared with women whose second child survived. By 1991 women whose first child died have 0.94 more children ever born than women whose first child survived, while women whose second child died have 1.13 more children ever born than women whose second child survived. From these numbers it appears that women who experience a child death also have more births, and that the strength of this phenomenon has increased over time.

Although the total number of births is consistently larger for women who lost a first or second child than for women whose first and second child survived, the number of surviving children is smaller for women whose first or second child died. Women who experience a child death early in their reproductive careers go on to have more births, but ultimately smaller numbers of living children than do their counterparts whose early children survive.

On average, the difference between the number of children ever born and the number of surviving children is more than two children among women whose

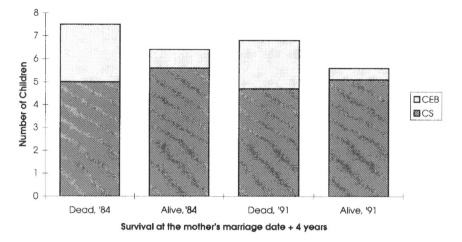

FIGURE 9-2 Children ever born (CEB) and children surviving (CS) by survival status of
the second child for women aged 41-46 with two births in the first 4 years of marriage.

first or second child died by the specified date. For women whose first or second
child survived to the specified date, the difference between the number of children ever born and the number of children surviving is considerably less than one
child. These differences suggest that mortality risks of children with the same
mother are correlated. Mortality is higher among the subsequent children of
women who experienced the death of a first or second child than among the
subsequent children of women whose first and second children survived to a
specified point.

I also present other measures of links between child mortality and subsequent fertility common in the demographic literature. Figure 9-3 displays parity
progression ratios by the number of children who survived until the birth of the
child at the specified parity. For example, at the birth of the second child (parity
two) a woman has had one previous child. If that child survived she has one
living child, if it died she has no living children. Rates are calculated for three
periods: 1971-1977, 1978-1984, and 1985-1991. A woman is counted as progressing to the next parity if she gives birth to her next child within 42 months of
attaining the parity recorded in Figure 9-3. I chose a cutoff date of 42 months
because I wanted an interval long enough to capture most women who progress to
the next parity (and so longer than mean length of birth intervals) but short
enough to guarantee an adequate number of women within the 6-year window. A
woman may contribute multiple observations to the figure, depending on which
dates she attained which parities.

At a general level, several of the patterns that emerge from Figure 9-1 reap-
pear in the parity progression ratios. Overall, the proportions of women in each

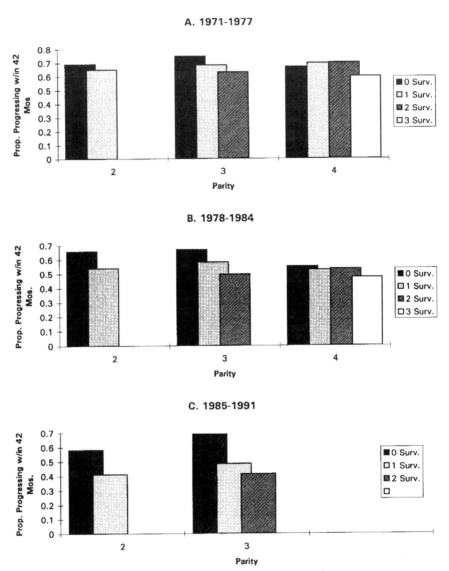

FIGURE 9-3 Parity progression by survival status of previous children.

succeding parity/surviving children category have declined over time, as expected in a setting where fertility is declining. For a given parity, the smaller the number of living children, the higher the proportion progressing to the next parity within 42 months. However, exceptions are found among parity-four women for whom two or three of the preceding children have died.

Patterns in the parity progression ratios over time are quite interesting. In 1971-1977, within a parity, changes in parity progression ratios with each additional surviving child tend to increase with parity. For example, for women of parity two, the proportion progressing to parity three within 42 months is 0.689 when the first child has died by the birth of the second, 0.649 when the first child survived to the birth of the second—a difference of around 6 percent. For women of parity three, the parity progression ratio for women with no surviving children is 8.7 percent greater than the parity progression ratio for women with one surviving child (0.746 versus 0.681), whereas for women with one surviving child the parity progression ratio is 7.5 percent greater than for women with two surviving children (0.681 versus 0.63). On the other hand, in 1985-1991 within-parity differences in parity progression ratios by one-child increments in the number of surviving children are greater at the lower parities than at the higher parities. For example, among parity-two women, the parity progression ratio is 0.58 when the first child died and 0.41 when the first child survived, a difference of 30 percent. A similar difference is observed between parity-three women with zero versus one surviving child. The differences are smaller for parity-three women with one versus two surviving children and much smaller for parity-four women.

Two statements can be made from these patterns. First, as desired family size shrinks and fertility falls, there is a corresponding decline in the parity at which differences in behavior by number of living children emerge. Second, within-parity differences in parity progression ratios by number of surviving children increase with time. Possibly these widening differentials mark an increase in women's ability to control their fertility through contraceptive use.

Birth intervals are another indicator of reproductive patterns that researchers typically investigate in efforts to learn about fertility responses to mortality. Table 9-3 summarizes the average length of time between births. Birth intervals are stratified by period, birth order, and survival status of the initiating (index) child at 1 month and at 12 months after birth. In constructing such a table one wants to avoid the issue of reverse causality. Specifically, it is possible that a woman becomes pregnant again quickly after the birth of the index child and that after this conception the index child dies. Such a phenomenon could occur if the subsequent conception causes the mother to stop breastfeeding the index child, who then dies during the vulnerable period of weaning. In this scenario the short subsequent interval causes the death of the index child, rather than the death of the index child causing a short subsequent interval. To avoid this problem I classify the index child as alive if it was alive 9 months before the birth of the subsequent child. That is, children who died within 9 months of the birth of the subsequent child (and so presumably after the conception of the subsequent child) were counted as alive.

The standard argument with respect to birth interval is that the interval after a child that dies in infancy will be shorter than the interval after a child that survives infancy. The shorter interval occurs either because the mother wants to

TABLE 9-3 Subsequent Birth Interval Lengths by Survival Status of Initiating Child

Birth Order	Survival Status at:	1971-1977		1978-1984		1985-1991	
		Dead	Alive	Dead	Alive	Dead	Alive
1	1 month	24.3	35.4	22	34.2	21.5	28.8
		(310)	(6,978)	(366)	(7,770)	(128)	(2,475)
	12 months	31.8	35.6	27.1	34.5	24.9	29
		(234)	(6,726)	(240)	(7,503)	(92)	(2,376)
2	1 month	27.5	37.6	24.9	36.7	22.6	30.9
		(212)	(5,533)	(235)	(6,005)	(59)	(1,645)
	12 months	32.1	37.8	30	36.9	26.5	31.2
		(176)	(5,346)	(161)	(5,835)	(91)	(1,550)
3	1 month	26	36.4	26.5	36.8	27	31.3
		(140)	(4,089)	(132)	(4,306)	(64)	(1,296)
	12 months	30.5	36.7	30.1	37.1	24.4	31.7
		(137)	(3,935)	(171)	(4,123)	(60)	(1,230)
4	1 month	24.9	36.2	27.2	36.1	21.4	30.6
		(96)	(2,987)	(108)	(2,904)	(32)	(918)
	12 months	31.7	36.5	33	36.2	24.9	31
		(112)	(2,866)	(113)	(2,801)	(44)	(873)

NOTE: Numbers in parantheses below birth interval lengths are sample sizes.

"replace" the child she has lost or because the death of an infant ends breast-feeding, which hastens the return of ovulation and thus increases the risk of a rapid subsequent conception.

The results in Table 9-3 demonstrate that birth intervals are considerably shorter after a child dies either as a neonate or as a postneonate than after a child who survives those periods, regardless of birth order or time period. The difference in interval lengths by survival status is much larger (25-30 percent) when one compares a neonatal death to a neonatal survival than when one compares a postneonatal death to postneonatal survival (10-15 percent).

Prior to the 1985-1991 period, birth intervals are remarkably similar in length when the index child survives. Regardless of birth order, subsequent intervals average 34-37 months. In the 1985-1991 period, however, subsequent intervals are consistently 29-32 months, indicating a fairly dramatic decline in average birth interval length over time. The average length of birth intervals after a child that died has also declined over time, but the decline is not so concentrated in the later period.

The differences between interval lengths after a child who died and interval lengths after a child who survived may arise because women who lose a child consciously try to replace the dead child by becoming pregnant again quickly, or because cessation of breastfeeding hastens conception, or because certain women are predisposed to high fertility (rapid childbearing) and high mortality.

One way to rule out the argument that cessation of breastfeeding causes a rapid subsequent conception is by moving forward an interval and considering how the survival status of the preceding sibling affects the interval between the next two children. Results from this exercise are displayed in Table 9-4.

Subsequent birth intervals are shorter when the preceding sibling died than when the preceding sibling survived. Absolute differences in interval lengths, however, are much smaller when it is the preceding sibling rather than the index child who died. No clear patterns emerge in differences in interval length by survival status of the preceding sibling. At birth order four, the proportionate difference in interval lengths by survival status declines over time. At other birth orders the proportionate difference is relatively constant with time.

All of the indicators considered here suggest that fertility patterns differ for women who have lost a child in comparison with women whose children have survived. Among older women, those who lose a first or second child soon after its birth go on to have more children than women whose early children survived. But despite larger numbers of births, the number of living children is lower for women who lost a child early on, suggesting that these women never "catch up" to their lower-mortality counterparts. At parities of four and below, the proportion of women having an additional child within 42 months rises with each prior

TABLE 9-4 Subsequent Interval by Survival Status of the Preceding Sibling

Birth	1971-1977		1978-1984		1985-1991	
	Dead	Alive	Dead	Alive	Dead	Alive
2	35	37.5	33	36.6	29.1	30.8
	(668)	(5,077)	(724)	(5,516)	(200)	(1,504)
3	33.6	36.4	34	36.8	28.5	31.5
	(457)	(3,772)	(496)	(3,942)	(156)	(1,204)
4	31.5	36.5	32.9	36.1	28.7	30.5
	(360)	(2,723)	(335)	(2,677)	(121)	(829)
5	29.9	34.6	34.8	34.3	29.5	30.2
	(274)	(1,782)	(253)	(1,848)	(68)	(563)

NOTE: Numbers in parantheses below birth interval lengths are sample sizes.

child that died. At parities of four and lower, subsequent intervals are shorter when the index child died than when the index child survived. At parities of two through five, subsequent intervals are shorter when the preceding sibling died than when it survived to the birth of the index child. These general patterns prevail across time, in the face of declining levels of fertility and child mortality and increasing availability of contraceptives.

The analysis of replacement rates and parity progression ratios suggest that differences in fertility outcomes by child survival experience have widened over time. This phenomenon is consistent with the idea that family planning and health programs make available to women knowledge and technologies that help them control their fertility. It may also be the case that as access to those technologies increases, differentials widen between women with characteristics that predispose them to high fertility and high mortality and women without these characteristics.

Accordingly, the question that remains unanswered, despite the results presented above, is whether the death of an infant or young child prompts a conscious, intentional fertility response in a woman. If her child had survived, would the woman's fertility be different? Or do her fertility patterns and the mortality experiences of her children arise from other factors? If other factors are the reason, then secular declines in mortality are not likely to affect fertility patterns unless they are accompanied by changes in other factors as well.

IS THERE A CAUSAL LINK BETWEEN
CHILD MORTALITY AND REPRODUCTIVE PATTERNS?

In this section I briefly summarize results from an attempt to pinpoint a conscious, behavioral response of one element of fertility patterns to a child death. The approach, which is described more fully elsewhere (Frankenberg, 1996) relies on birth intervals. The goal of the analysis is not to quantify the effect of child mortality on total fertility as measured by completed family size. Instead, the intent is to design and implement an approach that measures a behavioral response to a child death but is relatively free of the statistical problems described above that confound empirical work on this topic.

A multivariate counterpart of the bivariate results presented on birth interval length would involve a model of the determinants of the birth interval after the nth child. Such a model can be written as:

$$\log S_n = \alpha_n + \beta_n X + \delta_n D_{n-1} + \varepsilon_n + \varepsilon , \tag{1}$$

where

S_n = length of the interval after the nth child,
X = characteristics that might affect the interval length,
D_{n-1} = survival status of the $(n - 1)^{th}$ child,
ε_n = idiosyncratic error, and
ε = mother-specific error.

Similarly, for the interval after the $(n + 1)^{th}$ child, one could write:

$$\log S_{n+1} = \alpha_{n+1} + \beta_{n+1}X + \delta_{n+1}D_n + \varepsilon_{n+1} + \varepsilon. \qquad (2)$$

In both models, the parameter estimates are biased if ε is correlated with D_{n-1} or with X. For example, suppose women differ in their level of initiative with respect to use of health and family planning services. Level of initiative is difficult to measure, but is a likely determinant of both child mortality and fertility patterns. If level of initiative is excluded from the models, parameter estimates will be biased. One way to rid the parameters of this bias is to estimate the equation:

$$\log \left(\frac{S_{n+1}}{S_n} \right) = (\beta_{n+1} - \beta_n)X + (\delta_{n+1} - \delta_n)D_n + (\Sigma_{n+1} - \Sigma_n) + (\Sigma - \Sigma,) \qquad (3)$$

where the woman-specific errors drop out of the equation.

The intuition behind this model is that the relationship between the interval after the nth and the interval after the $(n + 1)^{th}$ child is a function of X characteristics and the survival status of the $(n - 1)^{th}$ child. The approach is one of differences in differences. I am comparing the difference between the nth and $(n + 1)^{th}$ interval when the $n - 1$ child died to that difference when the $n - 1$ child survived.

In stylized terms I consider two sequences:

and ask how the survival status of the $(n - 1)^{th}$ child in the interval between its birth and the birth of the nth child affects the relationship between the interval after the nth child and the interval after the $(n + 1)^{th}$ child.

Earlier results suggested that the interval after the nth child is shorter when the preceding sibling died than when it survived. Is this because the death causes women to become pregnant again more quickly than they would have had the child survived? Or do other "background" factors that predispose a woman to high mortality and high fertility explain both the short interval and the death of a child? If the explanation lies in other factors, the association between the interval after the nth child and the death of the child will be spurious. However, if the other factors have the same effect on the interval after $(n + 1)^{th}$ child as on the interval after the nth child, any difference in the relationship between those two intervals by the survival status of the $(n - 1)^{th}$ child is not a result of predisposing background factors.

It may be that these predisposing factors are relatively unimportant and that a simpler estimation strategy would be adequate. This question can be answered by computing a Hausman statistic that compares the results from the differences in differences to a simpler model.

A question that immediately arises is how to implement this approach with data. One could analyze the relationship between two adjacent intervals for any woman who experienced this sequence, controlling for factors such as birth order and survival status of children higher than order $n - 1$. However, it is difficult to construct a set of controls for reproductive history that parsimoniously captures differences in reproductive factors other than the survival status of the $(n - 1)^{th}$ child. Alternatively, I impose a series of conditions that force certain similarities on the women in the analysis.

The first condition is that women must have had at least four births at the time of the interview. The second condition is that the first four births must all be singletons. The third condition is that first child must have died before the birth of the second child or survived to the birth of the fourth child. The third and fourth conditions are that the second and third child must have survived to the birth of the fourth child. Together, the third and fourth conditions guarantee that the only mortality event the women have experienced over the period analyzed is the death of the first child before the birth of the second child. The last condition is that the birthdates of the children in question must be fully reported (the mother provides the year and month of birth). A total of 7,761 women of the 32,000 women interviewed met these criteria.

These conditions are equivalent to stringent controls with respect to reproductive patterns. Inevitably, the conditioning selects certain women for the analysis while excluding others. I compared the characteristics of the 7,761 women analyzed with the characteristics of other women in the sample who had at least two births by the time of the interview (25,674 women, pooled from the 1987 and 1991 DHS data). The women analyzed are on average about 3 years older and have 1.2 more children than the other mothers of at least two children. The main reason that the women I analyzed are older is that I require them to have at least four children, whereas the comparison group needed only two children. Levels of education and marital status are similar across the two groups. One might expect that the older, higher-fertility women would have less education than their counterparts. Instead, education levels are similar because I eliminated women with imputed birthdates, and these tend to be the less-educated women.

The women selected are relatively high-fertility women with relatively low-mortality children. The characteristics that lead to high fertility and low mortality will not affect my results to the extent that they have the same effect on all of a woman's birth intervals. By comparing two birth intervals from the same woman I obtained estimates free from biases caused by unobserved factors that affect both intervals the same way.

The hypothesis of interest is that the survival status of the first child affects the ratio of the interval after the third child to the interval after the second child. The death of the first child lowers by one the number of surviving children at subsequent parities and so might affect interval lengths if it interrupts a woman's desired schedule of childbearing. The death of the first child also changes the potential order of children by sex. The second child, which may be the opposite sex of the child who died, becomes the first surviving child. My model contains only three variables: whether the first child survives, the sex of the first surviving child, and the sex of the first surviving child interacted with the survival status of the first child.[2] The variables correspond to four categories of women: those whose first child survived and is female, those whose first child survived and is male, those whose first child died and whose second child is female, and those whose first child died and whose second child is male. Although evidence on fertility preferences in Indonesia suggest that Indonesians display a strong preference for balance in the overall sex composition of their offspring, it is possible that there are preferences for order (Cleland et al., 1983).

The model of interest is the model of log of the ratio of the two intervals (the interval after the third child divided by the interval after the second child). The predicted ratios of the interval lengths are shown in Figure 9-4. From the figure it is clear that the ratios vary by whether the first child survived, but that the effect of the first child's death on the ratio is strongly mediated by the sex of the second child (the first surviving child for these women). When the first child died and the second child is female, the ratio is lower than when the first child survived. When the first child died and the second child is male, the ratio is higher than when the first child survived. Ratios for women whose first child survived are lower when the first child is female than when the first child is male.

These results provide evidence of a causal effect of the first child's survival status on the timing of subsequent fertility, mediated by the sex of the first surviving child. The ratio for women whose first surviving child is female is significantly different from the ratio for women whose first surviving child is male. However, the ratio for women whose first child is female and survives is not statistically significantly different from the ratio for women whose first child

---

[2] I tested for the significance of additional covariates related to socioeconomic status, but none were significant. In one version of the model I included a term for survey year to test the appropriateness of pooling women from the 1987 and 1991 surveys. The term was not statistically significant and so was not retained in the final analysis. Although an earlier table suggested that the overall samples differ, the subsample of women who contribute to this analysis do not differ by sample membership.

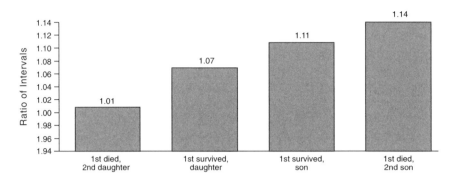

FIGURE 9-4 Ratio of interval after third to interval after second child.

dies and whose second child is female. Nor is the ratio for women whose first child is male and survives statistically significantly different from the ratio for women whose first child died and whose second child is male.

The ratio models provide a way to check for a causal relationship between the death of a child and timing of subsequent fertility under the assumption that unobserved woman-specific factors affect both fertility and mortality, so that estimates based on comparisons across women are biased. I can check the validity of this assumption, and thus the necessity of using the ratio approach, with a Hausman test. The Hausman test compares the results of the ratio model with the results from a model in which the two birth intervals of interest are pooled:

$$\log S = \alpha + \beta X + \delta D + \varepsilon, \tag{4}$$

where S is the interval after the second or the third birth and D indicates the survival status of the first child. Parameter estimates for the ratio model and the pooled model are presented in Table 9-5. The Hausman test yields a statistic of 27.7, which is highly significant.

SUMMARY AND CONCLUSIONS

This chapter reviews the relationship between infant and child mortality and fertility in Indonesia. Both fertility and child mortality have fallen dramatically since the late 1960s (the point after which national-level statistics are available). Evidence for periods prior to the 1960s suggests that a steady mortality decline began in the 1950s, as food supplies returned to their prewar levels and public health programs were initiated. The decline in mortality appears to have preceded the decline in fertility by 10-15 years. Accompanying and likely contributing to declines in fertility and mortality have been dramatic increases in the availability of health and family planning services since the mid-1960s.

TABLE 9-5 Coefficients from the Differences in
Differences and Pooled Models

Model	Coefficient	Standard Error
Differences in differences		
First child dead	−0.541	0.0399
First surviving child male	0.0351	0.0153
Male child x first child dead	0.0867	0.0561
F statistic	3.49	
Pooled estimates		
First child	0.0047	0.0215
First surviving child male	0.0122	0.0082
Male child x first child dead	−0.1036	0.0301
F statistic	7.38	
Hausman statistic	27.7	

I present a series of descriptive statistics as a means of charting the evolution of the relationship between infant and child mortality and subsequent fertility over time. A number of tentative findings emerge from this exercise. First, completed family sizes, in terms of number of children ever born have declined over time regardless of child survival experiences. However, the decline is steeper for women whose first two children survived their early years than for women whose first or second child died as an infant or toddler.

Second, the difference in fertility patterns by survival status of offspring appears to have widened over time. That is, differentials in parity progression ratios and in children ever born by survival experiences are larger in more recent periods. Such a result is consistent with the idea that the increasing availability of contraceptive and health technology has given couples more control over their fertility and thus more scope for responding to child's death or survival. But from these results one cannot tell whether differentials widen with time because all couples use newly available technology to respond to a child's death, or whether some couples assertively use this technology to alter both fertility and children's health, while other couples take a more laissez-faire approach.

Third, changes over time in parity progression ratios by the survival status of preceding offspring suggest that over time there has been a decline in the parity at which survival status of preceding children affects the decision to go on to the next parity. Again, this finding is not surprising in a context where fertility has been declining.

Analysis of subsequent birth interval lengths reveals that birth intervals are consistently shorter when either the index child or the preceding sibling of the index child died than when it survived. Differences in interval lengths by survival status are larger when it is the survival status of the index child that is monitored rather than the survival status of the preceding sibling. This difference almost certainly reflects the fact that the death of a child ends breastfeeding and so speeds the return of ovulation and thus the conception of the next child. This mechanism operates in the comparison of interval lengths stratified by the survival status of the index child, but not in the comparison of interval lengths stratified by the survival status of the preceding sibling. The results for birth interval lengths suggest that intervals were on average six months shorter in the late 1980s than they were in earlier periods. No clear time trends emerge in the differences in interval lengths by survival status of index or preceding children.

In the last section of the chapter I summarize results obtained from a model that attempts to establish a causal link between a child death and subsequent fertility patterns. These results provide evidence that for certain groups of women a child's death changes the pattern of subsequent interval lengths relative to that pattern when a child survives. However, the changes are small in magnitude and occur on average at interval lengths of more than 2 years. Consequently, it is extremely unlikely that these changes have any serious implications for completed levels of fertility. Given that the intervals are well within the range considered to be healthy for women and children, it is also unlikely that the changes contribute to poor health either for mothers or for their offspring.

ACKNOWLEDGMENTS

This work was supported by National Institute of Child Health and Human Development grant no. 5R29 HD32627-02. The author gratefully acknowledges comments from Barney Cohen, Irma Elo, Andrew Foster, Mark Montgomery, Samuel Preston, Duncan Thomas, and two anonymous referees.

REFERENCES

Ben-Porath, Y.
  1976   Fertility response to child mortality: Micro data from Israel. *Journal of Political Economy* 84(2):S163-S178.

Boerma, J.T., A.E. Sommerfelt, J.K. van Ginneken, G.T. Bicego, M.K, Stewart, and S.O. Rutstein
  1994   Assessment of the quality of health data in DHS-I surveys: An overview. Pp. 1-26 in *An Assessment of the Quality of Health Data in DHS-I Surveys.* DHS Methodological Reports, No. 2. Calverton, Md.: Macro International, Inc.

Central Bureau of Statistics [Indonesia], National Family Planning Coordinating Board [Indonesia], and Institute for Resource Development/Westinghouse
  1989   *National Indonesian Contraceptive Prevalence Survey, 1987.* Columbia, Md.: Institute for Resource Development/Westinghouse.

Central Bureau of Statistics [Indonesia], National Family Planning Coordinating Board [Indonesia], Ministry of Health [Indonesia], and Macro International, Inc.
  1992   *Indonesia Demographic and Health Survey, 1991.* Columbia, Md.: Macro International, Inc.

Central Bureau of Statistics [Indonesia], State Ministry of Population/National Family Planning Coordinating Board, Ministry of Health, and Macro International, Inc.

1995   *Indonesia Demographic and Health Survey 1994.* Calverton, Md.: Macro International, Inc.

Cleland, J., J. Verrall, and M. Vaessen

1983   Preferences for the Sex of Children and the Influence on Reproductive Behavior. World Fertility Survey Comparative Studies no. 27. Voorburg, Netherlands: International Statistical Institute.

Frankenberg, E.

1996   Child Death and the Timing of Subsequent Fertility. Unpublished manuscript, RAND, Santa Monica, Calif.

Heer, D., and H. Wu.

1978   Effects in rural Taiwan and urban Morocco: Combining individual and aggregate data. Pp. 135-159 in S.H. Preston, ed., *The Effects of Infant and Child Mortality on Fertility.* New York: Academic Press.

Hugo, G., T. Hull, V. Holland, and G. Jones

1987   *The Demographic Dimension in Indonesian Development.* Oxford, England: Oxford University Press.

Hull, T.H.

1989   Roots of primary health care institutions in Indonesia. Pp. 500-508 in J. Caldwell, S. Findley, P. Caldwell, G. Santow, W. Cosford, J. Braid, and D. Broers-Freeman, eds., *What We Know About The Health Transition: The Cultural, Social, and Behavioral Determinants of Health,* Vol. II. Canberra: Health Transition Centre, The Australian National University.

Knodel, J.

1978   European populations in the past: Family-level relations. Pp 21-45 in S.H. Preston, ed., *The Effects of Infant and Child Mortality on Fertility.* New York: Academic Press.

Lantz, P., M. Partin, and A. Palloni

1992   Using retrospective surveys for estimating the effects of breast feeding and child spacing on infant and child mortality. *Population Studies* 46(1):121-129.

Matthiessen, P.C., and J.C. McCann

1978   The role of mortality in the European fertility transition: Aggregate-level relations. Pp. 47-68 in S.H. Preston, ed., *The Effects of Infant and Child Mortality on Fertility.* New York: Academic Press.

Mauskopf, J., and T. Wallace

1984   Fertility and replacement: Some alternative stochastic models and results for Brazil. *Demography* 21(4):519-536.

Mensch, B.

1985   The effect of child mortality on contraceptive use and fertility in Columbia, Costa Rica, and Korea. *Population Studies* 39(2):309-327.

Nitisastro, W.

1970   *Population Trends in Indonesia.* Ithaca and London: Cornell University Press.

Olsen, R.

1980   Estimating the effect of child mortality on the number of births. *Demography* 17(4):429-443.

Pebley, A.R., and P.W. Stupp

1987   Reproductive patterns and child mortality in Guatemala. *Demography* 24(1):43-60.

Potter, J.E.

1988   Birth spacing and child survival: A cautionary note regarding the evidence from the WFS. *Population Studies* 42(3):443-450.

Preston, S.H.
    1978   Introduction. Pp. 1-18 in S.H. Preston, ed., *The Effects of Infant and Child Mortality on Fertility*. New York: Academic Press.
Rinehart, J., and S. Kols
    1984   Healthier mothers and children through family planning. *Population Reports*. Series J, no. 27., May-June.
Rodriguez, G., J. Hobcraft, J. McDonald, J. Menken, and J. Trussell
    1984   A comparative analysis of determinants of birth intervals. World Fertility Survey Comparative Studies no. 30. Voorburg, Netherlands: International Statistical Institute.
Ross, J., and E. Frankenberg
    1993   *Findings from Two Decades of Family Planning Research*. New York: The Population Council.
Sullivan, J., G. Bicego, and S. Rutstein
    1990   Assessment of the quality of data used for the direct estimation of infant and child mortality in the DHS surveys. Pp. 113-140 in *An Assessment of DHS Data Quality*. Columbia, Md.: Institute for Resource Development.
Trussell, J., L. Martin, R. Feldman, J. Palmore, M. Concepcion, and D. Abu Bakar
    1985   Determinants of birth-interval length in the Philippines, Malaysia, and Indonesia: A hazard-model analysis. *Demography* 22(2):145-168.
van Ginneken, J.K.
    1974   Prolonged breastfeeding as a birthspacing method. *Studies in Family Planning* 5(6):201-206.
Wolpin, K.
    1984   An estimable dynamic stochastic model of fertility and child mortality. *Journal of Political Economy* 92(5):852-874.
World Bank
    1984   *Population Change and Economic Development*. Washington, D.C.: The World Bank.
    1991   *Indonesia: Health Planning and Budgeting*. Washington, D.C.: The World Bank.
    1994   *Indonesia: Sustaining Development*. Washington, D.C.: The World Bank.

10

Micro and Macro Effects of Child Mortality on Fertility: The Case of India

P.N. Mari Bhat

The assumption that a secular fall in mortality would eventually lead to a fertility reduction is central to the propositions of demographic transition theory. But when mortality began to decline dramatically in most of the developing world in the 1950s and the 1960s, the lack of a quick fertility response puzzled many pundits and policy makers. Financial and technical assistance flowed in unprecedented quantities to help deal with the rapid growth of population in the world's poorest regions. Now that many countries have experienced declines in fertility, it is possible to investigate the degree to which improvements in survival chances, especially those of children, are responsible for the current declines in fertility. In this chapter I attempt such an exercise for India, the second-most populous country in the world, which contributes one-fifth of the global population increase.

Perhaps because of the increasing availability of survey data on individual couples, much of the recent analyses of the relationship between infant mortality and fertility has focused on the estimation of the replacement rate and on refining techniques to measure it. As the estimated replacement rates are generally significantly below unity, an increasing body of literature has concluded that declines in child mortality tend to accelerate population growth both in the short- and the long-run. But why would a large majority of couples choose a strategy that generally tends to undercompensate child loss in societies where children are valued for their economic contribution and for their support at old age? Because it is unlikely that the majority of couples would use a strategy that usually fails, the mean replacement rate of significantly below unity probably suggests infrequent use of the strategy rather than its inefficiency.

An alternative to replacement is hoarding, which is a response to perceived mortality risk not necessarily learned from one's own experience. Consequently, true understanding of the influence of child mortality on fertility is impossible without a thorough analysis at both the micro and the macro levels (Preston, 1978). In India I find that the macro relationship between child mortality and fertility is changing from a weak association to a strong bond. This shift appears to be occurring as a function of a growing preference for the replacement mechanism, increased access to family planning, and lags in the perception of mortality decline. As a consequence, it is contended that more than compensatory declines in fertility could result at certain phases of the mortality transition.

In this chapter I focus on three aspects of the mortality fertility relationship with respect to India. First, I investigate the changing relationship between child mortality and fertility in the context of large regional variations in fertility and mortality levels observed in India (Bhat, 1996). Second, I investigate the degree to which the fertility response is specific to the sex of the dead child. This has been a subject of several simulation studies in the past (May and Heer, 1968; Venkatacharya, 1978). Third, I investigate the implications for population policy of a family planning environment that emphasizes sterilization over reversible methods.

The empirical results presented in this chapter are obtained using household and macro-level data, aggregated for various levels of administrative divisions. Period-specific indicators from census and registration systems are employed, as well as cohort measures from sample surveys. Table 10-1 gives a brief description of the types of data employed, substantive themes addressed, and statistical methods employed at various levels of the analysis.

THEORETICAL FRAMEWORK

My conceptual framework rests on the useful distinction between hoarding and replacement effects of child mortality made by Ben-Porath (1978) and includes some of the elements of the family-building model discussed by Lloyd and Ivanov (1988). I assume hoarding, a family-building strategy based on the assumption that some children will not survive, is the typical form of behavior in high-mortality, high-fertility populations, whereas child replacement is the predominant characteristic of family building in low-mortality, low-fertility settings. Such a switch in strategy is consistent with the notion of the demographic transition as a process whereby individuals and households gain greater control over their vital events (see also Heer and Smith, 1968, and O'Hara, 1972).

Figure 10-1 portrays the expected relationship between total number of children ever born (B) and total child deaths (D) in cohorts that have completed their family-building process. Child deaths are represented on the horizontal axis and are assumed to reflect only the changes in child mortality (q) and not of live births. As child deaths fall, the number of births responds in a curvilinear fashion, as shown by the RH (replacement/hoarding) curve. The shape of the RH

TABLE 10-1 Overview of the Analysis

Level of Analysis	Data Employed	Issues Addressed	Statistical Methods	Dependent Variable	Key Explanatory Variables
Macro Analysis					
National level	Annual rates from 1970 to 1993 from the SRS	Lags in child mortality-fertility relationship	Distributed-lag model (Koyck)	Total fertility rate	Under-5 mortality rate, time
State level					
Analysis of period rates	SRS rates for major states for three periods: 1971, 1981, and 1991	Structural shift; estimation of RH rate	Pooled, time series cross-sectional analysis	Total fertility rate	Under-5 mortality rate, female literacy, time
Analysis of cohort data	Data from two national surveys in 1970 & 1993 for women aged 35-44	Structural shift; estimation of RH rate	Pooled, time series cross-sectional analysis	Children ever born	Child deaths, desired family size, time
District level	District-level data from the 1991 census	Estimation of RH rate	OLS regression	Total fertility rate	Under-5 mortality rate and a large number of covariates
Micro Analysis					
Cohort analysis	Data from the NFHS for women aged 35-49 in Karnataka and Uttar Pradesh	Separation of replacement and hoarding effects; gender differential	Olsen technique; OLS regression with multilevel analysis	Children ever born	Child deaths by sex, desired family size, district child mortality
Determinants of contraceptive use	Data from the NFHS for married women aged 13-49 in Karnataka	Estimation of volitional replacement rate; hoarding effects and contraceptive method choice	Logit analysis by method of use and number of children ever born, multilevel analysis	Contraceptive use status	Child deaths by sex, age of first child, district child mortality plus large number of covariates

NOTES: SRS, Sample Registration System; RH, replacement/hoarding; OLS, ordinary least squares; NFHS, National Family Health Survey.

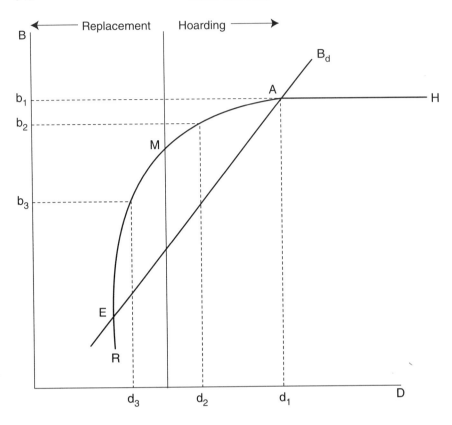

FIGURE 10-1 A macro model of the relationship between children ever born and child deaths in cohorts.

curve is determined by the rate of substitution between the hoarding and the replacement strategies.

At high levels of mortality, the RH curve is inelastic and the rate of substitution low for several reasons. Because hoarding is associated with expected mortality rather than actual experience, the substitution rate is determined partly by perceived changes in mortality risks. Because there may be significant lags in the perception of mortality decline (see Montgomery, in this volume), large reductions in mortality may be necessary before they are perceived and acted upon. Furthermore, if mortality declines are not accompanied by an increase in the cost of children, there would not be a strong motive to avoid unwanted births. An extreme example of this is the decline in child mortality until point A in the graph which will not elicit any fertility response. Note that at extremely high mortality levels a price effect may be operating to suppress fertility levels (Schultz, 1976). If few children survive, some may consider childbearing is not worth the effort.

Consequently, as mortality declines from this high level, some parents may revise upward their family size desires, and fertility levels may rise instead of falling. However, because the cost of contraception is typically high in these settings, it is doubtful that a significant price effect of mortality was actually present in preindustrial societies (see also Lloyd and Ivanov, 1988).

At low levels of mortality the RH curve is highly elastic. To see why this is so, Figure 10-1 includes a trend line for the desired number of births. This line (B_d) intersects the RH curve at points A and E. Beyond A and E, there is an unmet need for children, whereas unwanted fertility prevails between the region A and E. As mortality declines from point A in the RH curve, unwanted fertility (given by the vertical distance between the RH curve and the line B_d) begins to accumulate since desired family size falls, but substitution of replacement for hoarding does not occur at the desired speed. Unwanted fertility reaches its maximum at point M in the RH curve. But, as unwanted fertility rises, the cost of births also rises (implied by the fall in desired family size), and thus the total cost of inefficiency mounts in the hoarding regime. If now the cost of contraception also falls, more and more couples would consider switching to a replacement strategy. Consequently, unwanted fertility begins to decline and may reach point E where it totally disappears.

This conceptual framework informs the empirical analysis to follow. In high-mortality settings, say above point M in the graph, I would expect a relatively minor fertility response to child mortality variations, even though couples in those populations may be employing an insurance strategy that generally over-compensates actual child loss. On the other hand, for populations in the region under M, or who fall between the points A and E, I would expect a relatively larger impact of child mortality on fertility even though the majority of couples may be practicing the replacement strategy, which may undercompensate child deaths. This anomaly is due to the fact that the slope of the RH curve that measures the fertility response to child mortality is influenced by the changing rate of substitution between the two strategies, indicating the need to pay careful attention to the functional form posited for the relationship between fertility and child mortality in the empirical analysis.

TECHNICAL ISSUES IN ESTIMATION

In the analysis below, period measures of fertility and mortality, taken from censuses and registration systems for large geographic regions, are employed, as well as cohort measures available from sample surveys for individuals and for larger aggregates. The object of the analysis is to quantify, as far as possible, the effect of a reduction in child deaths (D) on children ever born (B) using multiple regression techniques. A number of limitations of the regression approach have been raised in the literature (see, for example, Brass and Barrett, 1978; Williams, 1977; Olsen, 1980). However, if the objective is to quantify both replacement and hoarding effects, the options available are quite limited. Therefore, I have pursued the regression approach, giving careful attention to the following questions: What are the appropriate indicators of fertility and mortality? What is the appropriate functional form? What can be done about the problem of endogeneity of both births and deaths? And, what additional controls should be employed in the regression?

For the cohort analysis, the information on the required variables (i.e., births and deaths) is directly available for cohorts at the end of childbearing. The problem is only one of defining an appropriate age cutoff. To have a sufficiently large sample, I use information on women aged 35 and older. For the analysis of period measures, the total fertility rate (TFR) is the appropriate choice for fertility because it is a surrogate measure of children ever born. For child mortality, the choice of an appropriate variable is less obvious because the relevant age interval changes as parents shift from a hoarding to a replacement strategy. Fortunately, because mortality levels at different intervals are strongly correlated, it should be sufficient to employ an age range that includes the majority of child deaths. I have used the under-5 mortality rate (q_5), given that there is significant mortality beyond infancy in India.

In the cohort analysis, the coefficient of child deaths in a linear regression of births and deaths (plus other appropriate controls) would give an estimate of the fertility response rate to a child death. To measure hoarding effects, one must add community-level measures of mortality as additional regressors. However, when cohort data refer to an aggregate, then the coefficient on the child death variable would capture a mixture of replacement and hoarding rates, and hereafter it is referred to as the RH rate, or simply as r. The RH rate may not be a constant, and is likely to increase as mortality declines. To model this relationship, I have regressed children ever born on the logarithm of child deaths. This functional form carries the implicit assumption that the effect of a child death on fertility is inversely proportional to total child deaths ($\partial B = \beta \partial D/D$, where β is the regression parameter). I refer to this functional form as the variable-rate form and the linear function as the constant-rate form.

In the analysis of period measures, it is useful to employ a functional form that provides a direct estimate of the RH rate as a regression parameter. Because the regressor here is the mortality rate rather than the number of deaths, a regression of logarithm of the TFR on under-5 mortality rate would give a direct estimate of the RH rate ($\partial TFR/TFR = \beta \partial q$, or $\partial TFR = \beta \partial D$). This is the constant-rate function. The variable-rate form in this case involves a regression of the logarithm of the TFR on the logarithm of the under-5 mortality rate. This functional form assumes that the effect of a reduction in child death on fertility is inversely proportional to child mortality rate ($\partial TFR = \beta TFR \partial q/q = \beta \partial D/q$).

While regressing children ever born on child deaths, however, a serious problem of simultaneity arises because child deaths may be higher for a woman simply because she bore many children, even though her children's mortality rate was the same as that of others. This problem can be remedied with a two-stage least-squares (TSLS) approach, using the proportion of children dead as an instrument for child deaths (Olsen, 1980). However, if fertility also influences the child mortality rate, this estimator can also be inconsistent.

In the case of period measures, the problem of reverse or joint causation can also be addressed by the instrumental variable method, but appropriate instruments for child mortality are hard to find. As a partial remedy, I have used the child mortality variable lagged by several years. In this case, the lag structure was estimated using a distributed-lag model applied to annual time series data on fertility and mortality rates for the country as a whole.

Because of my failure to fully address the problem of endogeneity of both births and deaths, my estimates of replacement and hoarding effects are subject to a potential upward bias. However, this bias is likely to be small because the effect of fertility on child survival is smaller than often claimed (Bongaarts, 1987). Moreover, my regressions suggest that the existence of a strong correlation between the two is of recent origin, and there is no reason to expect the effect of fertility on child mortality to increase with time. Therefore, I am confident that the measured effects of child mortality on fertility are largely genuine.

Because fertility levels are influenced by family size desires in addition to child mortality, it is essential to control for changes in the former so as to obtain an unbiased estimator of the effect of the latter on fertility. A question arises as to whether factors influencing unwanted fertility should also be used as covariates in the regression. An important insight on this can be obtained by examining the following identity for a cohort:

$$B = D + C \tag{1}$$

$$= D + C_d + C - C_d$$

$$= D + C_d + C_u ,$$

where C is the number of surviving children, C_d is the desired number of children, and C_u is the number of unwanted children. Essentially, the above equation states that children ever born is the sum of child deaths, surviving children desired, and surviving children unwanted. Note that the coefficient of all the terms on the right-hand side of the equation are equal to 1. Because of singularity, the model cannot be estimated from a regression analysis if all three variables are present. Suppose I drop unwanted fertility and impose the following model on the data:

$$B = \alpha + rD + pC_d + u , \tag{2}$$

where u is the stochastic disturbance term, and α is a constant representing the average unwanted births. By subtracting equation (1) from equation (2) and rearranging terms, I obtain

$$C_u = \alpha + (r - 1)D + (p - 1)C_d + u .$$ (3)

From equation (3) it is obvious that unwanted fertility is a direct consequence of r and p being different from 1. When the two parameters are less than 1, child deaths and desired family size are inversely related to unwanted fertility. When r is more than 1 (in the region below M in the RH curve in Figure 10-1), child deaths and unwanted children will be positively correlated. It is, however, difficult to visualize a situation in which p is larger than 1, which would imply that desired family size and unwanted fertility are positively related. Note that, as the nonstochastic variation in unwanted fertility is implicit in the parameters of child mortality and desired family size variables, unwanted fertility, or its proxies, should not be used as controls in the regression.

Factors that influence desired family size such as female literacy could also be influencing unwanted fertility. Hence, the desired family size variable is used directly in the regressions wherever possible. This eliminates indirect effects of child mortality on fertility through changes in reported desired family size. Because these effects are expected to have a net positive value, I could be underestimating the total effect of child mortality on fertility. This should act to partly suppress the upward bias resulting from not fully accounting for the endogeneity of fertility and mortality.

The above arguments are equally applicable to the analysis of period measures. I would have preferred to use period measures of desired family size or wanted fertility in these regressions (see Bongaarts, 1990 and references therein). But data on these measures are hard to obtain, and I have been forced to use proxies such as female literacy to control for variations in desired family size. Consequently, I am unable to interpret unambiguously the child mortality coefficients from these regressions as unconditional estimates of the RH rate.

EMPIRICAL RESULTS

National Trends

Child mortality in India began to fall around 1921 and accelerated downward in the 1950s. The evidence for this, however, is largely indirect and based mainly on data from the decennial censuses (Bhat, 1989). Fertility began its downward course in the 1960s, especially in certain pockets such as Kerala and Punjab (Bhat et al., 1984). By the beginning of the 1970s, when the Sample Registration System (SRS) began to track annual trends in vital rates, the total fertility rate had fallen to fewer than six births per woman, and the infant and child (under-5) mortality rates were below 140 and 230 per 1,000 live births, respectively.

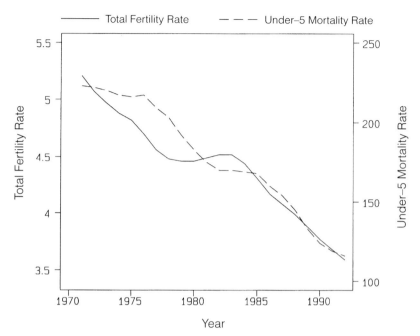

FIGURE 10-2 Trends in the total fertility rate and the under-5 mortality rate, 3-year moving averages, all India, 1971-1991.

Figure 10-2 shows the annual trends in fertility and child mortality (q_5) since 1971 as recorded by the SRS, plotted as 3-year moving averages. The figure shows that, by the time the SRS began to keep records, fertility had already begun to fall rapidly. The TFR declined from 5.3 births per woman around 1971 to 4.4 in 1978, whereupon the decline came to a sudden halt and remained at that level until the downward trend resumed around 1983. Since then, the TFR has fallen continuously to reach 3.7 births per woman by 1991. Meanwhile, under-5 mortality fell slowly initially, but the pace picked up after 1976 to reach a level of 170 in 1982. After remaining at this level until 1985, it began to fall again rapidly to reach a level of 120 by 1991.[1]

---

[1]There is evidence to suggest that, because the SRS was just taking root in many areas at the beginning of 1970s, it was probably underestimating vital rates, especially fertility levels. After examining all available evidence, a Panel on India constituted by the Committee on Population and Demography of the U.S. National Academy of Sciences, put the TFR at 5.6 in 1971-1972 instead of 5.3 births per woman recorded by the SRS (Bhat et al., 1984). On the other hand, the panel concluded that SRS death rates, including child mortality, did not require any corrections at the national level. The logistical problems that cause greater underenumeration of births than deaths has, how-

To what extent are these two trends related and what do they imply for the lag between changes in mortality and fertility? These issues are explored below by fitting a distributed-lag model to national-level data on fertility and child mortality using figures supplied by the SRS for the period 1970-1993. Table 10-2 shows the results obtained when a geometric-lag function (also known as a Koyck lag) is employed. This infinite lag function assumes that the effect of child mortality on a given period of fertility decays geometrically with time, a reasonable approximation of the delayed fertility response to reductions in child mortality. The distributed-lag form of the variable-rate function can be written as

$$\ln \mathrm{TFR}_t = \alpha + \beta(1-\lambda)\ln q_{5,t} + \beta(1-\lambda)\lambda \ln q_{5,t-1} + \ldots + u_t, \qquad (4)$$

$$= \alpha + \beta(1-\lambda)\sum_{i=0}^{t} \lambda^i \ln q_{5,t-i} + u_t,$$

where u_t is the random disturbance term. However, the model has been estimated in its simpler autoregressive form, wherein the fertility level of a given year is regressed against its level in the previous year and the level of child mortality in the same year.[2]

$$\ln \mathrm{TFR}_t = \alpha(1-\lambda) + \lambda \ln \mathrm{TFR}_{t-1} + \beta(1-\lambda)\ln q_{5,t} + v_t, \qquad (5)$$

where $v_t = u_t - \lambda u_{t-1}$.

When the model is estimated in this form, the coefficient of lagged fertility provides an estimate of the parameter λ, from which the implied mean lag of fertility response to child mortality can be computed as $\lambda/(1-\lambda)$. The coefficient of the mortality rate gives information required for the computation of the RH rate.

In the first specification, the under-5 mortality rate is employed as the only regressor apart from the lagged fertility variable. This specification suggests an RH rate of 2.8 births for the death of a child under-5 and a mean lag in the fertility response of 3.8 years (see Table 10-2). This estimate of r may be high due to the

---

ever, remained unclear. It could have arisen from the Indian custom of the mother returning to her natal home for delivery, if such births were not being properly recorded by the SRS enumerators in the early years of the SRS operation. The SRS performance appears to have improved markedly after the SRS sample units were replaced from those drawn using the 1961 census frame to those based on the 1981 census results. As such, fertility in India may have declined more rapidly than Figure 10-2 suggests (see Bhat, 1996).

[2]An attempt was also made to fit directly the distributed-lag form of the model through maximum likelihood procedures. However, it yielded less meaningful results, possibly because of autocorrelation in residuals.

TABLE 10-2 Ordinary Least-Squares Regression Results of Fitting Geometric-Lag Model to the Relationship between Total Fertility Rate and Child Mortality (q_5) in Autoregressive Form, India, 1970-1993

Explanatory Variable	Specification 1		Specification 2		Specification 3	
	Coefficient	t-Ratio	Coefficient	t-Ratio	Coefficient	t-Ratio
Lagged TFR[a]	0.793	5.74	0.729	4.47	0.775	5.68
Log (q_5)	0.103	1.57	0.067	0.84	0.014	0.20
Time	—	—	-0.002	0.77	-0.003	1.27
Time × dummy[b]	—	—	—	—	0.025	3.06
Constant	0.471	1.48	0.325	1.61	0.371	1.32
Estimated parameters:						
Mean lag of q_5	3.84	1.19	2.69	1.21	3.44	1.28
Elasticity of q_5	0.496	5.04	0.249	0.90	0.061	0.21
RH rate	2.84	—	1.43	—	0.35	—
Adjusted R^2	0.97		0.96		0.97	
D–W statistic	1.65		1.62		2.17	
N	23		23		23	

[a]Logarithm of total fertility rate lagged by a year.
[b]Dummy variable for the years 1978-1984.

omission of some relevant variables that may change along with child mortality. When time is used as an additional regressor, the estimated RH rate falls to 1.4 and the estimated mean mortality lag is 2.7 years.

In the final specification in Table 10-2, I examine the effect of the stagnation in fertility between 1978-1984 on parameter estimates. A time variable was interacted with a dummy variable for this period and used as an additional regressor. Note that a linear time variable would not capture this effect if the stagnation were caused by extraneous factors such as changes in family planning effort during and following the Emergency Period (1975-1976) or from a change of sampling units in the SRS. The interaction dummy is very statistically significant and the implied level of RH rate falls to 0.35, with a mean lag of 3.4 years.

Thus, the estimates of the mean lag of fertility with respect to a change in mortality derived from the national data are fairly stable at around 3 years, even though the lag coefficient is not statistically significant in any of the above specifications. On the other hand, estimates of the RH rate vary considerably under different model specifications from 2.8 to 0.4. Clearly not much confidence can be placed in the estimates of the RH rate from this analysis. However, the estimated mean lag of 3 years seems quite reasonable and, more importantly, is the only estimator I have. As such, it is accepted without further scrutiny. Its statistical insignificance has not been given undue importance because the analysis was based on only 23 observations.

State-Level Analysis

Two types of data are available at the state level, both of which help to clarify the changing nature of the mortality-fertility relationship. Annual estimates of the total fertility rate and of child mortality are available for 15 major states of India from the SRS from 1970 onward. Furthermore, cohort data are available from two national surveys conducted in 1970 and 1992-1993.

Analysis of Period Measures

Although the SRS began to provide state-level information in 1970, its performance initially was not very satisfactory in some states. Only after its sampling units were overhauled in the 1980s did the SRS reach near completeness in its reporting of vital events (Bhat, 1996). However, by using census and survey data, it is possible to construct an adjusted set of demographic estimates for 13 major Indian states at the beginning of the 1970s. These are used here in conjunction with the SRS estimates for later years. Partly because of the changing quality of the SRS data, and partly because information on other indicators such as literacy are unavailable on an annual basis, I examine the state-level data at three discrete points in time: 1970-1972, 1980-1981, and 1990-1992.

In Figure 10-3, I have plotted the estimates of the TFR (in log scales) against

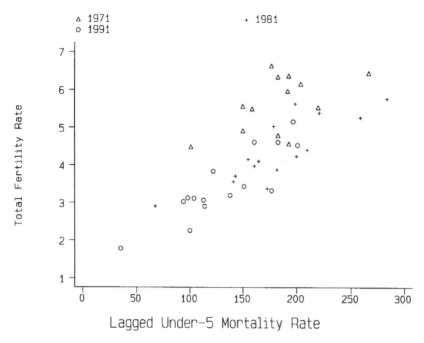

FIGURE 10-3 Relationship between the total fertility rate and lagged under-5 mortality
rate for major states of India, 1971, 1981, and 1991.

the under-5 mortality rate, the latter lagged by 3 years, as suggested by the
analysis of national data. A clear positive association between the two is visible,
but it does not appear to be as strong as the one observed in the case of time series
data for all of India. A striking feature of the graph is that the estimates for the
early 1970s stand apart from others, suggesting that the relationship might have
undergone a structural modification in the 1970s.

Table 10-3 presents the results of ordinary least-squares (OLS) regressions
for each of the three time periods. In all these regressions, the child mortality
variable was lagged 3 years as suggested by the analysis of national-level data.
When child mortality was used as the sole regressor, its coefficient increased
from 1.9 in 1970-1972 to 3.3 in 1980-1982, and further to 5.4 in 1990-1992. As
estimates of the RH rate, these are almost certainly biased upward because of the
omission of certain variables that influence the desire for children. When female
literacy (measured as the proportion of females aged 7 and older who are literate)
is included as an additional regressor, the implied RH rate falls substantially. The
new estimates of r are 0.1 around 1971, 1.9 around 1981, and 2.7 around 1991.
Interestingly, the coefficient of female literacy shows no clear pattern of change
over time (see Table 10-3).

TABLE 10-3 Results of Ordinary Least-Squares Regressions of Log of Total Fertility Rate on Child Mortality (q_5) and Female Literacy Using Data for Major States of India, 1970-1972, 1980-1982, and 1990-1992

Model and Year of TFR	Constant	q_5 Lagged by 3 Years	Female Literacy	N^a	R^2	SSE	Structural Change Test χ^2	df
Model 1								
1970-1972	1.375 (8.41)	1.893 (2.16)		13	0.23	0.120	27.34	2
1980-1982	0.849 (7.80)	3.313 (5.76)		15	0.70	0.111	(reference period)	
1990-1992	0.490 (4.40)	5.420 (6.79)		15	0.76	0.137	5.38	2
Model 2								
1970-1972	1.863 (5.77)	0.117 (0.09)	-0.637 (1.71)	13	0.35	0.111	24.68	3
1980-1982	1.294 (5.11)	1.922 (2.14)	-0.587 (1.91)	15	0.75	0.101	(reference period)	
1990-1992	1.214 (3.37)	2.711 (1.83)	-0.870 (2.09)	15	0.81	0.122	6.03	3

NOTES: Numbers in parentheses next to coefficient are T ratios. SSE, sum of squares due to error. df, degrees of freedom.

^{a}Bihar and West Bengal were excluded from the analysis of 1970-1972 because data were unavailable.

A likelihood ratio test is used to check for the possibility of structural change. It rejects the hypothesis of no structural change between 1971 and 1981 but fails to confirm a change over the subsequent decade. Because the quality of my data for the period 1970-1972 is relatively poor, the statistical inference of structural change during the 1970s may be attributable to data problems. However, the continuity of a rising trend in the mortality rate coefficient over the 1980s (though this is statistically insignificant) and the absence of a clear trend in the coefficient on female literacy, argue strongly in favor of a structural change in the mortality-fertility relationship.

If one accepts the hypothesis of structural change, however, the suggested level of the RH rate in the 1980s appears to be too high. Unfortunately, multi-colinearity problems prevented me from including additional regressors in the analysis apart from female literacy. However, to make optimal use of the available information, I combine the state-level data from all three periods and subject them to a pooled cross-sectional time series analysis. The standard errors of the estimates presented in Table 10-3 show that there is no reason to suspect that the error variance has changed significantly over time, and hence there appears to be no serious violation of the usual regression assumptions if the analysis is performed on the pooled data.

There are two principal methods of pooling. The first approach, known as the fixed-effects model, assumes that the intercept terms represent time-invariant effects on the dependent variable and differ for each cross-sectional unit. This model is estimated through OLS using dummy variables for each of the cross-sectional units. A second approach, known as the random-effects model, assumes that the residuals of the same cross-sectional units are correlated because of the random nature of the intercept term (possibly because of omission of relevant variables that are uncorrelated with those included in the model). This model is estimated using two-step generalized least squares. The random-effects model has the advantage of making greater use of the total variation in fertility, which results in savings in the degrees of freedom because only one intercept term must be estimated. On the other hand, it is more vulnerable to biases arising from omission of relevant variables.

Results of the two methods of pooling are shown in Table 10-4. In the case of constant-rate function, it can be seen that the time-child mortality interaction dummies are significant under both the fixed-effects and the random-effects models, which confirms the hypothesis of structural change. In particular, note that the interaction dummy for 1990-1991 is significant, showing that the change was not simply confined to the 1970s but carried forward to the subsequent decade. On the other hand, with one exception, when the variable-rate function is used, the interaction dummies are all insignificant. The implication is that the logarithmic function adequately captures the transformation that occurs in the fertility response to child mortality declines during the transition. The functional fit, however, is not perfect. The interaction dummy is negative for the period 1970-

TABLE 10-4 Results of Pooled Time Series and Cross-Sectional Regressions of Log of Total Fertility Rate, Major States of India, 1970-1972, 1980-1982, and 1990-1992

Explanatory Variable	OLS, Fixed-Effects Model				GLS, Random-Effects Model			
	Specification 1		Specification 2		Specification 1		Specification 2	
	Parameter	t-Ratio	Parameter	t-Ratio	Parameter	t-Ratio	Parameter	t-Ratio
Constant-Rate Function								
Lagged q_5	1.567	1.82	1.257	1.78	1.518	2.07	1.309	2.07
Female literacy	-2.828	3.98	-0.950	1.25	-0.965	3.58	-0.805	3.01
Time dummies[a]								
1970-1971 (D1)	0.064	1.03	0.454	3.20	0.210	6.20	0.475	4.73
1990-1992 (D2)	0.100	1.35	-0.276	2.17	-0.078	2.12	-0.295	3.79
Interactions:								
q_5 x D1	—	—	-1.326	2.24	—	—	-1.383	2.59
q_5 x D2	—	—	1.383	2.68	—	—	1.443	3.13
Constant	n.a.		n.a.		1.037	9.70	1.476	8.10
N	43		43		43		43	
R^2	0.97		0.98		0.82		0.88	
Variable-Rate Function								
Lagged log (q_5)	0.387	4.37	0.242	1.92	0.410	5.03	0.208	1.84
Female literacy	-1.732	2.72	-1.280	1.89	-0.538	1.96	-0.799	2.71
Time dummies[a]								
1970-1971 (D1)	0.140	2.62	-0.065	0.38	0.233	8.00	-0.107	0.65
1990-1992 (D2)	0.054	0.97	0.115	1.04	-0.512	1.71	0.105	0.97
Interactions:								
log (q_5) x D1	—	—	-0.142	1.35	—	—	-0.188	2.05
log (q_5) x D2	—	—	0.074	1.14	—	—	0.097	1.64
Constant	n.a.		n.a.		2.344	20.94	2.075	12.85
N	43		43		43		43	
R^2	0.98		0.98		0.84		0.87	
Mean RH rate	2.35		—		2.48		—	

NOTES: n.a., not applicable; instead there are 15 intercepts (fixed effects), one for each state. OLS, ordinary least squares. GLS, generalized least squares.
[a] 1980-1982 has been used as the reference period.

1972 and positive for the period 1990-1992, suggesting that the rise in the fertility response rate is sharper than is implicit in the logarithmic functional form.

In the case of the constant-rate function, the estimates on the interaction dummies imply that the RH rate increased from a value close to zero in the period 1970-1972 to 1.3 in the period 1980-1981, and further to 2.7 in the period 1990-1992. There is no significant difference in the estimates of the RH rate from the fixed- and random-effects models, and the results are similar to those presented in Table 10-3 for the regressions that included female literacy as a covariate. In the variable-rate function, the implied mean level of the RH rate can be computed from the estimated coefficient of child mortality from the regression that excluded the interaction dummies by dividing it by the sample mean of the under-5 mortality rate. The estimates so derived are 2.4 and 2.5 under the fixed-effects and the random-effects models, respectively. These certainly are very large effects and could suggest rapid substitution of replacement for hoarding. Alternately, the estimated effects could be high due to insufficient controls for changes in desired family size or because of simultaneity problems. It is necessary to examine estimates from alternate sources before commenting on their reliability.

Analysis of Cohort Measures

Cohort data have two distinct advantages over period measures. First, with cohort data, there is no need to worry about lags in the mortality-fertility relationship because the cohort measures reflect the cumulative fertility response to child mortality experience by the end of the reproductive period. Second, a cohort analysis allows us to control explicitly for variation in desired family size, circumventing the need to use proxies such as female literacy, which may also partly capture some portion of unwanted fertility.

Below I analyze state-level information on children ever born, children dead, and desired family size for married women aged 35-44 from two national surveys conducted in 1970 and 1992-1993. The 1970 survey was carried out by the Operations Research Group (1970) and covered the entire country, but the relevant data are available only for 10 major states (Srinivasan et al., 1984). The 1992-1993 information comes from the National Family Health Survey and is available for all 23 states (International Institute for Population Sciences, 1995), but I have confined the analysis to 15 major states for which the sample sizes are relatively large. Further details on the data used in the analysis are available in an unabridged version of this chapter (see Bhat, 1997).

As discussed above, the analysis involves the regression of number of children ever born (B) with number of child deaths (D) and desired family size (C_d). Because the number of child deaths would depend partly on the number of children ever born, the OLS estimate of the RH rate is biased upward. Hence I also estimate the model using two-stage least squares with the proportion of children who have died and desired family size as instruments for the number of child deaths. Results are presented in Table 10-5.

When child deaths are used as the sole regressor, the 1970 survey data suggest an RH rate of 0.18 when the model is estimated through OLS and 0.07 when it is estimated through TSLS. These rates are slightly higher when desired family size is added as an additional regressor (0.40 for OLS and 0.22 for TSLS). The effect of desired family size on children ever born in 1970 is estimated to be negative and negligible under both procedures. Because these estimates are based on only ten observations, none of the coefficients are large enough to be statistically significant. On the other hand, the data for 1992-1993 show substantially larger effects of both child deaths and desired family size on children ever born. A parsimonious specification of child deaths on children ever born suggests an RH rate of 2.3 under OLS and 2.0 under TSLS procedures. When desired family size is introduced as an additional regressor, these estimates fall to 1.8 and 1.5, respectively. On the other hand, a reduction in desired family size by one child is estimated to reduce ever-born children by 0.4 of a child under the OLS procedure and by 0.5 of a child under the TSLS procedure. These estimated effects are statistically significant. Furthermore, the difference in the estimated effects of child mortality and desired family size between 1970 and 1992-1993 conforms with my notion of structural change.

To throw further light on these changes, information from the two surveys can be compared over time for the same state. The data show that, in India as a whole (more specifically in the 10 states used in this analysis), completed family size declined from 5.7 children in 1970 to 4.3 children in 1992-1993, or by 1.4 children during a period of about 22 years. At the same time, child deaths declined by 0.6 children and desired family size declined by 1.2 children. Thus, the total demand for children declined by 1.8 children, whereas the actual decline in total fertility was only 1.4 children. My conceptual diagram shows that this typically happens when a country is above point M on the RH curve (see Figure 10-1). The implied increase in unwanted children from 0.3 in 1970 to 0.7 in 1992-1993 would seem surprising at first sight as it coincided with the rapid expansion of family planning services in India. However, this increase could be the result of excessive reliance on sterization as a method of fertility control, the low cost of unwanted fertility, and unanticipated declines in child mortality while pursuing an insurance strategy.

From the data presented in Table 10-6, a quick estimate of the RH rate can be made by assuming that changes in child deaths and desired family size elicit identical fertility responses. This is an unsatisfactory assumption, but it provides a minimum bound on the RH rate in the population. Using this assumption, the fertility response rate can be computed by dividing the change in children ever born by the sum of the changes in child death and desired family size. For all of India, this estimate equals 0.78. However, it would be incorrect to equate a change in the number of child deaths with a change in the desired family size,

TABLE 10-5 Regression Results of Children Ever Born with Child Deaths and Desired Family Size Using State-Level Data on Married Women Aged 35-44

| | OLS Regressions | | | | TSLS regressions | | | |
| | Specification 1 | | Specification 2 | | Specification 1 | | Specification 2 | |
Explanatory Variable	Coefficient	t-Ratio	Coefficient	t-Ratio	Coefficient	t-Ratio	Coefficient	t-Ratio
Operations Research Group Survey, 1970								
Child deaths, D	0.183	0.72	0.399	1.19	0.073	0.31	0.222	0.76
Desired family size, C_d	—		-0.217	0.99	—		-0.141	0.74
Constant	5.624	17.73	6.260	8.68	5.759	19.84	6.162	10.00
Adjusted R^2	-0.056		0.061		-0.081		-0.103	
SSE	0.183		0.183		0.166		0.157	
N	10		10		10		10	
National Family Health Survey, 1992-1993								
Child deaths, D	2.284	7.48	1.801	5.04	1.987	6.41	1.540	4.54
Desired family size C_d	—		0.425	2.09	—		0.522	2.75
Constant	2.876	12.73	1.943	2.09	3.083	13.52	1.836	4.80
Adjusted R^2	0.797		0.839		0.782		0.831	
SSE	0.295		0.263		0.285		0.241	
N	15		15		15		15	

NOTES: OLS, ordinary least squares; TSLS, two-stage least squares.

TABLE 10-6 Change in Average Number of Children Ever Born (B), Child Death (D), Desired Family Size (C_d), and Unwanted Children ($C - C_d$), in Two Cohorts of Married Women Aged 35-44, 1970 and 1992-1993

Variable	India (10-state average)			North India (3-state average)			South India (4-state average)		
	1970	1990-1993	Change	1970	1992-1993	Change	1970	1992-1993	Change
B	5.7	4.3	-1.4	5.6	5.1	-0.5	5.7	3.8	-1.9
C	4.4	3.6	-0.8	4.2	4.2	-0.0	4.6	3.3	-1.3
D	1.2	0.7	-0.6	1.4	0.9	-0.5	1.2	0.5	-0.6
C_d	4.1	2.9	-1.2	4.6	3.5	-1.1	4.0	2.7	-1.3
$C - C_d$	0.3	0.7	0.4	-0.4	0.7	1.1	0.6	0.6	0.1
RH rate:									
E.1			0.77			0.34			0.97
E.2			0.97			0.54			1.17

NOTE: The first estimate of the RH rate (E.1) assumes that changes in child loss and desired family size elicit identical fertility responses, whereas the second (E.2) assumes that the compensatory response for child loss is higher by 0.3.

SOURCE: Srinivasan et al. (1984) and state-level reports of the National Family Health Survey. The 1970 estimates have been adjusted slightly to exclude women with less than two surviving children.

since this ignores any biological response. Given prolonged breastfeeding in India, one can expect a biological replacement of about 30 percent of child deaths to occur virtually automatically (Preston, 1978). If I assume that a child death would elicit a response rate of 0.3 over and above the response to changes in desired family size, the above data imply an RH rate of 0.97. Actually, the true level of the RH rate implied by the data is even higher because I have not yet allowed for the effects of a switch in strategy.

The data on regional variations presented in Table 10-6 show that over the intersurvey period, the demand conditions changed about equally in north and south India. Desired family size fell by 1.1 children in the north and by 1.3 children in the south. By contrast, children ever born declined by 0.5 births in the north and by 1.9 births in the south. The reason for the anomaly can be found in the trends in the number of unwanted children in the two areas. In north India there has been a sharp increase in the number of unwanted children, where a situation of unmet need for children had existed previously. Thus, north India has moved from a point beyond A on the RH curve to a region between points A and M (see Figure 10-1). In south India, where a significant amount of unwanted childbearing was already present in 1970, the situation had remained more or less stable during the intersurvey period. However, it is quite possible that south India has traversed to a distance below M on the RH curve from an equidistant point above M. Consequently, unwanted fertility has remained more or less the same in south India, and the level of unwanted children in 1992-1993 is about the same in the two regions.

Again using the assumption that child loss and desired family size have the same effect on fertility, the implied RH rates are 0.34 in north India and 0.97 in south India. If I allow for a biological response, the implied levels are 0.54 in north India and 1.17 in south India. The higher response rate in the case of south India is in keeping with its position on the RH curve.

These estimates of RH rate are derived without explicitly taking into account the possibility of structural change and are computed by imposing restrictions on the effects of child loss and desired family size. It is possible to derive alternate estimates, allowing for structural change and without imposing the restrictions on the model parameters by conducting a pooled cross-sectional time series analysis, as I did in the case of period measures (see Table 10-7). However, in this case, I have data to pool for only two periods and ten cross-sectional units. The fixed-effects model is estimated using both OLS and TSLS procedures. In the latter, the instrumental regression for child deaths included the proportion of dead children and other exogenous variables in the model.

The results of the constant-rate form suggest an RH rate for 1992-1993 of 1.9 under the OLS fixed-effects model, 1.6 under the TSLS fixed-effects model, and 1.7 under the random-effects model. On the other hand, the effect of a change in desired family size on children ever born during the same period is estimated to be 0.7 under OLS and TSLS fixed-effects models, and 0.5 under the random-

TABLE 10-7 Results of Pooled Time Series and Cross-Sectional Regression of Children Ever Born to Married Women Aged 35-44, 1992-1993 and 1970 Using Constant-Rate Function

Variable	OLS, Fixed Effects		TSLS, Fixed Effects		GLS, Random Effects	
	Coefficient	t-Ratio	Coefficient	t-Ratio	Coefficient	t-Ratio
D	1.868	2.86	1.610	2.32	1.700	4.36
C_d	0.662	1.71	0.703	1.75	0.477	2.06
Time dummy[a]	3.387	2.38	3.584	2.44	4.121	4.04
Time dummy $\times D$	−1.609	2.68	−1.607	2.56	−1.372	2.48
Time dummy $\times C_d$	−0.466	1.19	−0.489	1.22	−0.636	1.86
Constant	n.a.		n.a.		1.810	3.22
R^2	0.983		0.982		0.954	
N	20		20		20	
T Ratio[b]	1.43		1.02		2.18	

NOTES: n.a., not applicable; instead, there are 10 intercepts, one for each state. OLS, ordinary least squares. TSLS, two-stage least squares. GLS, generalized least squares.

[a]The year 1992-1993 is used as the reference period.
[b]For the equality of the coefficients of D and C_d.

effects model. The implied difference in the effects of child death and desired family size is substantially larger than 0.3, indicating that additional forces must be inflating the size of the fertility response. Statistically, however, the difference between the two coefficients is significant only in the random-effects model, perhaps due to the fact that the results are based on only 20 observations.

The significance of the interaction dummy of child mortality in all three models supports the hypothesis of structural change with respect to child mortality. The implied level of the RH rate for 1970 is close to zero in all three models. In the case of desired family size, there is also an indication of a structural shift, but its interaction dummy, though negative, is not statistically significant.

The results of the variable-rate form (not shown) reveal the following (see Bhat, 1997, for further details):

• The logarithmic form for the changing effects of child mortality is an adequate but imperfect representation of reality.
• The mean RH rate implied by the analysis was 1.4 under the OLS fixed-effects model, 1.2 under the TSLS fixed-effects model, and 1.0 under the random-effects model. These estimates are significantly lower than the ones obtained from the analysis of period measures using the variable-rate form.

In summary, the state-level analysis strongly suggests the possibility of a structural shift in the relationship between child mortality and fertility. An indication to this effect comes from the pooled cross-sectional time series analyses of both period and cohort measures of fertility and child mortality, controlling for changes in desired family size. The fertility response rate appears to rise sharply but is adequately captured by expressing child mortality in proportionate terms. The cohort analysis suggests a mean response rate of about one birth for a decline of one child death. The period analysis suggests an even higher response rate, which is consistent with the evidence that the response rate is rising as child mortality declines. However, the response rate for changes in family size desires is also rising, perhaps reflecting a general increase in couples' ability to exercise their reproductive choices.

District-Level Analysis

Thanks to some special questions in the 1981 census, for the first time it became possible to estimate reliably fertility and child mortality at the district level. Although similar data were collected in the 1991 census, much of them are yet to be published. However, using the data on children enumerated in the age interval 0-6 years, I have derived elsewhere estimates of the birth rate and total fertility rate from the 1991 census at the district level (Bhat, 1996), which should serve as fairly good approximations to the levels of fertility that prevailed during the period 1984-1990. Where data for some explanatory variables are unavailable for 1991, and if intercensal changes are expected to be small, the data from the 1981 census have been used to supply the missing information.

Table 10-8 presents the results of OLS regressions on district-level estimates of the TFR derived from the 1991 census. Briefly, four categories of variables were considered for the analysis: structural elements of the economy that bear on fertility behavior; social, religious, and gender differentials that affect fertility; factors that govern ideational change and individual modernity; and, indicators of child health and family planning program effort. Conceptually, I view the first two categories of variables as representing the superstructure that, although slow to change, can facilitate or regulate the impact of the more direct forces of change represented by the third and fourth categories of variables. A brief description of the variables employed in the regression, along with sample means, standard deviations, and the expected sign of the coefficients in the multivariate context are available in the Appendix table.

In the first specification of the model, I include all relevant variables. This regression is found to explain 90 percent of the variation in the log of the TFR. All variables, except for a few proxies for economic development and family planning effort, are statistically significant and show the expected relationship to fertility. Because the economic variables are highly correlated, their separate influences cannot be estimated from the data. The same is true for the family planning variables, which are available only at the state level and are strongly correlated with the media exposure variables. When the powerful media variables are dropped, family planning variables, especially the unmet need for contraception, show strong statistical significance (see Bhat, 1996). As can be seen from Table 10-8, the under-5 mortality rate is highly significant, and implies an RH rate of 0.63.

In the second specification of the model, the family planning variables—unmet need for contraception and sterilization target achievement—are dropped on the grounds that they could be capturing part of unwanted fertility. Female and child labor force participation rates and age at marriage are also dropped because their inclusion could be objected to on the grounds of endogeneity. In addition, the child mortality rate is employed in logarithmic form. As can be seen from Table 10-8, these changes have little influence on the estimated effects of either child mortality or other covariates. The implied mean RH rate, computed by dividing its coefficient by the sample mean of under-5 mortality rate, is 0.65 instead of 0.63 suggested earlier.

On the whole, the district-level data suggest an RH rate in the neighborhood of 0.65 under different model specifications. However, the use of a 10-year lag in mortality may have biased the estimates of the RH rate downward. If the true lag is only 3 years, then my estimate of the RH rate would be about 0.8, which is still substantially lower than the state-level analyses suggest. At the same time, it is not at all clear how much of the variation in desired family size the covariates used in the district regressions captured and how much unwanted fertility they

TABLE 10-8 Results of Ordinary Least-Squares Regressions with District-Level Estimates of the Total Fertility Rate, 1984-1990

Explanatory Variable	Specification 1		Specification 2	
	Parameter	t-Ratio	Parameter	t-Ratio
Economic Structure				
Male workers in agriculture	−0.1024	1.15	−0.0995	1.15
Agricultural laborers	0.1255	2.41	0.1211	2.40
Female work participation	−0.1150	1.13	—	—
Child laborers	0.5586	1.95	—	—
Banks per population[a]	−0.0662	2.79	−0.0617	2.58
Social Structure				
Joint family	1.4521	8.39	1.6017	11.02
Female age at marriage[a]	−0.3649	2.77	—	—
Population sex ratio[a]	0.2735	1.75	0.2445	1.81
Muslims	0.6009	7.76	0.6135	8.32
Scheduled tribes	0.1469	2.73	0.1400	3.17
Ideational Factors				
Female literacy	−0.4633	5.07	−0.5508	6.90
Media exposure[b]	−0.6874	4.16	−0.6938	5.46
Cinema exposure[b]	−0.2814	2.13	−0.2568	2.14
Transportation and communication workers[a]	−0.0081	0.43	−0.0086	0.46
Population density[a]	−0.0347	3.17	−0.0383	4.16
Health and Family Planning				
Under-5 mortality[c]	0.6309	4.50	0.1339	5.34
Target achievement[b]	0.0666	0.80	—	—
Unmet need for contraception[b]	0.0888	0.42	—	—
Constant	0.8302	0.71	0.4648	0.49
Adjusted R^2	0.895		0.892	
N	326		326	

[a]Used in logarithmic form.

[b]Information was available only at the state level.

[c]Lagged by 10 years; used in logarithmic form in Specification 2.

omitted. Unfortunately data on desired family size are not available at the district level.

Individual-Level Analysis

In macro-level analyses, hoarding and replacement effects become con-founded, but micro-level data provide an opportunity to separate these two ef-fects. Micro-level data can be used in several different ways to investigate the effect of child mortality on fertility, for example, through the analyses of parity progression ratios or birth intervals. However, to be consistent with the macro analysis presented above, I have employed a multiple regression approach. The data come from the National Family Health Survey of 1992-1993 for two states, Karnataka in the south and Uttar Pradesh in the north. Uttar Pradesh serves as a case study of a population at an early stage of demographic transition (TFR = 5.2, infant mortality rate = 94), while Karnataka presents the case of an area at a fairly advanced stage of the transition (TFR = 2.9, infant mortality rate = 67). The data have been analyzed for cohorts at the end of their reproductive lives, as well as for all women of reproductive age. The cohort analysis employed data on chil-dren ever born, children dead, and desired family size, whereas the analysis of all married women examined data on contraceptive practice with child loss as one of the key determinants. In addition, in both analyses an indicator of community-level mortality was included to check for the presence of hoarding behavior.

Cohort Analysis

The data examined here refer to married women aged 35-49 at the time of the survey who have had at least one live birth. The data were analyzed using the Olsen technique (Olsen, 1980; Trussell and Olsen, 1993). This technique incor-porates two estimators of the replacement rate, one based on the OLS regression of children ever born on child deaths and the other derived from the TSLS regression using proportion of dead children as an instrument for child deaths. Although the former estimate is always biased, Olsen and Trussell note that the latter can be consistent in some cases but needs adjustment under certain circum-stances. Trussell and Olsen have suggested ways to correct both estimates using various diagnostic tools. The main diagnostic criterion is the implied within-parity variance of the child mortality rate, which indicates whether the probabil-ity of a child death is constant for all women or correlated with their fertility. The results of this procedure are reported in Table 10-9.

The unadjusted estimate of the replacement rate from the OLS procedure is 1.19 for Karnataka and 0.94 for Uttar Pradesh. The TSLS procedure implies significantly lower estimates, 0.75 and 0.59, respectively, for the two states. When the diagnostic criteria suggested by Trussell and Olsen are examined for Karnataka, the implied within-parity variation in mortality is negative (which is

TABLE 10-9 Results of Applying the Olsen Technique to Estimate the Effect of Child Mortality on Fertility from the Data of the National Family Health Survey for Karnataka and Uttar Pradesh, 1992-1993

Model Parameter	Assumed Distribution[a]	Karnataka, Ages 35-49 (N = 1,209) OLS-based	IV-based	Uttar Pradesh, Ages 35-49, (N = 3,504) OLS-based	IV-based
Diagnostic criterion		D		C	
Replacement rate r					
Unadjusted estimate		1.19	0.75	0.94	0.59
Adjusted estimate	A				
	B	0.66[b]	—	0.02	0.00
Correlation between fertility (n) and mortality rate (q)	A	—	—		0.64
	B	—	—		0.70
Standard deviation of mortality (σ_q)	A	—	—		0.10
	B	—	—		0.11
Hoarding rate h[c]	A	—	—		2.45
	B	—	—		2.40

NOTE: OLS, ordinary least squares. IV, instrumental variables.

[a]A. Adjusted by assuming bivariate log normal distribution for n and q; B, adjusted by assuming normal lognormal distribution for n and q.

[b]Corrected under the assumption that mortality rate (q) is random and uncorrelated with fertility (n).

[c]Computed on the assumption that the entire estimated correlation between n and q is due to hoarding.

theoretically impossible), and the mortality rate is random (diagnostic D). Trussell and Olsen advise that under these circumstances the confidence attached to the estimates should not be very high; however, the OLS estimates can be corrected using their formula and compared with the uncorrected TSLS estimates. The closer the two estimates, the higher the degree of confidence that they capture the true replacement rate. The corrected OLS estimate for Karnataka was 0.66, which was reasonably close to the uncorrected TSLS estimate of 0.75. However, the observed variance on child death was substantially higher than that computed using Olsen's formula, which implies that both estimates may be overstating the true replacement effect (see Trussell and Olsen, 1983).

When the diagnostic tests are applied to Uttar Pradesh, the results suggest that the child mortality rate cannot be assumed to be constant across women, nor can it be assumed to be uncorrelated with fertility (diagnostic C). The estimated correlation between the mortality rate and the fertility rate under two different distributional assumptions is in the range of 0.64-0.70. Adjusted estimates of the replacement rate are close to zero, which is implausibly low in the presence of lengthy breastfeeding. Hence, Olsen's technique appears to overcorrect for the correlation between fertility and mortality. In his original paper, Olsen suggested a way to estimate the hoarding rate under the assumption that the entire correlation between mortality rate and fertility is due to hoarding (Olsen, 1980). This will, of course, provide an upper-bound estimate of the hoarding effect. Under this assumption, the hoarding rate is about 2.4 births per child death in Uttar Pradesh. For Karnataka, a similar estimate could not be derived because the computed within-parity variance of the child mortality rate was negative.

When desired family size is directly controlled in the regression, as in the state-level analysis, a problem arises. As many as 20 percent of women gave nonnumeric responses to the question on desired family size. Because these women could belong to a nonrandom group, their exclusion could bias the results. To circumvent this problem, I create a dummy variable for these women (*GOD*), which takes the value of 1 if they failed to report a desired family size and zero otherwise. And on the desired family size variable they were assigned a value of zero.

To use the individual-level data to check for hoarding, I added the community-level mortality rate, measured as the proportion of dead children among children ever born to women aged 35-49 by district of residence as an additional regressor. Because the National Family Health Survey was a sample survey, it was not possible to use geographic subdivisions smaller than the district level. Thus, the variable is measured with a large error (though of random nature) that could result in a downward bias in my estimated coefficient. In the regression analysis I test two functional forms. In the first specification I assume that fertility responds linearly to the changes in community-level mortality; in the second I use a logarithmic form on the assumption that the hoarding response to child mortality is inelastic at high levels.

Tables 10-10 and 10-11 show the results of this analysis for Karnataka and Uttar Pradesh, respectively. For the sake of brevity, only the results of the TSLS regressions are presented. When child deaths is the sole regressor, the results are fundamentally the same as those reported in connection with the Olsen technique. The inclusion of desired family size variable, along with the dummy for nonnumeric responses, reduces the implied replacement rate from 0.75-0.62 in the case of Karnataka, and from 0.59-0.52 in the case of Uttar Pradesh. Interestingly, the coefficient of desired family size (0.62 for Karnataka and 0.60 for Uttar Pradesh) is about the same as the coefficient on the child death variable. Even more significant is the fact that the coefficient on the desired family size variable is not substantially different from the estimate I obtained using macro-level co-hort data, whereas there is a large difference in the estimated effects of child mortality from the two data sets. This is consistent with my belief that the macro-level effects of a reduction in child mortality are larger because it is influenced by the substitution of replacement for hoarding over the course of the transition.

It can also be noted that the dummy variable for nonnumeric response is also strongly significant in my micro-level regressions. The estimated coefficient on this variable suggests that women who gave nonnumeric responses to the question on desired family size have an average desired family size of 4.6 in Karnataka and 4.9 in Uttar Pradesh. This was computed by dividing the coefficient on the dummy variable *GOD* by the coefficient on the desired family size variable. Those women who provided a numeric response reported an average desired family size of 2.7 in Karnataka and 3.7 in Uttar Pradesh, suggesting that women who failed to provide a numeric answer to the question on family size desires were indeed different.

When the district-level mortality variable is introduced into the regression in linear form, it is significant in Karnataka but not in Uttar Pradesh. The coefficient of the variable is substantially different in the two states (4.9 in Karnataka and 0.7 in Uttar Pradesh). However, when the variable is employed in logarithmic form, it is significant in Uttar Pradesh as well, and the difference in the coefficients is substantially smaller (0.7 in Karnataka and 0.3 in Uttar Pradesh). Again, these results conform to my a priori expectations that lags in the perception of mortality decline tend to weaken fertility response to community-wide changes in child mortality at higher levels.

From these results it is also possible to obtain a rough idea of the relative size of replacement and hoarding effects. At the sample mean, the estimated coefficients of district-level mortality imply a hoarding response of 0.9 and 0.2 births per child death in Karnataka and Uttar Pradesh, respectively. It is important to recognize that these rates do not reflect the absolute level of hoarding; they show the change in hoarding response in response to declines in community-level mortality. One could expect this response to be relatively weak in a high-mortality state such as Uttar Pradesh. As noted above, for the two states, the estimates of replacement rate are 0.6 and 0.5, respectively. Thus, the total effect of a

TABLE 10-10 Two-Stage Least-Squares Regression Results of Children Ever
Born with Child Deaths and Desired Family Size Using Individual-Level Data
on Married Women Aged 35-49, National Family Health Survey, Karnataka,
1992-1993

	Specification 1		Specification 2	
Variable	Parameter	*t*-Ratio	Parameter	*t*-Ratio
Any child deaths	0.752	13.5	0.623	11.6
Male child deaths	—	—	—	—
Female child deaths	—	—	—	—
Desired family size	—	—	0.626	12.7
District child mortality	—	—	—	—
District child mortality (in logarithmic scale)	—	—	—	—
Dummy variables[a]				
GOD	—	—	2.865	14.5
SEX	—	—	—	—
DFS × SEX	—	—	—	—
Constant	4.077	58.4	2.268	15.7
Adjusted R^2	0.306		0.393	
N	1,209		1,207	

[a]*GOD* is a dummy variable for women who gave a nonnumeric response to the question on
desired family size. For these women, the desired variable has been set at zero. *SEX* is a dummy
variable for sex preference.   Women who had the desired sex combination of children when their

change in child loss experience works out to be 1.5 in Karnataka and 0.7 in Uttar
Pradesh. As levels of fertility and mortality in Karnataka are fairly close to the
all-India average, and those of Uttar Pradesh significantly higher, these estimates
appear to be consistent with the RH rates derived from the cohort analysis of
state-level data.

Two additional model specifications examine the extent to which sex preference affects the mortality-fertility relationship. First, I test the possibility that
boys who die are replaced more frequently than girls. This appears to be the case,
although the difference is not statistically significant in either state. The estimated replacement rates are 0.60 and 0.51, respectively, for male and female
children in Karnataka and 0.50 and 0.47 in Uttar Pradesh. As expected, the sex
difference is larger in Karnataka where volitional replacement is greater.

In a final specification I examine the effect of sex-specific reproductive goals
by introducing a dummy variable for the sex composition of children (*SEX*) and
interacting it with the desired family size variable. This dummy variable equals
1 for all women fortunate enough to have their desired sex composition of chil-

Specification 3		Specification 4		Specification 5		Specification 6	
Parameter	t-Ratio	Parameter	t-Ratio	Parameter	t-Ratio	Parameter	t-Ratio
0.567	10.0	0.574	10.2	—	—	—	—
—	—	—	—	0.599	6.7	0.610	6.8
—	—	—	—	0.513	5.7	0.509	5.6
0.623	12.6	0.627	12.7	0.565	11.0	0.301	3.5
4.875	4.2	—	—	—	—	—	—
—	—	0.671	3.8	0.639	3.5	0.574	3.2
2.832	14.3	2.849	14.4	2.722	13.3	1.655	5.0
—	—	—	—	—	—	−1.420	4.0
—	—	—	—	—	—	0.367	3.4
1.548	7.0	3.570	9.6	3.995	10.4	4.939	11.1
0.390		0.390		0.384		0.394	
1,207		1,207		1,013		1,013	

first *n* births were equal to the total desired family size were coded as 1. All others were assigned a value of 0. DFS, desired family size.

dren when they attain their desired family size and 0 otherwise. Only about 60 percent of the women in Karnataka and 50 percent of women in Uttar Pradesh had attained their desired sex composition when they reached their desired family size. The results of my analysis (Tables 10-10 and 10-11) show that failure to attain the preferred sex composition reduces the effect of desired family size on fertility by about 15 percent in Karnataka and 17 percent in Uttar Pradesh. But even in a situation where sex-specific targets are attained, my results imply that only about two-thirds of the change in desired family size is reflected in children ever born in both the states (see Bhat, 1997, for details).

In sum, the cohort analysis of individual-level data has shown that the replacement rate is much below 1. My estimates may be slightly high because I have only partially taken into account the problem of simultaneity. The replacement rate is marginally higher for male deaths than for female deaths. Also evident is a hoarding effect, measured in terms of a fertility response to variations in district-level mortality. In an environment of high mortality risk, hoarding behavior is insensitive to small changes in mortality. The estimated coefficients

TABLE 10-11 Two-Stage Least-Squares Regression Results of Children Ever Born with Child Deaths and Desired Family Size Using Individual-Level Data on Married Women Aged 35-49, National Family Health Survey, Uttar Pradesh, 1992-1993

Variable	Specification 1		Specification 2	
	Parameter	t-Ratio	Parameter	t-Ratio
Any child deaths	0.586	26.5	0.524	23.2
Male child deaths	—	—	—	—
Female child deaths	—	—	—	—
Desired family size	—	—	0.602	24.4
District child mortality	—	—	—	—
District child mortality (in logarithmic scale)	—	—	—	—
Dummy variables [a]				
GOD	—	—	2.955	24.1
SEX	—	—	—	—
DFS × SEX	—	—	—	—
Constant	5.048	108.1	2.761	28.6
Adjusted R^2	0.337		0.431	
N	3,504		3,498	

[a]See footnote to Table 10-10.

of district-level mortality suggest that a decrease in child mortality of one child death reduces hoarding by 0.9 births in Karnataka and 0.2 births in Uttar Pradesh. Thus, the total effect of a decrease in one child death is estimated to be around 1.5 in Karnataka and 0.7 in Uttar Pradesh. These estimated total effects compare favorably with those derived from the analysis of state-level data but are higher than those derived from district-level data. Interestingly, my estimates suggest that the experience of own-child mortality and desired family size have fertility effects of roughly the same order of magnitude, even though there is an additional biological component to the former. The effect of the latter could be overstated by a rationalization in the reports of family size desires, but this is partly offset by the desire to have children of a particular sex.

Determinants of Contraceptive Use

From the individual-level analysis of data on children ever born, children dead, and desired family size I distinguished between hoarding and replacement effects, but I could not separate volitional from physiological components of the

Specification 3		Specification 4		Specification 5		Specification 6	
Parameter	t-Ratio	Parameter	t-Ratio	Parameter	t-Ratio	Parameter	t-Ratio
0.518	22.2	0.512	22.0	—	—	—	—
—	—	—	—	0.502	11.9	0.527	12.4
—	—	—	—	0.470	11.1	0.446	10.3
0.589	24.0	0.594	23.9	0.492	19.8	0.299	8.1
0.688	1.1	—	—	—	—	—	—
—	—	0.319	2.3	0.309	2.2	0.317	2.3
2.932	23.6	2.909	23.4	2.468	19.8	1.522	8.8
—	—	—	—	—	—	−1.567	7.7
—	—	—	—	—	—	0.328	6.7
2.624	16.8	3.281	13.2	3.933	15.6	4.892	17.5
0.429		0.428		0.406		0.417	
3,498		3,498		3,140		3,140	

replacement effect. Such a distinction is possible from an analysis of deliberate fertility regulation. From the timing and methods used to regulate fertility, it is also possible to throw light on hoarding behavior.

The data analyzed here pertain to 3,585 married women of Karnataka aged 13-49 in 1992-1993 with at least one living child. The National Family Health Survey, from which these data are derived, did not collect information on complete contraceptive history and cannot be subjected to an event-history analysis. Instead, logit models were used to analyze the determinants of contraceptive status of women at the time of the survey. A multinomial logit analysis model was used to predict whether women are nonusers of contraception, users of reversible methods, or users of nonreversible methods (i.e., sterilization). The parameter estimates of the model were normalized on the nonusers. Covariates included in the analysis were of three types: demographic characteristics of women and their children, socioeconomic variables, and community characteristics. The key variables of interest are the number of dead sons, the number of dead daughters, the age of the first surviving child, and the contextual child mortality level, measured at the district level. Results of the analysis are presented in Table 10-12.

Loss of a boy is inversely related to the acceptance of sterilization, after controlling for the number of boys ever born. However, loss of a girl makes little difference to sterilization acceptance. A Wald test showed that the sex difference in the response to a child death experience is statistically significant at the 1 percent level. Interestingly, the experience of a child loss of either sex is not a statistically significant predictor of the use of a reversible method of contraception. Perhaps I obtain confounding results in this case because of the presence of two opposing forces: users of reversible methods tend to be self-selected for their higher child mortality experience (as the positive sign of the coefficients seem to suggest), but continuity of use is affected adversely by subsequent child mortality because of the replacement motive. The regression based on the current status measure cannot capture this dynamic aspect, but indicates the underlying heterogeneity through a large standard error of the estimate. Nevertheless, from the estimated net effect of near zero, it would not be wrong to conclude that greater access to reversible methods would help lower fertility levels in relatively high child mortality settings.

Wolpin (in this volume) has proposed a measure of the replacement rate based on a comparison of birth probabilities of women during a fixed time period who start out with the same number of live births but differ in their past child mortality experience. My logit analysis achieves much the same objective indirectly, except that it is based on the comparison of contraceptive behavior and therefore reflects only the volition component of the replacement. The similarity can be made clearer by directly controlling for the number of live births by running separate logistic regressions on different groups of women classified according to their number of children ever born. The results of this analysis are also presented in Table 10-12 for women who have borne 1, 2, 3, 4, and 5+ children. Because of sample size limitations, here I have used only the binary logit model that considered two groups: users and nonusers of any method of contraception at the time of the survey.

The results of this analysis show that the effect of child loss experience is quite large and negative at parities below 5. The coefficient on male child death is strongly significant at parities 3 and 4 whereas that of female child loss is significant only at parity 3. The coefficients of child loss experience are also quite large and negative at parities 1 and 2 but are not statistically significant. It is interesting to note that, unlike the analysis on all women, parity-specific analysis indicates that the death of a girl also tends to reduce the rate of contraceptive adoption, though not to the same extent as the death of a boy.

The marginal effect of a child death on the contraceptive prevalence rate can be evaluated at each parity by multiplying the respective coefficient by the cross product of proportion of users and proportion of nonusers at that parity. My estimates imply that, by elimination of a child death, the contraceptive prevalence rate would rise by 16, 20, and 9 percent at parities 2, 3, and 4, respectively. However, the combined result of these changes is expected to cause an increase of only 4 percent in the level of contraceptive practice of all married women (5 percent from the elimination of a male child death and 3 percent from a female child). This is because a large percentage of child deaths in the population is accounted for by women with five or more births who respond only weakly to their own child mortality experience, possibly because they are self-selected for higher family size desires or for greater reliance on an insurance strategy.

A rough estimate of the mean replacement rate can be derived by multiplying the expected increase in the contraceptive practice by the total fertility rate and dividing by the proportion of nonusers of contraception. As the TFR was about 3.0 and about 50 percent of the married women (including childless women) were not using contraception in Karnataka, the average increase of 4 percent in the contraceptive prevalence rate implies a volitional replacement rate of 0.24 births per child death (0.30 for boys and 0.16 for girls). In addition, if a biological component of 0.3 is associated with prolonged breastfeeding, the implied total replacement rate would be 0.54, almost identical to the estimate derived from the cohort analysis using desired family size as a control (0.56). However, the cohort analysis indicates a smaller sex differential in the response rate than suggested here.

Because an overwhelming majority of women (87 percent in my sample) who use contraceptives use sterilization, a nonreversible method, children's survival after acceptance of contraception could be a real concern. To test for its possible effects, age of the first surviving child at the time of the survey was used as an additional covariate. The results obtained in the case of all women show that the age of the first child and its square are strongly significant in the sterilization equation and marginally significant in the case of reversible methods (see Table 10-12). The older the child is, the more likely that his or her parents would accept sterilization. As one would expect, the effect of child's age is nonlinear; the estimated age function implies that prevalence of sterilization peaks when the first surviving child is 24 years old. Because the mean interval between sterilization acceptance and the survey was about 8 years, the result suggests that acceptance of contraception rises until the child is 16 years old. Thus, parents appeared to be concerned about child survival to ages much beyond infancy, and it is in such conditions that hoarding behavior flourishes.

Although the coefficient of age of the first child is marginally significant in the case of women who use a reversible method, a Wald test reveals that the estimated effect is substantially smaller than that on sterilization acceptance (significant at the 0.001 level). Thus, my empirical results support the contention that sterilization tends to promote hoarding behavior.

By demonstrating the importance of age of the child on contraceptive acceptance I can demonstrate the existence of an insurance motive, but it is difficult to quantify a hoarding rate. The use of contextual child mortality as an additional

TABLE 10-12 Results of Logit Analysis of Covariates of Current Use of Contraception by Method and Number of Children Ever Born, Karnataka, 1992-1993

	All Married Women		Use of any Method, by Number of Children Ever Born				
Explanatory Variable	Sterilization	Reversible Methods	1	2	3	4	5+
Demographic Variables							
Age of woman	0.245***	0.377***	0.484**	0.358**	0.296*	0.382*	0.280
Age of woman squared	−0.005***	−0.006***	−0.008**	−0.006**	−0.005*	−0.006*	−0.005*
Male children ever born	1.329***	−0.078	−0.075	0.806*	2.117***	0.595	0.553***
Male children ever born squared	−0.211***	−0.003	—	−0.080	−0.469***	−0.038	−0.103***
Female children ever born	0.353***	−0.267	—	—	—	—	—
Female children ever born squared	−0.073***	0.022	—	—	—	—	—
Male child deaths	−0.348***	0.029	−1.209	−0.838	−1.178***	0.659**	0.011
Female child deaths	0.030	0.036	−11.129	−0.497	−0.653*	−0.243	0.023
Age of first surviving child	0.324***	0.105*	—	0.268***	0.385***	0.167	0.188*
Age of first child squared	−0.007***	−0.003	—	−0.007**	−0.012***	−0.003	−0.003
Socioeconomic Variables							
Religion and caste							
Muslims	−1.037***	0.094	−0.899	−0.891**	−0.958***	−1.027**	−0.663**
Scheduled caste	−0.295*	−0.124	−0.731	−0.152	−0.044	−0.927**	−0.153
Scheduled tribe	−0.061	−0.236	−0.401	−0.162	0.139	0.351	−0.324
Others[a]							
Wife's schooling	0.038	0.112*	0.034	0.085	0.037	0.019	0.001
Wife's schooling squared	−0.001	0.002	0.004	−0.004	0.001	−0.001	0.009
Husband's schooling	0.059*	0.047	0.080	0.019	0.019	0.005	0.137*
Husband's schooling squared	−0.002	−0.003	−0.002	0.002	−0.000	−0.003	−0.008

	(1)	(2)	(3)	(4)	(5)	(6)	(7)
Woman's work status							
Agricultural work	0.159	-0.628*	-0.117	0.079	-0.048	0.041	0.292
Nonagricultural work[a]	0.051	-0.112	-0.245	0.187	0.179	0.509	-0.119
Nonworker[a]							
Own landholding	-0.003	0.012	-0.034	-0.026	0.032	-0.030	0.006
Own landholding squared[b]	-0.000	-0.000	0.000	0.000	-0.000	0.001	-0.000
Household assets[b]	-0.014	0.105*	-0.012	0.024	-0.028	0.062	0.024
Exposure to mass media[c]	0.262***	0.047	0.009	0.348***	0.150	0.174	0.223*
Community Variables							
Current residence							
Urban	-0.087	-0.144	0.081	-0.175	0.020	-0.451	-0.072
Rural[a]							
Childhood residence							
Urban	-0.244*	0.066	-0.144	-0.298	0.081	-0.157	-0.201
Rural[a]							
District child mortality[d]	-0.665***	-1.273***	-0.390	-0.636*	-0.510	-1.407***	-0.662*
Constant	-8.395***	-10.802***	-9.908***	-8.836***	-8.818***	-9.509***	-7.738***
Log-likelihood	-2,452		-206.8	-443.6	-368.4	-272.1	-539.4
χ^2	1,579	104.4	268.7	218.8	102.9	118.6	
N	3,585		582	836	768	551	881
Proportion of current users	0.478	0.073	0.163	0.530	0.686	0.726	0.582

NOTES: *, $p \leq 0.05$. **, $p < 0.01$. ***, $p < 0.001$.

[a]Reference group for the dummy variables.

[b]Number owned by the household out of a list of 11 consumer durables.

[c]Regular exposure of married women to radio, television, and cinema as defined in the National Family Health Survey. The variable was constructed by giving a score of one for each media exposure.

[d]Proportion of children dead among women aged 35–49 in logarithmic form.

regressor provides a means by which one can not only detect hoarding behavior but can also quantify the fertility response. As in the case of cohort analysis presented above, the level of contextual mortality was measured at the district level. As seen in Table 10-12, this variable was strongly significant in both sterilization and reversible method equations. Interestingly, the effect is larger in the case of reversible method use; the Wald test confirmed this at a 5 percent level. The greater sensitivity of reversible method use to variations in contextual mortality is in line with my expectation that mortality decline induces a switch from a predominantly hoarding to a predominantly replacement regime. Clearly, as more couples adopt a replacement strategy, use of reversible methods should increase. I also find an increase in the use of sterilization associated with declines in community-level mortality because it reduces the number of children required for insurance.

The results of parity-specific analysis also conform to my a priori expectations. The district-level child mortality variable is significant at most parities, but its effect is nearly three times larger at parity four than at any other parity (see Table 10-12). Because the average desired family size in Karnataka is about three children, many have a fourth child primarily for insurance. Thus, contextual mortality has greater bearing on contraceptive acceptance at this parity.

By multiplying by the contraceptive prevalence rate and dividing by the mean child mortality rate, the coefficient of contextual mortality can be converted to an estimate of the hoarding response to a change in community-level mortality. The weighted average of method-specific effects implies a hoarding response of 2.1 births per child death, whereas the weighted average of parity-specific coefficients implies a response rate of 2.0 births. If I add to this the replacement effect of 0.54, estimated earlier, I obtain a total RH rate of 2.6 children per child death, which is significantly higher than the estimate of 1.5 derived from the cohort analysis of women aged 35-49. The difference in the estimates obtained from period and cohort analyses suggests a rising trend in the RH rate, an indication consistent with the hypothesis of a structural shift.

The almost exclusive reliance on sterilization in the Indian family planning program tends to promote hoarding behavior. This point becomes even clearer when the timing of sterilization is examined. Due to certain social as well as technical reasons, most women find it advantageous to accept sterilization immediately after delivery. The data for Karnataka imply that the interval between the last live birth and the acceptance of sterilization is less than a month in 58 percent of cases and 1 month in another 14 percent of the cases (Table 10-13). This obviously raises questions as to the parents' concern about the survival of the last child. The question becomes even more intriguing when one observes that the sex ratio of the last live birth is highly skewed with 144 male births for 100 female births among sterilized couples. Thus, there is a clear indication that couples waited to have a son before accepting a nonreversible method. Most likely, couples do not accept sterilization as soon as the desired family size is

TABLE 10-13 Percentage Distribution of Sterilized Couples by Interval Between Birth of Last Child and Date of Sterilization and According to Sex of Last Child, Karnataka, 1992-1993

	Sex of Last Child		
Interval in Months	Male	Female	Either Sex
0	59.0	56.6	58.0
1	14.6	14.1	14.4
2-3	7.0	7.6	7.2
4-6	2.6	3.1	2.8
7-11	1.6	2.8	2.1
12+	9.8	9.9	9.8
Inconsistent/not reported	5.4	5.9	5.6
Sterilized couples	1,020	710	1,730

SOURCE: National Family Health Survey, Karnataka.

reached but they wait until after the next birth to decide whether to discontinue childbearing. If the next child is a boy, the survival safeguard is considered complete and couples accept sterilization immediately after the child is born. Perhaps parents would have accepted contraception after the preceding birth if reversible methods were easily accessible. The strong influence of the sex combination of children on sterilization acceptance seen in Table 10-12 partly reflects this sex-specific hoarding behavior.

In short, the analysis of contraceptive acceptance patterns shows that the prevalence rates for sterilization, a method used by a overwhelming majority of couples in India to control their fertility, is lower because of their experience of child loss and their concerns about the survival of their living children. The estimated reduction in sterilization prevalence because of child loss implies a volitional response of about 0.25 for a child death in Karnataka. The strong presence of hoarding is indicated both by the significance of first child's age to contraceptive acceptance and by the timing of sterilization, which suggests that the last child born is a hoarded child and in many cases is insurance against the death of a son. The analysis unambiguously shows that the almost exclusive reliance on sterilization, and its provision mainly as a postpartum service, has accentuated the hoarding response, increased inefficiency (in the form of unwanted fertility), and enhanced the effect of son preference on fertility.

CONCLUDING REMARKS

The analysis presented in this chapter is based on the premise that as individuals gain increasing control over their fertility and mortality risks, they switch from a hoarding to a replacement strategy to cope with the uncertainties of child survival. The shift occurs because over the transition mortality risks beyond infancy reduce substantially, the amount and cost of unwanted fertility increase, and improved access to family planning methods make it more feasible to use a replacement strategy. However, at initial stages of the transition, the substitution of replacement for hoarding occurs at a sluggish pace because of lags in individual perception of community-wide mortality declines, the low cost of unwanted fertility, and the lack of access to family planning services. Consequently, the relationship between fertility and child mortality is generally weak at this stage.

As conditions change, couples increasingly switch to a replacement strategy. Because replacement can be less than fully compensatory, and hoarding often results in excess fertility, the switch tends to accelerate the fertility decline. Even though replacement is incomplete at the family level, at the macro level, the mortality-fertility relationship is characterized by increasing returns to scale.

My data for India show that the replacement rate is substantially below 1, about 0.5-0.6, of which about one-half is a volitional component. I interpret the low rates of volitional replacement as evidence that the majority of Indian women have still not adopted a replacement strategy. This is supported by the significance of variations in community-level mortality as demonstrated in the multivariate analysis of household-level data and the analysis of macro-level data that suggest that declines in child mortality currently bring more than compensatory changes in fertility. This is a different situation than two decades ago when the magnitude of the fertility response indicated deceasing returns to scale. Thus, the strategy shift appears to have begun. The implication of this result to health policy is fairly obvious. Whatever the fertility response in the past, structural changes have occurred, and current investments in child survival programs would trigger more than compensatory effects on fertility and thus contribute significantly in reducing global population growth. To maximize this effect, it is essential to strengthen fertility control programs, focusing mainly on reversible methods. As my analysis of Indian data shows, almost exclusive reliance on sterilization has favored the insurance strategy and delayed the adoption of a pure replacement mechanism.

APPENDIX

Appendix tables begin on following page.

APPENDIX TABLE Description, Mean, Standard Deviation, and Expected Signs of Explanatory Variables Used in the Regression Analysis of District-Level Estimates of Total Fertility Rate

Variable	Description	Mean	Standard Deviation	Expected Relationship
Economic Structure				
Male workers in agriculture	Proportion of agricultural workers among total male workers (main), 1991 census	0.663	0.158	+
Agricultural laborers	Proportion of agricultural laborers among total agricultural workers (main), 1991 census	0.387	0.170	?
Female labor force participation	Proportion of main workers among females aged 7 years and over, 1991 census	0.200	0.130	–
Child laborers	Proportion of main and marginal workers among children age 5-14, 1981 census	0.081	0.047	+
Bank offices	Bank offices per 100,000 population, March 1986	6.8	2.5	–
Social Structure				
Joint family	Proportion of linearly or collaterally joint households, 1981 census	0.204	0.054	+
Female age at marriage	Mean age at first marriage of ever-married females as reported in the 1981 census	16.63	1.35	–
Population sex ratio	Males per 1,000 females, 1991 census	1080	68	+
Muslims	Proportion of Muslims in the population, 1981 census	0.098	0.091	+
Scheduled tribes	Proportion of scheduled tribes in the population, 1991 census	0.090	0.152	?

Ideational Factors

Female literacy	Female literacy rate at ages 7 and over, 1991 census	0.359	0.176	—
Media exposure[a]	Proportion of couples regularly exposed to mass media (either newspaper, radio, television, or cinema), Operations Research Survey Group, 1988	0.493	0.142	—
Cinema exposure[a]	Proportion of married women who see a movie at least once in 3 months, Operations Research Group, 1988	0.127	0.121	—
Transport and communication	Transport and communication workers per 1,000 population, 1991 census	8.4	5.7	—
Population density	Population density per square kilometer, 1991 census	622	2123	—

Health and Family Planning

Under-5 mortality	Under-5 mortality rate derived from 1981 census	0.205	0.068	+
Target achievement[a]	Proportion of sterilization targets achieved, 1984-1991	0.809	0.126	—
Unmet need	Unmet need for contraception for limiting and spacing, National Family Health Survey, 1992-1993	0.196	0.063	+

[a]State-level data only are available. In the regression analysis the districts were assigned a value equal to their respective state average.

SOURCE: See Bhat (1996).

REFERENCES

Ben-Porath, Y.
   1978   Fertility response to child mortality: Microdata from Israel. Pp. 161-180 in S.H. Preston,
           ed., *The Effects of Infant and Child Mortality on Fertility*. New York: Academic Press.
Bhat, M.
   1989   Mortality and fertility in India, 1881-1961: A reassessment. In T. Dyson, ed., *India's
           Historical Demography: Studies in Famine, Disease and Society*. London: Curzon Press.
   1996   Contours of fertility decline in India: A district-level study based on the 1991 census. Pp.
           96-177 in K. Srinivasan, ed., *Population Policy and Reproductive Health*. New Delhi:
           Hindustan.
   1997   Micro and Macro Effects of Child Mortality on Fertility: The Case of India. Population
           Research Center Report no. 94. Dharawad, India: JSS Institute of Economic Research.
Bhat, M., S.H. Preston, and T. Dyson
   1984   *Vital Rates in India*. Report no. 24, Committee on Population and Demography. Wash-
           ington, D.C.: National Academy Press.
Bongaarts, J.
   1987   Does family planning reduce infant mortality rates? *Population and Development Re-
           view* 13(2):323-334.
   1990   The measurement of wanted fertility. *Population and Development Review* 16(3):487-
           506.
Brass, W., and J.C. Barrett
   1978   Measurement problems in the analysis of linkages between fertility and child mortality.
           Pp. 209-233 in S.H. Preston, ed., *The Effects of Infant and Child Mortality on Fertility*.
           New York: Academic Press.
Heer, D.M., and D.O. Smith
   1968   Mortality level, desired family size and population increase. *Demography* 5(1):104-121.
International Institute for Population Sciences (IIPS)
   1995   *National Family Health Survey, India, 1992-93*. Bombay: IIPS.
Lloyd, C.B., and S. Ivanov
   1988   The effects of improved child survival on family planning practice and fertility. *Studies
           in Family Planning* 19(3):141-161.
May, D.A., and D.M. Heer
   1968   Son survivorship motivation and family size in India: A computer simulation. *Population
           Studies* 22(2):199-210.
O'Hara, D.J.
   1972   Mortality risks, sequential decisions on births, and population growth. *Demography*
           9(3):485-498.
Olsen, R.
   1980   Estimating the effect of child mortality on the number of births. *Demography* 17(4):429-
           443.
Operations Research Group
   1970   *Family Planning Practices in India*. Baroda, India: Operations Research Group.
Preston, S.H.
   1978   Introduction. Pp. 1-18 in S.H. Preston, ed., *The Effects of Infant and Child Mortality on
           Fertility*. New York: Academic Press.
Schultz, T.P.
   1976   Interrelationship between mortality and fertility. Pp. 239-289 in R.G. Ridker, ed., *Popu-
           lation and Development: The Search for Selective Interventions*. Baltimore, Md.: Johns
           Hopkins University Press.

Srinivasan, K., S.J. Jeejeebhoy, R.A. Easterlin, and E.M. Crimmins
   1984   Factors affecting fertility control in India: A cross-sectional study. *Population and Development Review* 10(2):273-296.
Trussell, J., and R. Olsen
   1983   Evaluation of the Olsen technique for estimating the fertility response to child mortality. *Demography* 20(3):391-405.
Venkatacharya, K.
   1978   Influence of variations in child mortality on fertility: A simulation model study. Pp. 235-257 in S.H. Preston, ed., *The Effects of Infant and Child Mortality on Fertility.* New York: Academic Press.
Williams, A.D.
   1977   Measuring the impact of child mortality on fertility: A methodological note. *Demography* 14(4):581-590.

11

Child Mortality and the Fertility Transition: Aggregated and Multilevel Evidence from Costa Rica

Luis Rosero-Bixby

INTRODUCTION

Is decreasing child mortality a prerequisite—a necessary condition—for decreasing fertility? Can decreasing child mortality alone trigger the fertility transition? These questions have important policy implications. If improving child survival is a precondition for birth control, family planning programs in the least developed regions are unlikely to succeed, especially if these programs have a vertical organization independent of child health interventions. In turn, if reducing child mortality is a sufficient condition, family planning programs may be somewhat superfluous: "Development is the best contraceptive." In this chapter I address the issue of whether reduced child mortality is crucial for the fertility transition by examining the empirical evidence from Costa Rica, a developing country that managed to decrease both child mortality and birth rates. Here I examine Costa Rica's record at the aggregate and the individual level.

A strong association between child mortality and fertility is well documented in the literature. Countries with low infant mortality almost always have low birth rates (Heer, 1966; Mauldin et al., 1978). Couples that have lost a child are, in turn, less likely to use contraception, tend to have more children, and have shorter birth intervals (Taylor et al., 1976). However, this association is neither proof of causation nor indicates the direction of causation. The association may have three closely linked origins: First, child mortality and fertility share a common set of determinants, such as mother's education, access to health services, breastfeeding practices, and less observable traits such as a preference for "high-quality" children or a less fatalistic outlook on life (Hanson et al., 1994). Second, lower fertility may lessen child mortality by acting on such potential mechanisms as maternal depletion associated with pregnancies and lactation (Trussell and Pebley, 1984), sibling competition for scarce family resources and maternal care including breastfeeding (Pebley and Millman, 1986), and transmission of infections in child-crowded environments (Blacker, 1987; Haaga, 1989). The third possibility—the one addressed in this chapter—is that the direction of causation runs from child survival to fertility. Although disentangling these three types of causal links is an impossible task with the data available, by statistically controlling the effect of particular variables and by paying attention to the sequence of events over time, I try to reach some conclusions about the third causal link: the role of child mortality on contemporary fertility transitions.

There are several explanations for the postulated effect of child mortality on fertility. In the classic demographic transition theory, high fertility is in part a response to high levels of infant and child mortality (Notestein, 1953; Davis, 1955). Parents have many children to replace those who have died (replacement effect) or parents set excess fertility goals in anticipation of their children's deaths (insurance effect) (Lloyd and Ivanov, 1988). Increased probabilities of child survival may thus be a necessary condition for fertility decline: Parents will not control their fertility unless they have assurance their children will survive (Taylor et al., 1976). Moreover, improvements in child survival may be a sufficient condition for fertility decline as soon as parents realize that it is no longer necessary to have many children or to suffer the economic consequences of larger families (Preston, 1978). Under these circumstances, fertility transition would be merely an adjustment process to conditions brought about by reduced child mortality (Carlsson, 1966). Where long periods of breastfeeding are the norm, a physiological mechanism may also be important: The death of an infant may substantially reduce the breastfeeding period and, consequently, the period of temporary infecundity after childbirth, which would result in shorter birth intervals and more children born by the end of the reproductive life (Cochrane and Zachariah, 1983).

Two earlier studies of the Costa Rican record show significant effects on reproductive behavior of couples whose children have died (Rutstein and Medica, 1978; Mensch, 1985). The replacement strategy is the most likely effect of one's own children's deaths. This effect seems reasonable and is well documented in populations that already control fertility, as it was in the Costa Rican samples analyzed in these two studies. In pretransition societies, however, it is hard to believe that couples turn on and off their fertility in response to child deaths. Data for European populations in the past usually do not show significant replacement effects (Knodel, 1978).

A third Costa Rican study, based on the 1976 World Fertility Survey, does not find a significant effect of child mortality in the community upon the reproductive behavior of individual women (Heer and Rodríguez, 1986). The insurance strategy is the most likely causal mechanism for the postulated effect of community-level child mortality. This effect has been seldom studied in other countries because of the lack of reliable multilevel data. One of the problems for building multilevel data sets is the definition of community and then having reliable estimates of child mortality or other contextual variables. The study of Heer and Rodríguez used the *cantón* as the unit for computing contextual variables. This Costa Rican administrative unit is, however, in many cases too large and internally too heterogeneous to be considered a meaningful entity; its boundaries are often arbitrary and the relevant context for the *cantón*'s edges may be that of neighboring *cantones*. In this chapter I overcome these limitations by using geographic information system data to obtain a precise and compact definition of "context" (the area within a radius of 5 kilometers in rural areas and 1 kilometer in urban areas from the index household). In addition, in this chapter I focus on the crucial event, adoption of family planning for the first time, as the dependent variable. In the studied cohorts, which grew up in a natural fertility environment, this represents a breaking point with the past.

After a brief analysis of Costa Rican national trends during this century, I examine the role of child mortality on the fertility transition at the macro- and the micro-level. The analysis at each level looks first at bivariate associations and then moves into multivariate associations with the purpose of isolating net effects. The macro-level analysis is based on data from 89 Costa Rican counties, which are small geographic entities defined on the basis of the country's administrative division in *cantones* and *distritos*. The multivariate analysis of this data set includes traditional regression models of the effect of child mortality on fertility at three points in time and between these points. It also models the event "fertility transition," as operationalized by two dependent variables: onset and pace of decline. The multivariate analysis of the onset of the fertility transition is carried out using Cox regression. The individual-level analysis uses a survey conducted in 1984 that included a lifetime calendar of contraceptive use. The analysis tests the hypothesis that contextual child mortality patterns influence the adoption of fertility control. This analysis focuses on the individual-level equivalent of fertility transition—the timing in the adoption of birth control—rather than on reproductive behavior in general, and it is restricted to the cohorts that lived through the fertility transition (i.e., women aged 15-34 in 1960). Given that the analysis combines contextual or macro-level indicators of child mortality and other variables to explain individual-level reproductive behavior, this analysis is referred to as "multilevel."

SECULAR TRENDS IN COSTA RICA

Costa Rica experienced one of the earliest and fastest, although incomplete, fertility transitions in the developing world. The total fertility rate fell from 7.3 to 5.5 between 1960 and 1968, the year an energetic national family planning program started, and then to 3.7 by 1976, the year the decline abruptly stopped (United Nations, 1985). After fluctuating erratically around 3.7 births, the rate began to decline again by 1986, although at a slow pace. According to the most recent estimate, the total fertility rate is 2.7 births per woman in 1995 and the contraceptive prevalence rate is 75 percent in 1993 (Caja Costarricense de Seguro Social, 1994).

There is no unique and simple explanation for the fertility transition in Costa Rica. Some authors stress the role of education, especially among women (Stycos, 1982). Other authors note the pervasiveness of the decline across all regions and social sectors to stress the role of the government in erasing differentials and redistributing income (Behm and Guzmán, 1979). Others underscore the explosive increase in the supply of contraceptives by the private sector and later by the public sector that took place in the 1960s (Tin Myaing Thein and Reynolds, 1972). It is obvious that the official family planning program, launched in 1968, had nothing to do with the early fertility decline, which occurred mostly among the urban, middle class. It is, however, accepted that the rapid propagation of the process to rural and urban working classes was catapulted by the energetic family planning program launched in 1968 (Rosero-Bixby et al., 1982). Recent literature also stresses diffusion, or social interaction, processes as one of the key determinants of the transition (Rosero-Bixby and Casterline, 1994, 1995; Knight, 1995).

Although most studies mention child mortality decline among the socioeconomic transformations that may have brought some of the fertility transition, none considers it a crucial factor.

At the fertility transition onset, the country's infant mortality rate was 76 per 1,000 and the child mortality risk (the probability of dying before the age of 5 years) was 96 per 1,000, which are high levels at current standards but were not in the late 1950s. In absolute terms, most of the possible reduction in child mortality rate had already taken place by 1960. It had declined by two-thirds from levels of about 300 per 1,000 observed by the 1910s (Figure 11-1). In relative terms, however, the fastest infant and child mortality reductions occured in the 1970s. The child mortality rate of about 18 per 1,000 in 1990 is one-fifth that of 1960. This acceleration in the pace of child and infant mortality decline in the 1970s has been linked to three factors (Rosero-Bixby, 1991a): public health interventions, which probably were the most important; development, including social improvements and a vigorous and sustained growth in the economy (Figure 11-3), and the fertility decline.

Figure 11-1 compares the evolution during the twentieth century of the general fertility rate, the child mortality rate, and an indicator of the economy (imports per capita, one of the few indicators with a series covering the entire period). The data for this figure come from official statistics, which in Costa Rica are reasonably reliable. The only apparent association between the general fertility rate and the child mortality rate is the acceleration in the relative decline in the latter during the fertility transition.

Actually, this acceleration starts a few years after the fertility transition

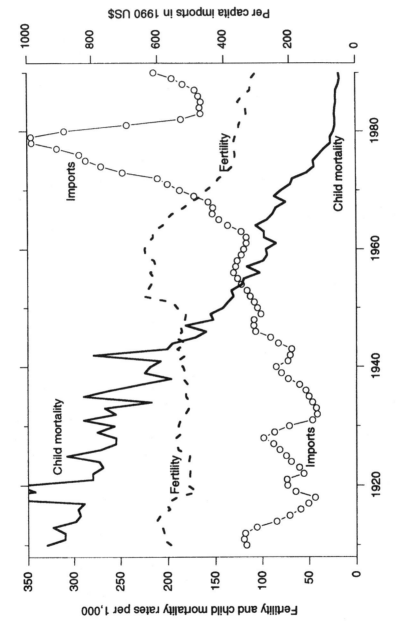

FIGURE 11-1 Child mortality rate, general fertility rate, and per capita imports, Costa Rica, twentieth century.

onset. This temporal sequence suggests that the direction of causation, if any, may run from fertility to child mortality. The rapid, concurrent economic growth suggests, in turn, that both child mortality and fertility declines were part of a broader transformation process in society and living standards.

Figure 11-1 hardly supports the thesis that child mortality decline was key for the fertility transition in Costa Rica. In particular, the record until 1964 is that neither the secular decline nor the short-term fluctuations (mostly due to measles epidemics) in child mortality was sufficient to alter fertility or start the transition. The small fluctuations in fertility during those early years are mostly linked to marital disruption, a marriage boom in the 1950s, and declines in widowhood. The only way that Figure 11-1 could be compatible with the "sufficient condition" thesis would be if the effect of child mortality requires long lags, or threshold doses, to act.

The data in Figure 11-1 are not conclusive as to whether a certain minimal level of child survival is required for fertility transition—the necessary condition thesis. If such a prerequisite exists, the Costa Rican experience indicates a child mortality rate threshold of 100 per 1,000 or higher.

The rate did not need to be as low as, say, 50 for people to adopt family planning; the fertility transition started at levels substantially higher than this. In turn, it would not be appropriate to conclude that the fertility transition is not possible at a rate of, say, 200 per 1,000. The transition did not start in Costa Rica in 1945 when the child mortality rate was approximately 200 per 1,000 either because of prevailing mortality conditions or because of the absence of other conditions, such as the availability of contraceptives or the rising costs of childbearing.

MACRO-LEVEL BIVARIATE ASSOCIATIONS

The covariations in fertility and child mortality across geographic units may cast some light on the nature of the association between these two variables. These covariations may be studied in a rich data set for 89 Costa Rican counties. The unit of analysis, the county, is a small geographic unit usually on the order of 20,000 inhabitants, defined on the basis of the Costa Rican administrative divisions, *cantones* and *distritos*. Indicators available in this data set are the marital fertility rate (births per married woman aged 15-44) in 1965, 1975, and 1985; and the child mortality rate (probability of dying before the fifth birthday) lagged 2 years. The numerator for computing the marital fertility rate is a 5-year average from the country's vital statistics; the denominator is an estimate based on the 1963, 1973, and 1984 censuses. The data on births were validated with estimates obtained by projecting the census populations backward. The child mortality rates in 1963 and 1973 were estimated using a variation of the Brass method (United Nations, 1983) on data from the 1973 and 1984 censuses on the proportions of surviving children by mother's age. The child mortality rate in 1983 is a

5-year average from vital statistics corrected by the ratio between the census-based estimate and a vital statistics estimate in 1973 (no correction was larger than 20 percent). Eleven counties with seemingly unreliable estimates were excluded from the original pool of 100 counties (details reported in Rosero-Bixby, 1991b).

Bivariate Macro-Level Associations

Figure 11-2 shows a hypothetical scatterplot for interpreting the data of bivariate covariations in fertility and child mortality levels. The figure's four quadrants result from combining high and low child mortality levels with high and low fertility rates. Most populations should fall in quadrants II and IV, the

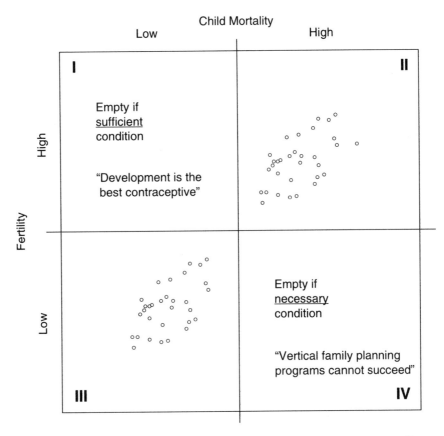

FIGURE 11-2 Expected scatterplot for the causal associations of child mortality on fertility.

high-high and low-low quadrants. Quadrant I of low child mortality and high fertility is expected to be nearly empty if a decreasing child mortality is a sufficient condition to bring down fertility rates. Quadrant III of high child mortality and low fertility should not contain observations if lowering child deaths is a precondition for fertility decline. If real data show a substantial number of observations in quadrants I or III, the corresponding hypotheses should be rejected (although the contrary does not mean that the hypotheses are true). A few observations in quadrants I and III may occur in real data as a consequence of measurement errors or effect lags.

How do the Costa Rican counties behave in comparison with this hypothetical association? Figure 11-3 shows the scatterplots for 1965, 1975, and 1985. The 1985 marital fertility rate is also plotted against the child mortality rate 22 years earlier to give an impression of the effect of considering lengthened lags. A striking feature in the figure is the fast pace of change in both fertility and child mortality. In just 10-year intervals, there are remarkable shifts in the cloud of observations toward the origin. Although the expected positive correlation occurs in the four cross sections, the correlation becomes weak by 1985.

By 1965, although most counties lay in the high-high zone (quadrant II), some have moderate child mortality and high fertility rates as counter evidence for the "sufficient condition" thesis: Birth rates continued to be high in spite of moderate infant mortality. By 1975, counties with either high mortality or high fertility are extinct species for practical purposes. Very few counties ever fall in the region of low fertility and high mortality (quadrant IV). The "necessary condition" thesis is neither supported nor rejected by these data.

By the mid-1980s, all counties but one had a low child mortality rate of less than 50 per 1,000. The variation in fertility rates is somewhat broader and the correlation coefficient is a modest 0.31—a suggestion that at these low levels there may be little connection between the two variables.

To what extent do child mortality levels in the past influence current fertility levels? An effect may come about if knowledge of the chances of child survival acquired in childhood and adolescence (news of child deaths heard at home from parents and other adults) is what make couples pursue an insurance reproductive strategy later on life (i.e., have as many children as possible to ensure that some will survive). Figure 11-3 examines this point by plotting the 1985 marital fertility rate against a 22-year lagged child mortality rate. The new correlation coefficient (0.65) is substantially higher than that for the 2-year lagged child mortality rate (0.31). This higher association may be, however, just an artifact of other variables such as the county's level of socioeconomic development. In particular, less developed counties, which tended to have a high fertility rate in 1985, had high child mortality in the 1960s; these counties, however, do not have high child mortality in the 1980s, thanks to health programs implemented in Costa Rica in the 1970s (especially primary health care interventions), which

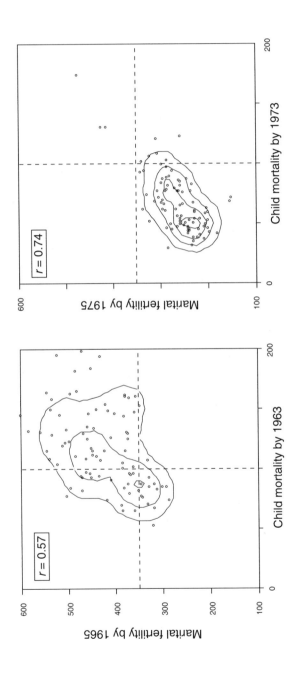

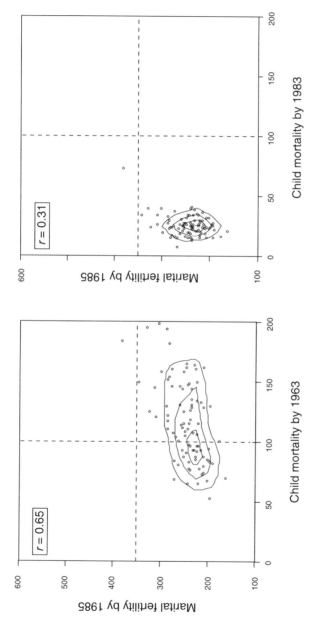

FIGURE 11-3 Relationship between marital fertility and child mortality, Costa Rican counties, 1965-1985. (*N* = 89 counties, *R* = correlation coefficient weighted by county's population.)

erased most of the socioeconomic differentials in infant mortality (Rosero-Bixby, 1986).

The scatterplot for the 22-year lagged effect shows a substantial number of counties in quadrant III, which can be taken as evidence against the thesis that low child mortality during childhood and adolescence is a precondition for controlling fertility later in life.

Multivariate Macro-Level Effects on Fertility Rates

To what extent are the bivariate association examined so far and its fluctuations over time a manifestation of third determinants shared by both child mortality and fertility? I addressed this question by statistically controlling the effect of potential confounders in multivariate regression models. In addition to child mortality, regression equations explaining the general marital fertility rate include seven indicators of socioeconomic, programmatic, diffusionist, and geographic conditions at the aforementioned three points in time (unless otherwise indicated, these indicators are lagged 2 years from the marital fertility rate and come mostly from the 1963, 1973, and 1984 censuses). Given that these indicators are considered only to control their potentially confounding effects on the relationship between child mortality and fertility, neither a theoretical construct nor details about their meaning and operationalization are given here (details in Rosero-Bixby, 1991b).

Multiple regression models estimated for the three cross sections of child mortality and marital fertility rates (1965, 1975, and 1985) show relatively modest net effects of child mortality lagged 2 and 12 years on marital fertility (Table 11-1). The net elasticities (i.e., the percentage of change in the marital fertility rate resulting from a 1 percent change in the child mortality rate) range between 0.02 and 0.18. All but the elasticity for the 2-year lagged child mortality rate in 1985 are statistically significant. As with the bivariate correlation coefficient, the association weakens in the cross sections before and after the fertility transition.

Although these estimates do control the potentially confounding effect of other variables in the model, there is no guarantee that the model is fully identified and thus that all spurious associations have been purged; there is always the possibility that the child mortality rate is picking up the effect of a confounding variable that was not included in the model. Regression models on change rates, rather than on levels, ameliorate this possibility by purging all of a county's characteristics and residuals that do not vary over time, such as systematic registration errors or cultural constants influencing both fertility and child mortality. (Random and other errors in the data are, however, magnified by the computation of changes, and the "regression to the mean" phenomenon may introduce considerable noise in the variance of changes (Bohrnstedt, 1969) and can bias toward zero the estimated effects (Freedman and Takeshita, 1969).)

TABLE 11-1 Multiple Regressions on the Marital Fertility Rate, Costa Rican Counties, 1965-1985

Explanatory Variable	Elasticity				
	1965[a]	1975[a]	1985[a]	1965-1975[b]	1975-1985[b]
Child mortality					
Lagged 2 years	0.05*	0.18*	0.02	0.10	−0.04
Lagged 12 years	—	0.08*	0.08*	—	−0.11
Development index	−0.02	0.16*	0.13*	−0.96*	−0.46
Social security coverage	0.00	−0.04*	−0.04	−0.03	−0.07*
Legal union proportion	0.33*	−0.01	0.09*	−0.38	0.22
Family planning supply[c]	—	−0.01	−0.04	0.02	0.17*
Diffusion: out-county					
fertility	0.73*	0.70*	1.11*	2.92*	−0.01
Pretransition fertility	0.49*	0.19*	−0.05	—	—
Travel time to San Jose	0.10*	−0.01	0.08*	—	—
Constant	−11.23*	−8.06*	−8.87*	−1.13*	0.14*
Pseudo R^2	0.62	0.39	0.38	0.30	0.20

NOTES: All regressions weighted by the square root of the county's population. N = 89 counties.
*indicates significant effect at $p < 0.05$.

  [a]Poisson regression on the natural logarithm of the explanatory variables.

  [b]Ordinary least-squares regression on proportional changes computed as $(X1 - X2)/(X1 + X2)$.

  [c]For "family planning supply" in 1965-1975, the change is in absolute terms (from zero by 1965).

The estimate based on change rates in 1965-1975 shows a modest, positive elasticity of 0.10 of child mortality rate on marital fertility rate. This effect is not statistically significant ($t = 1.1$). The change rates in 1975-1985 show perverse negative effects of child mortality on fertility, but these effects are not statistically significant either. There is thus no support for the thesis that child mortality has been an important determinant of fertility in Costa Rican counties above and beyond socioeconomic and other conditions.

The results for other explanatory variables in the regressions on change rates merit brief comment. In 1965-1975, when most of the Costa Rican fertility transition took place, two strong and significant effects were socioeconomic development (elasticity of 7–1) and diffusionist influences from other relevant counties (elasticity of about 3). The family planning program (measured by the per capita density of services in a radius of 30 kilometers) does not appear as a significant factor during this period, which is not a surprise given that the program started somewhat late. These results conform to most explanations of the fertility transition. Between 1975 and 1985, although fertility rates for the country as a whole did not conform to a clear trend, fertility continued to decline in backward counties but increased in some of the more developed counties. According to the results from the 1975-1985 regression, these changes appear to be related to only two factors: a policy of "universalization" of social security coverage launched by the government in 1976 and the strength of government family planning services. The diffusionist process ceased to act, and the negative effect of development on fertility weakened.

Macro-Level Effects on the Onset and Pace of Fertility Transition

The pattern of variation over time in the aggregated associations suggests that the causal link between child mortality and fertility may be weak or nonexistent in pre- and post-transition equilibria. The causal connection, if any, emerges or strengthens only in cross sections taken halfway through the transition process. These patterns suggest that there is no general causal relationship, but a one-time, irreversible event that constitutes the fertility transition. The effect of child mortality on the fertility transition event could be that of a true causal agent that promotes the transition (the sufficient condition hypothesis), that of a precondition for the transition, or that of a mild facilitator of other determinants. Onset year and pace are two dependent variables that characterize the fertility transition. The onset year of the transition in the county is defined as the first year of a mean decline in the marital fertility rate of 3 percent per year over 6 years. The pace of the fertility transition is defined as the rate of reduction in the marital fertility rate over the 8 years following the onset of the transition.

In about 90 percent of Costa Rican counties, fertility started to fall between 1959 and 1968 (median is 1965)—before the government established the family planning program in 1968. What was the child mortality level by the onset of the fertility transition in these counties? It ranges between 50 and 190 per 1,000 for all counties, with an inter-quartile range from approximately 90 to 130 (see the box in the lower part of Figure 11-4). In one-fourth of the counties the fertility transition onset occurred when child mortality levels were 130 or more. A level of 130 means that couples with five children have a 50 percent probability of experiencing the death of a child. In spite of this close contact with children's deaths, fertility started to decline—suggesting that low child mortality often is not a prerequisite for the fertility transition.

Does the child mortality rate correlate with the timing of the fertility transition onset? Given the positive correlation between fertility and child mortality, I would expect an earlier transition onset in counties with lower child mortality. Interestingly enough, those counties with child mortality rates of 130 or higher were not the laggards for the transition onset. The late adopters (1969 or later) actually had somewhat lower child mortality rates when the transition started. This, however, is an artifact of the time trends in child mortality: The laggards benefited from the substantial fall in child mortality that occurred in the 1970s. Looking at the child mortality rate at a fixed point in time (1963) shows that counties with higher child mortality rates lag behind in the fertility transition.

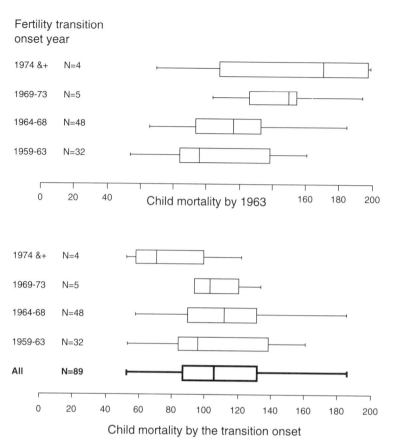

FIGURE 11-4 Child mortality by the fertility transition onset, Costa Rican counties.

The median 1963 mortality rate is about 150 among counties with transition onset in 1968 or later, whereas it is about 100 among the early adopters. The data are thus consistent with the expectation that high child mortality rates may delay the fertility transition.

   With regard to the pace of the fertility transition, the expectation is that lower child mortality may facilitate or promote faster declines. Data for the 89 Costa Rican counties do not support this expectation. The marital fertility rate fell by 56 percent in the 8 years following the transition onset independently of the child mortality rate in the county (data not shown).

   As with previous bivariate covariations, the association between the child mortality rate and the transition onset may be contaminated by interrelated county characteristics. To check this possibility, a Cox multiple regression model was estimated. Cox regression gives estimates of the proportional rate of occurrence

TABLE 11-2 Multiple Regressions on the Fertility Transition Onset Year and the Following Transition Pace, Costa Rican Counties, 1960-1988

	Elasticity	
Explanatory Variable	Onset Risk[a]	Pace[b]
Child mortality (interval)	−0.67	0.05
Socioeconomic development index	1.97*	0.23*
Social security coverage	−0.06	−0.02
Legal marital union proportion	−1.95*	0.03
Family planning service supply	—	0.03
Diffusion, out-county fertility	−7.65*	−0.48
Pretransition, in-county fertility	3.58*	0.78*
Travel time to San Jose	−0.23	−0.02
Onset year (1959 = 0)	—	−0.011
Constant	—	8.34
Pseudo R^2	0.06	0.26
Proportional effects for child mortality categories		
<75	2.64	1.02
75-99	1.24	0.95
100-124	0.60	0.94
125-149	0.95	1.00
150+	1.00	

NOTES: All regressions weighted by the square root of county's population. N = 89 counties.
* indicates significant effect at $p < 0.05$.

[a]Cox regression on the onset risk and the natural logarithm of the explanatory variables measured by 1963.

[b]Ordinary least-squares regression on the percent fertility decline in the 8 years following the transition onset. Elasticity measured at the mean. Explanatory variables measured by the transition onset, lagged 2 years.

of a discrete event given some observed time-to-response variable (Cox, 1972). In the present analysis the time-to-response variable was the onset year of the fertility transition. Table 11-2 shows the elasticity in the risk of "transition onset," estimated by the Cox regression coefficients for explanatory variables entered in the model as natural logarithms. The table also shows the elasticities for the pace of fertility decline during the first 8 years of transition. These elasticities were evaluated at the variable's means using regression coefficients estimated by ordinary least squares. Note that the explanatory variables in the model for the onset are measured at the early 1960s, whereas in the pace model they are measured at the onset year.

Each percent increase in the child mortality rate would decrease the likelihood of starting the fertility transition by 0.7 percent. This effect, however, is not statistically significant. The child mortality effect on the transition pace is nil and not significant. Both the onset and pace are significantly accelerated by socioeconomic development (a summary index of seven indicators) and by reduced fertility in other relevant counties. These effects are much stronger for the onset of fertility transition than for the pace. For the latter, there is also a small, marginally significant effect of the family planning program.

To allow curvilinear effects, the child mortality rate was re-entered into the regression models as a categorical variable. The lower panel in Table 11-2 shows the risk ratio and the relative pace. There is now a marginally significant effect on the transition onset. Counties with a child mortality rate below 75 per 1,000 by 1963 are two or three times more likely to begin the fertility transition than counties with a rate of 150 or more. The pace of fertility decline, however, continues to be unrelated to child mortality.

MULTILEVEL ANALYSIS: INDIVIDUAL-LEVEL FERTILITY AND CONTEXTUAL CHILD MORTALITY

Nations, counties, or other aggregated units do not make reproductive decisions: couples do. Families (or women) are thus the right unit of analysis for studying the relationship between child mortality and fertility. The social dynamics implicit, however, is multilevel in nature: Specific individuals are the ones who make reproductive decisions but these decisions may be influenced by others' experience with child deaths, that is contextual child mortality rates. This effect of aggregated child survival experiences on individual reproductive decisions is at the core of the so-called hoarding or insurance strategy against likely child deaths. To test whether this reproductive strategy influenced the fertility transition in Costa Rica, I examine the record of adoption of family planning among the agents of fertility change, women born between 1927 and 1946. Older and younger cohorts added little to the fertility decline brought about by these cohorts (Rosero-Bixby and Casterline, 1995).

The event of interest, or dependent variable, for this analysis is the individual-level equivalent of the fertility transition onset, the timing for adopting contraception for the first time. The individual-level data come from a nationally representative sample of women gathered for a 1984 study of cancer and contraception (Lee et al., 1987; Rosero-Bixby et al., 1987; Irwin et al., 1988; Rosero-Bixby and Oberle, 1989). This sample is well suited for the present study because it includes the cohorts of interest as well as a lifetime calendar of reproductive events that provides reliable information on the first use of contraception and a migration history that identifies the place of residence during adolescence. The analysis is restricted to women aged 37-58 at the time of the survey who reported having ever been sexually active. The time until adoption of family planning was measured as the time between first sexual intercourse and first use of contraception. Observations were censored at 1981, 25 years since first intercourse or the 45th birthday, whichever came first. The sample size usable in the analysis was only 470 women, which means a limited statistical power for detecting small associations (this sample size has less than 80 percent statistical power for detecting relative rates in the range of 0.6-1.7).

The "exposure" variable—contextual child mortality—comes from the 1973 and 1984 censuses, coded into a geographic information system. Although mortality estimates were readily available at the county or even *distrito* level, conventional geographic units were not considered because of the large heterogeneities between and within them and the frequent changes in their boundary layout. Instead, a standard definition of "context," independent of administrative boundaries, was adopted, namely, the area within a radius of 1 kilometer in urban areas and of 5 kilometers in rural areas from the index women's reported place of residence during most of adolescence. The contextual child mortality was defined as the cumulative proportion of children who had died to women aged 40-49 who belong to the respondent's cohort and live in the previously defined context. Therefore, the proportion of children dead among women aged 40-49 in the 1973 census were assigned to respondents born in 1926-1936 and the proportion from the 1984 census, to respondents born in 1937-1947.

Other contextual indicators used in the multilevel analysis were:

• Completed fertility. Children ever born per woman aged 40-49 in the aforementioned census, cohorts, and radius.
• Proportion of households under the poverty line in the aforementioned radius. Poverty defined with unmet basic needs criteria (absence in a household of any two of seven minimum items, including running water, sanitation, electricity, dwelling's materials, a kitchen, bedrooms, and a radio or TV set).
• Family planning supply estimated as the per capita density of services (weighted by the inverse of distance) in a radius of 30 kilometers from the index household.

At the individual level, the following respondent's characteristics were considered:

• Completed years of formal education.
• Wealth index, number of commodities existing in the household by 1984.
• Calendar year at first sexual intercourse, which defines the starting point of the exposure and also time-trend effects.
• Age at first sexual intercourse.
• Whether the respondent has ever married (a time-varying covariate).

Bivariate and Multilevel Effects

Does the pattern of adoption of family planning differ with contextual child mortality levels? The presence of censored observations in the data calls for the use of life table techniques to estimate the adoption curves. Figure 11-5 shows the cumulative adoption curves for six contextual levels of child mortality. These are cumulative "survival" curves estimated by the Kaplan-Meier method (Kaplan and Meier, 1958). It is evident that women from low-mortality contexts adopt contraception quicker and in higher proportions than women in high-mortality contexts. The curves suggest three child mortality levels for differentiating the incidence of contraception: less than 75 per 1,000, 75 to 124, and 125 and higher. The Kaplan-Meier median waiting time for adopting family planning by these three groups is 4, 10, and 25 years since first intercourse, respectively (Table 11-3). The association could not be clearer.

There are large differences in the timing of the adoption of family planning related to other macro- and micro-level characteristics, but none appears to be as important or large as that observed between various child mortality groups (Table 11-3). However, the level of contextual child mortality itself seems strongly associated to these other characteristics. For example, the median family planning adoption time varies from 21 years since first sex among the poor to 3 years among the wealthy, but the child mortality proportion also varies greatly from

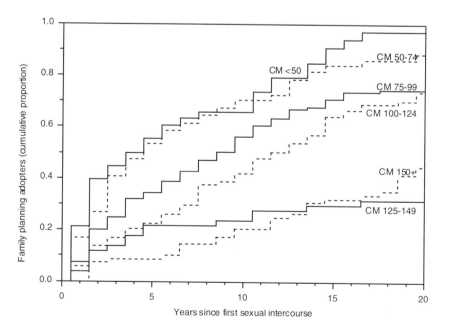

FIGURE 11-5 Family planning adoption curve by level of contextual child mortality (CM).

TABLE 11-3 Contextual Child Mortality and Median Duration until Adoption of Family Planning by Selected Variables

Variable and Categories	N	Median Adoption Year[a]	Contextual Child Mortality
Total	469	10.2	102
Contextual-level			
Child mortality			
29-74	140	4.0	57
75-124	209	9.9	98
125-290	120	24.9	164
Family planning supply 1968-1972			
Moderate	200	12.7	123
High	269	9.0	87
Completed fertility			
2.7-3.9	108	3.4	59
4.0-5.4	160	8.0	88
5.5-8.9	201	18.4	137
Households under poverty line			
<10%	309	6.5	82
10% or more	160	20.3	143
Individual-level			
Education (years)			
0-2	135	18.4	125
3-6	231	9.6	99
7 or more	103	2.6	81
Wealth group			
Poor	121	20.6	128
Low	216	11.2	102
Medium/high	132	3.2	80
Birth cohort			
1926-1936	231	18.1	130
1937-1947	238	5.9	76
Year first sex			
1937-1959	293	15.3	115
1960-1969	139	4.9	83
1970-1983	37	1.9	73
Age at first sex			
11-16	98	18.4	112
17-24	274	10.0	103
25-47	97	3.8	92

[a]Kaplan-Meier estimate. Time counted since first sexual intercourse (women aged 38-58 years in 1984, ever sexually active).

128 to 80 per 1,000, respectively. Child mortality variation overlaps substantially with all these other variables, and it is thus quite possible that most of the bivariate association is attributable to these confounding factors. Thus, statistical control of these confounding effects with multivariate models appears to be mandatory.

Multivariate and Multilevel Effects

Adjusted effects of contextual child mortality on the individual-level rate of adoption of family planning were estimated with Cox multivariate regression. The explanatory variables in the model were categorized to accommodate curvilinear effects. Two of the explanatory variables were allowed to vary over time: contextual family planning supply (zero until 1968 and the average for 1969-1979 thereafter) and individual marital status. Because preliminary models showed interaction between cohort and child mortality, the two variables were combined. Table 11-4 shows the estimated effects as rate ratios of adopting family planning.

Among the older cohorts of women born in 1926-1936, a contextual child mortality rate under 125 per 1,000 increases the rate of adoption of family planning by 51 percent. For the younger cohorts born in 1937-1947, crossing a child mortality threshold of 75 per 1,000 increases the likelihood of adopting family planning by 36 percent (2.38 ÷ 1.75 = 1.36). Net child mortality effects are statistically significant. The extreme shifts in mortality levels over time makes them, however, a moving target. For example, studying the effect of crossing the line of 125 deaths per 1,000 only makes sense for older cohorts because virtually no one among the younger cohorts has been exposed to a contextual mortality rate of 125 or higher.

Other variables with significant net effects on the adoption of birth control are marital status, the year when the observation started, and household wealth, as well as the contextual level of family planning supply. In contrast with previous results, there are no significant diffusion effects from contextual fertility in this data set, perhaps because the explanatory variable is cohort-based, rather than the period-based total fertility.

Is a moderate contextual child mortality rate a precondition for the adoption of family planning? The cumulative adoption curves in Figure 11-6 show that a contextual child mortality rate of 125 or higher may be a serious obstacle for adopting family planning but it is not an absolute impediment: About 20 percent of couples in this category have adopted birth control after 10 years of sexual activity. More interestingly, a Cox model estimated only for contexts where child mortality is 100 or higher shows that the adoption rate may increase sharply in these contexts with the supply of family planning services or with the household's wealth (Table 11-5). Thus, the obstacle of high child mortality can be circumvented.

TABLE 11-4 Rate Ratio of Adopting Family Planning Estimated with a Cox Regression Model

Variable	N	Rate Ratio	95% Confidence Interval
Contextual-level			
Child mortality,			
mothers' cohort			
≥125, old	109	1.00	Reference Group
<125, old	122	1.51	1.00-2.27
≥75, young	128	1.75	1.08-2.82
<75, young	110	2.38	1.39-4.06
Family planning supply[a]			
None	527	1.00	Reference Group
Moderate	158	1.76	1.20-2.60
High	176	1.59	1.09-2.34
Completed fertility			
2.7-3.9	108	1.00	Reference Group
4.0-5.4	160	0.88	0.64-1.21
5.5-8.9	201	0.99	0.64-1.53
Households under poverty line			
<10%	309	1.00	Reference Group
10% or more	160	0.80	0.56-1.13
Individual-level			
Education (years)			
0-2	135	1.00	Reference Group
3-6	231	1.19	0.90-1.57
7 or more	103	1.33	0.93-1.91
Wealth group			
Poor	121	1.00	Reference Group
Low	216	1.50	1.10-2.03
Medium/high	132	2.57	1.77-3.73
Age at first sex			
11-16	98	1.00	Reference Group
17-24	274	1.20	0.87-1.64
25-47	97	1.13	0.68-1.87
Marital status[a]			
Premarital	259	1.00	Reference Group
Ever married	602	2.47	1.79-3.40
Year first sex		1.04	1.00-1.07

NOTE: N indicates number of observed segments for these variables.

[a]Time-varying covariate.

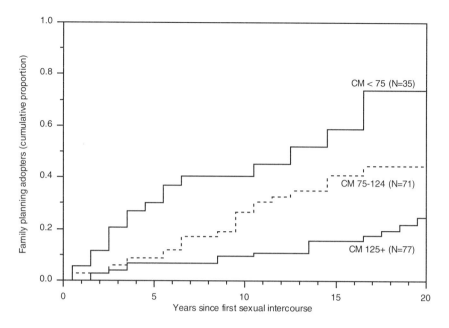

FIGURE 11-6 Family planning adoption curve among unlikely adopters by level of child mortality (CM).

Conversely, lowering child mortality seems by itself a factor for increasing the adoption rate of birth control. Figure 11-6 shows the adoption curves for women who, according to the regression estimates, were unlikely adopters of contraception, women with minimum wealth and education and no family planning services. Among these unlikely adopters, the cumulative adoption curve clearly shifts upward with lower contextual child mortality.

DISCUSSION

In a series of focus group discussions conducted with Costa Rican women in their 50s in 1993 (i.e., from the cohorts that lived through the fertility transition), high child mortality was not perceived as a reason for having large families in the past nor was its reduction seen as a reason for the shift to the small family of today (Rosero-Bixby and Casterline, 1995). Although these discussions focused on the diffusion of the family planning message, the child survival hypothesis was explicitly raised by the moderators in all groups. The suggestion that a decline in child mortality may have played an important role in the fertility transition did not resonate in the focus groups. However, two possible links with low child mortality emerged spontaneously in the discussions. Namely, (1) that

TABLE 11-5 Rate Ratio of Adopting Family Planning Estimated with a Cox Regression Model for Contexts with Child Mortality of 100 or Higher

Variable	N	Ratio	95% Confidence Interval
Family planning supply			
None	260	1.00	Reference Group
Moderate	97	1.92	1.04-3.51
High	57	1.91	0.99-3.72
Wealth group			
Poor	81	1.00	Reference Group
Low	92	1.63	1.09-2.44
Medium/high	36	2.20	1.33-3.66
Marital status[a]			
Premarital	120	1.00	Reference Group
Ever married	294	1.84	1.08-3.17
Year first sex		1.05	1.01-1.09

NOTES: N indicates number of observed segments for this variable.

[a]Time-varying covariate.

the family planning message often diffused in waiting rooms of health centers where increasing numbers of mothers were taking their children for preventive or curative care:

> I heard about family planning for the first time when I brought my sick daughter to the clinic. I started to listen to the other women. They would say, "Did you hear from Carmen that they are going to offer family planning here, that they are going to bring pills." Once I heard a woman telling that she used condoms and got pregnant. She didn't know what had happened inside, or if the condom was torn, the thing was that she got pregnant. Those women came from everywhere (Rosero-Bixby and Casterline, 1995:65).

(2) that the burden of helping their mothers to rear a large family was a motivation for wanting a small family. Increased child survival is an obvious reason for larger families:

> My mother had two pairs of twins and a lot of other kids. I would come home from school and had to go pick coffee and help my mother to sew because we needed the money to raise so many kids. It was changing diapers and washing all the time. And I got the idea that having lots of kids was a kind of slavery (Rosero-Bixby and Casterline, 1995:74).

Neither the focus group discussions nor the statistical record at the aggregate and individual levels support the claim that decreasing child mortality is critical for decreasing fertility. However, decreasing child mortality may facilitate the fertility transition, and high child mortality may delay the transition.

Just as there are developing countries that, in spite of moderate infant mortality, continue having high birth rates, the decline of child mortality in Costa Rica during several decades did not affect fertility trends. The data show that one cannot expect that crossing a child mortality threshold of 200 or 150 per 1,000 will automatically bring about fertility decline. Not even falling below 100 per 1,000 child deaths will generate an automatic response. In short, decreasing child mortality does not appear to be a sufficient condition for fertility decline, nor can the Costa Rican fertility transition be explained solely in terms of an adjustment process to moderate child mortality rates.

The data are inconclusive regarding the thesis that reduced child mortality is a condition for fertility decline. Supporting the thesis is the fact that practically no Costa Rican county, nor for that matter population in the world (Hanson et al., 1994), has experienced low fertility and high child mortality simultaneously. This statement is, of course, conditional on what one considers high child mortality. If one draws the line at a child mortality rate of 100 per 1,000 or higher, it is indeed almost impossible to find populations with controlled fertility. A closer look at the data show that in a substantial number of Costa Rican communities the onset of the fertility transition occurred at child mortality levels above 130 per 1,000. Moreover, individual-level data of the cohorts that changed fertility in Costa Rica show that the rates of adoption of family planning in contexts of high child mortality were far from zero. More interestingly, the data for those contexts show that adoption of family planning increases sharply with the presence of such conditions as family planning services and higher living standards. The obstacle of high child mortality does not seem impossible to beat.

Evidence suggesting that moderate child mortality may facilitate the fertility transition comes from the significantly earlier transition onset in counties with lower child mortality, as well as from the earlier adoption of family planning among women from low-mortality contexts. These effects persist after controlling for the potentially confounding effect of standards of living, education, supply of family planning services, and the like.

To discuss the causal mechanisms behind this association one should first understand how reproductive decisions are made before and during the fertility transition. Following Fishbein's theory of reasoned action, reproductive behavior may be shaped by "the person's beliefs that the behavior leads to certain outcomes and his evaluation of these outcomes," and "the person's beliefs that specific individuals or groups think he should or should not perform the behavior and his motivation to comply with the specific referents" (Fishbein and Middlestadt, 1987:363). The discussion about replacement and insurance strategies for having children (or before this, for having sex or using contraceptives) assumes the perfectly rational type of behavior implicit in the belief that behavior leads to predictable outcomes. It is probable, however, that reproduction, like many human actions, is not based mainly on day-to-day conscious decisions but guided by cultural norms and reference groups. High fertility as a response to high mortality may be implicit in these cultural norms. The distinction between replacement and insurance strategies does not seem meaningful at this collective level. Under a routine-dictated behavior, situations may occur in which an individual's self-interest clashes with the prevailing cultural precepts and leads the person to exercise conscious decision making. The onset of fertility transition could be one of these situations. Enlarged families resulting from improved child survival rates could be one of the reasons for questioning routine reproductive behavior. The second quote above from a Costa Rican woman suggests this possibility.

Although the Costa Rican experience cannot be extrapolated uncritically, the findings in this chapter suggest the following three policy considerations:

1. It would be a mistake for a government to expect an automatic fertility decline to follow a fall in child mortality. The latter does not seem to be a sufficient condition for the former.

2. High child mortality is not a good reason for not providing family planning services since a sizable proportion of couples may adopt family planning in contexts of high child mortality.

3. Fertility reductions are more likely to occur and family planning programs more likely to succeed in contexts where child mortality is low. A family planning intervention coupled with a child survival program will probably have more effect than a vertical program of only family planning services.

REFERENCES

Behm, H., and J.M. Guzmán
　　1979　Diferencias socioeconómicas del descenso de la fecundidad en Costa Rica 1960-1970. Pp. 158-183 in *Sétimo Seminario Nacional de Demografía*. San José, Costa Rica: Dirección General de Estadística y Censos.

Blacker, J.G.
　　1987　Health impacts of family planning. *Health Policy and Planning* 2(3):193-203.

Bohrnstedt, G.W.
　　1969　Observations on the measurement of change. Pp. 1113-1136 in E.F. Borgatta, ed., *Sociological Methodology*. San Francisco: Jossey-Bass.

Caja Costarricense de Seguro Social
　　1994　*Fecundidad y Formación de la Familia. Encuesta Nacional de Salud Reproductiva 1993*. San José, Costa Rica: Caja Costarricense de Seguro Social.

Carlsson, G.
　　1966　The decline of fertility: Innovation or adjustment process. *Population Studies* 20(2):149-174.

Cochrane, S.H., and K.C. Zachariah
　　1983　Infant and Child Mortality as a Determinant of Fertility: The Policy Implications. World Bank Staff Working Paper no. 556. The World Bank, Washington, D.C.

Cox, D.R.
　　1972　Regression models and life tables. *Journal of the Royal Statistical Society* Series B 34:187-202.

Davis, K.
   1955   Institutional patterns favoring high fertility in underdeveloped areas. *Eugenics Quarterly*
           2(1):33-39.
Fishbein, M., and S.E. Middlestadt
   1987   Using the theory of reasoned action to develop educational interventions: Applications to
           illicit drug use. *Health Education Research* 2(4):361-371.
Freedman, R., and J.Y. Takeshita
   1969   *Family Planning in Taiwan: An Experiment in Social Change.* Princeton, N.J.: Princeton
           University Press.
Haaga, J.G.
   1989   Mechanisms for the association of maternal age, parity and birth spacing with infant
           health. Pp. 96-139 in A.M. Parnell, ed., *Contraceptive Use and Controlled Fertility*:
           Health Issues for Women and Children. Committee on Population, National Research
           Council. Washington, D.C.: National Academy Press.
Hanson, L.A., S. Bergstrom, and L. Rosero-Bixby
   1994   Infant mortality and birth rates. Pp. 37-48 in K.S. Lankinen, ed., *Health and Disease in
           Developing Countries.* London: MacMillan Press.
Heer, D.
   1966   Economic development and fertility. *Demography* 3(2):423-444.
Heer, D., and V. Rodríguez
   1986   The Impact of Child Mortality Levels on Fertility Behavior and Attitudes in Costa Rica.
           Unpublished research report, The Population Council, New York.
Irwin, K.L., L. Rosero-Bixby, M.W. Oberle, N.C. Lee, A.S. Whatley, J.A. Fortney, and N.G.
Bonhome
   1988   Oral contraceptives and cervical cancer risk in Costa Rica: Detection bias or causal
           association? *Journal of the American Medical Association* 259(1):59-64.
Kaplan, E.L., and P. Meier
   1958   Nonparametric estimation from incomplete observations. *Journal of the American Statis-
           tical Association* 53:457-481.
Knight, R.
   1995   The Diffusion of Information and Adoption of Contraception in Costa Rica. Chapter
           presented at the International Seminar on the Population in Central America. Universidad
           de Costa Rica, San Jose, Costa Rica, October 21.
Knodel, J.
   1978   European populations in the past. Family-level relations. Pp. 21-45 in S.H. Preston, ed.,
           The Effect of Infant and Child Mortality on Fertility. New York: Academic Press.
Lee, N.C., L. Rosero-Bixby, M.W. Oberle, C. Grimaldo, A.S. Whatley, and E.Z. Rovira
   1987   A case-control study of breast cancer and hormonal contraception in Costa Rica. *Journal
           of the National Cancer Institute* 79(6):1247-1254.
Lloyd, C.B., and S. Ivanov
   1988   The effects of improved child survival on family planning practice and fertility. *Studies
           in Family Planning* 19(3):141-161.
Mauldin, W.B, B. Berelson, and Z. Sykes
   1978   Conditions of fertility decline in developing countries, 1965-1975. *Studies in Family
           Planning* 9(5):89-147.
Mensch, B.
   1985   The effect of child mortality on contraceptive use and fertility in Colombia, Costa Rica,
           and Korea. *Population Studies* 39(2):309-327.
Notestein, F.W.
   1953   Economic problems of population change. Pp. 13-31 in *Proceedings of the Eight Interna-
           tional Conference of Agricultural Economists.* London: Oxford University Press.

Pebley, A., and S. Millman
    1986   Birth spacing and child survival. *International Family Planning Perspectives* 12(3):71-79.
Preston, S.H.
    1978   Introduction. Pp. 1-18 in S.H. Preston, ed., *The Effects of Infant and Child Mortality on Fertility.* New York: Academic Press.
Rosero-Bixby, L.
    1986   Infant mortality in Costa Rica: Explaining the recent decline. *Studies in Family Planning* 17(2):57-65.
    1991a   Socioeconomic development, health interventions, and mortality decline in Costa Rica. *Scandinavian Journal of Social Medicine* 46(Suppl. N):33-42.
    1991b   Interaction Diffusion and Fertility Transition in Costa Rica. Unpublished Ph.D. dissertation, University of Michigan, Ann Arbor.
Rosero-Bixby, L., and J. Casterline
    1994   Interaction diffusion and fertility transition in Costa Rica. *Social Forces* 73(2):435-462
    1995   Difusión por interacción social y transición de la fecundidad: Evidencia cuantitativa y cualitativa de Costa Rica. *Notas de Población* 61:29-78.
Rosero-Bixby, L., and M.W. Oberle
    1989   Fertility change in Costa Rica 1960-84: Analysis of retrospective lifetime reproductive histories. *Journal of Biosocial Science* 21(4):419-432.
Rosero-Bixby, L., M. Gómez, and V. Rodríguez,
    1982   *Determinantes de la Fecundidad en Costa Rica. Análisis Longitudinal de Tres Encuestas.* Costa Rica: Dirección General de Estadística y Censos, World Fertility Survey, International Statistical Institute.
Rosero-Bixby, L., M.W. Oberle, and N.C. Lee
    1987   Reproductive history and breast cancer in a population of high fertility, Costa Rica, 1984-5. *International Journal of Cancer* 40(6):747-754.
Rutstein, S.O., and V. Medica
    1978   The Latin American experience. Pp. 93-112 in S.H. Preston, ed., *The Effects of Infant and Child Mortality on Fertility.* New York: Academic Press.
Stycos, J.M.
    1982   The decline of fertility in Costa Rica: Literacy, modernization, and family planning. *Population Studies* 36(1):15-30.
Taylor, C., J. Newman, and N. Kelly
    1976   The child survival hypothesis. *Population Studies* 30(2):263-278.
Tin Myaing Thein, and J. Reynolds
    1972   *Contraception in Costa Rica. The Role of the Private Sector, 1959-1969.* San José, Costa Rica: Asociación Demográfica Costarricense.
Trussell, J., and A. Pebley
    1984   The potential impact of changes in fertility on infant, child, and maternal mortality. *Studies in Family Planning* 15(6):267-280.
United Nations
    1983   *Manual X: Indirect Techniques for Demographic Estimation.* New York: Department of International Economic and Social Affairs.
    1985   *Socio-economic Development and Fertility Decline in Costa Rica.* New York: Department of Economic and Social Affairs.

Index

411

E

East Asia, 19
  see also specific countries
Economic factors and models, 2, 22, 41,
    42, 45, 75-110, 339
  AIDS, 144
  birth spacing, 262-263
  contraception, 128
  diffusion models, 128
  East Asia, 19
  family planning *vs* health programs,
    261-262
  fertility, general, 5, 148
  India, 342, 362
  Indonesia, 317
  optimization models, 75-76, 82, 90, 96,
    97
  Southeast Asia, 19
  standard analysis, inadequacy, 7
  sub-Saharan Africa, 148-151, 287
  utility maximization models, 76-77,
    80-88, 114-115
  see also Cost factors; Employment and
    occupational status; Hazard
    models; Household data and
    models; Human capital
    investment; Insurance behavior;
    Replacement behavior;
    Socioeconomic status
Education and training
  AIDS, household model, 174
  contraception, 273
  Costa Rica, 387, 400
  developing countries, national curricula,
    129
  Europe, country studies, 203, 206, 209
  Indonesia, 317
  Malaysia, 19-20
  mass media, 122, 129, 209
  mortality risk, perception of, 113, 322
  Philippines, 19-20
  replacement behavior and, 105
  school-age morbidity, human capital
    aspects, 10
  social *vs* formal learning, 113, 117,
    124-125, 128-129

temporal order of information, 124-125
United States, 129
women, 9, 19-20, 41, 42, 45, 51, 272-
    273, 279, 283, 384, 387, 400
  see also Bayesian learning; Literacy
    level; Social learning
Emigration, *see* Migration
Employment and occupational status
  Africa, country studies, 273-274, 283
  Europe, country studies, 193, 197, 200,
    203-207
England and Wales, 23, 127, 196(n.14),
    197, 198, 200-203
Estimation issues, 11, 88-99, 190-195,
    303, 343-346
  approximate decision rules, 105-106
  birth/death history data, 99-103
  birth/death totals, 103-105
  developing countries, general, 11
  population-invariant mortality risk, 88-
    95
  population-variant mortality risk, 95-99
  structural/non-structural, 90, 107-109,
    353, 359
  two-stage techniques, 24
  see also Hazard models; Reverse
    causality statistics
Ethnicity
  Africa, 273, 283
  Germany, 203, 206
  Malaysia, 20
  Middle East, 21
  United States, 229-231, 232, 235, 241-
    242, 244, 245
Europe, country studies, 24, 182, 190,
    195-215, 227
  adult mortality, 192
  aggregate analysis, 187-222
  birth spacing, 190, 192
  bivariate analyses, 182, 184, 195(n.14),
    207
  breastfeeding, 184, 190, 215
  community-level analysis, 187-215
  cross-sectional analysis, 182, 183, 189,
    191, 208-215
  demographic transition theory, classic,
    23, 138